LITERATURE AND AGING

LITERATURE AND AGING
An Anthology

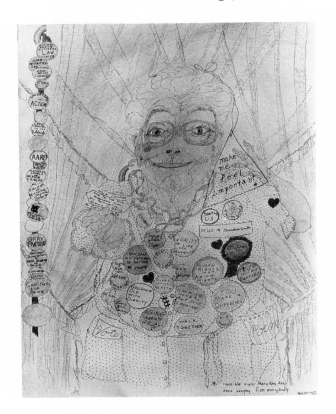

EDITED BY
MARTIN KOHN, CAROL DONLEY, AND DELESE WEAR

The Kent State University Press
KENT, OHIO, AND LONDON, ENGLAND

© 1992 by The Kent State University Press, Kent, Ohio 44242
All rights reserved
Library of Congress Catalog Card Number 92-7855
ISBN 0-87338-466-0
Manufactured in the United States of America

Illustrations are reproduced through the courtesy of the artist,
Elizabeth Layton, and her agent, Don Lambert.

Due to the length of the permissions acknowledgments, a
continuation of the copyright page appears on pages 427–32.

Library of Congress Cataloging-in-Publication Data

Literature and aging : an anthology / edited by Martin Kohn, Carol
    Donley, and Delese Wear.
        p.   cm.
    Includes index.
    ISBN 0-87338-466-0 (pbk. : alk. paper) ∞
    1. Aging—Literary collections.   2. Aged—Literary collections.
3. American literature.   4. English literature.   I. Kohn, Martin.
II. Donley, Carol C.   III. Wear, Delese.
PS509.A37L58   1992
810.8′0354—dc20
                                                                92-7855

British Library Cataloging-in-Publication data are available.

To Aunt Gertrude whom I embrace from afar. M.K.

To my parents. C.D.

To my mother and father. D.W.

Contents

Preface   xiii

Editors' Statements   xv

1. AGING AND IDENTITY
   Introduction   3

   Monet Refuses the Operation
   LISEL MUELLER   5

   Next Day
   RANDALL JARRELL   7

   A Worn Path
   EUDORA WELTY   9

   A Clean, Well-Lighted Place
   ERNEST HEMINGWAY   16

   The Workhouse Ward
   LADY GREGORY   20

   The Space Crone
   URSULA K. LE GUIN   31

   Mr. Flood's Party
   E. A. ROBINSON   35

   An Old Man's Winter Night
   ROBERT FROST   37

   Provide, Provide
   ROBERT FROST   38

CONTENTS

A Woman Alone
DENISE LEVERTOV   39

Virginia Portrait
STERLING BROWN   41

Miss Rosie
LUCILLE CLIFTON   43

A Lady
AMY LOWELL   44

On A Winter Night
MAY SARTON   45

How to be Old
MAY SWENSON   46

Old
ANNE SEXTON   47

Fortitude
KURT VONNEGUT, JR.   48

The Jilting of Granny Weatherall
KATHERINE ANN PORTER   74

2. AGING AND LOVE
Introduction   85

The Pleasures of Old Age
MICHAEL BLUMENTHAL   87

Medicine
ALICE WALKER   88

Now, Before the End, I Think
EDWIN HONIG   89

The Bean Eaters
GWENDOLYN BROOKS   90

CONTENTS

Crazy Jane Talks with the Bishop
W. B. YEATS   91

from Asphodel, That Greeny Flower
WILLIAM CARLOS WILLIAMS   92

We Are Nighttime Travelers
ETHAN CANIN   96

Grandma's Got a Wig
HENRY DUMAS   108

In Retirement
BERNARD MALAMUD   109

Epstein
PHILIP ROTH   117

The Linden Tree
ELLA LEFFLAND   134

Fallback
PHILIP BOOTH   146

3. AGING AND THE FAMILY
Introduction   151

Tell Me A Riddle
TILLIE OLSEN   153

Porte-Cochere
PETER TAYLOR   184

Everything That Rises Must Converge
FLANNERY O'CONNOR   192

The Jewbird
BERNARD MALAMUD   205

Maggie of the Green Bottles
TONI CADE BAMBARA   213

CONTENTS

from The Joy Luck Club
AMY TAN
219

Grandfather in the Old Men's Home
W. S. MERWIN
236

My Father-in-Law's Contract
PETER HARRIS
237

Stroke
SUSAN IRENE REA
239

Grandmother and Grandson
W. S. MERWIN
240

A Conversation with My Father
GRACE PALEY
242

The Sandbox
EDWARD ALBEE
247

The 90th Year
DENISE LEVERTOV
257

The Stroke
RITA DOVE
259

Strokes
WILLIAM STAFFORD
260

Grandmother's Stroke
STEPHEN DUNN
261

Sequel
L. J. SCHNEIDERMAN
262

Appropriate Affect
SUE MILLER
271

Spelling
ALICE MUNRO
281

CONTENTS

4. AGING AND THE COMMUNITY
Introduction   295

from Emperor of the Air
ETHAN CANIN   297

The Very Old
TED KOOSER   308

Near the Old People's Home
HOWARD NEMEROV   309

He Makes a House Call
JOHN STONE   310

Ancient Gentility
WILLIAM CARLOS WILLIAMS   312

To Hell with Dying
ALICE WALKER   315

Toenails
RICHARD SELZER   321

Misery
ANTON CHEKHOV   326

A Visit of Charity
EUDORA WELTY   331

Dillinger in Hollywood
JOHN SAYLES   336

Idiots First
BERNARD MALAMUD   347

What You Hear From 'Em?
PETER TAYLOR   355

Old Doc Rivers
WILLIAM CARLOS WILLIAMS   368

CONTENTS

Leaving the Yellow House
SAUL BELLOW
388

The Black and White
HAROLD PINTER
415

About the Authors
421

Permissions Acknowledgments
427

Index
433

Preface

This anthology is the culmination of a number of years of joyful work. Our task has been to find literature that best conveys the experience of aging, of being old. We selected primarily modern American writers, many of our most distinguished, who represent the American experience and vision of aging. Seeking variety, we included stories, poems, plays and an essay written by persons of diverse color, ethnicity, and experience.

During the selection process, patterns of thematic emphasis emerged which suggested the organization of the anthology. That model can best be visualized as concentric circles. The first, at the core, is the individual and one's personal search for identity and love. The second circle includes the family in its multi-varied forms—those who most often accompany us in our individual pursuits. The widest band and final circle is the larger context in which we live and grow old with others, the community.

What, one may ask, is the value of reading literary representations of the aging process, especially accounts of old age? Several beliefs motivated us to create this volume. First, we believe that students in preprofessional and professional education need a nongeneralized understanding of aging and older persons to complement their generalized knowledge. Second, persons seeking to understand their parents or their own aging (a dramatically increasing number of us in North America) can do so vicariously by listening attentively to the stories of others. Third, we can experience literary works not only in our private spaces, but in the public classroom or discussion group as well. Plays and poems can and should be read aloud. All the works can be transformed into reader's theater presentations.

We want readers of this anthology to experience these fine works without the interference of editorial comment and interpretation. We have, however, included introductory remarks for each section. Their purpose is to raise questions, to prepare the table for the feast that follows. For those who want guidance and critical commentary about each work, a comprehensive reader's/instructor's guide is available.

Many people deserve our grateful acknowledgment of their contributions to this project.

First, we have worked with several colleagues who volunteered their time to participate in two Literature and Aging courses we team-taught at Hiram College in the summers of 1990 and 1991. These include Eugene Hirsch, M.D., who taught both courses with us and brought wonderful expertise and experience to the classes. Also participating the first summer were Marcia Silver, M.D.; Sandra Stephan, R.N. Ph.D.; Jeanne Novotny, R.N., M.S.,C.; and Ellen Whiting, B.A.

First, we have worked with several colleagues who volunteered their time to participate in two Literature and Aging courses we team-taught at Hiram College in the summers of 1990 and 1991. These include Eugene Hirsch, M.D., who taught both courses with us and brought wonderful expertise and experience to the classes. Also participating the first summer were Marcia Silver, M.D.; Sandra Stephan, R.N. Ph.D.; Jeanne Novotny, R.N., M.S.,C.; and Ellen Whiting, B.A.

Second, we wish to thank our students, both those from Northeastern Ohio Universities College of Medicine (NEOUCOM) and those from Hiram College, who taught us which stories and poems and plays were most effective. Our students not only responded to the works we provided but also made many suggestions of other appropriate stories and poems, several of which we have included in this collection.

Third, we thank both our institutions for their support, and, in particular, Colin Campbell, M.D., president and dean, NEOUCOM; Edward Smerek, Ph.D., professor of Mathematics and former dean at Hiram College; and Nancy Moeller, M.Ed., dean of Hiram's Weekend College.

Several sponsors at NEOUCOM deserve thanks for their help in providing funding for copyright permissions. These include Western Reserve Geriatric Education Center at NEOUCOM and Office of Geriatric Medicine/ Gerontology; Area Health Education Center; Division of Basic Medical Sciences, Director's Office; and MEFCOM, Medical Education Foundation of the College of Medicine. Our appreciation also goes to those working in the NEOUCOM Word Processing Center who steadfastly put the manuscript into shape.

Very special thanks go to Mona Adorni whose organizing skills kept our project on track.

Finally, we wish to express our special thanks to our spouses, Marcia Silver, Alan Donley, and Steve Broderick, who have given us their patient support and encouragement, and to our families, children and parents, who kept their senses of humor and our spirits buoyed throughout this project.

Editors' Statements

MARTIN KOHN

What does it mean to age, to become old? What happens to our *self* as our body begins to outlive its usefulness? What becomes of the person we once were, knowing that we simultaneously exist as a being in the process of becoming? Gerontology, the study of the aging process, can provide some of the general and theoretical answers to these and other questions. Literature provides different paths to understanding the aging process and old age. Paths of particularity and poignancy. Paths down which you, the reader, vicariously will travel.

Lives ripened by age are what unfold in the pages ahead. Each story, poem, or play reveals to us the particular context of a life. Therein lies one of the important values of literature. For each of us, whether alive on the page or in the flesh, chooses how to live, chooses the story he or she becomes, chooses how to spend one's time (to use a crass economic metaphor).

The act of reading good literature is a dynamic process involving many voices—most importantly one's own. Exercise your voice well as you read these pages. Take advantage of this opportunity to find your own voice—your own identity—whether you count yourself among the elderly or are just a younger version of an older person.

And as you discover the voice of your older self, share it with another. Together we create a community of voices.

Welcome to our anthology, to our community.

CAROL DONLEY

The great cellist, Pablo Casals, was still giving concerts in his nineties in spite of his problems with arthritis. When asked how he managed such a long, productive career, Casals replied, "I am perhaps the oldest musician in the world. I am an old man but in many senses a very young man. And this is what I want you to be—young, young all your life, and to say things to the world that are true."

This anthology of literature and aging gathers together many different voices who say things to the world that are true. The voices speak of the experiences of older people; they express the hopes and fears of people struggling with retirement, with failing health, with recognitions of their own mortality. The voices complain of prejudice against the elderly, they celebrate the closeness of family and friends, they grieve over losses of loved people and places. Good literature is a reservoir of truths about life; that is why it is so valued in every culture.

Literature about aging is also one of the most fruitful resources for understanding interactions between the experiences of clinicians, health care providers, family and friends of the elderly, and the aging person. This anthology of literature and aging serves several purposes. A story or play gives us empathy for the older person, an understanding which sometimes is hard to achieve in any other way. Good literature about aging is perhaps our best entrance into the world of the aging. It allows us to participate in their experiences, to see through their eyes instead of looking at them from a distance, to recognize that what we may have thought about them is not necessarily the truth as they know it. It also lets us see the older person from the point of view of family members who may experience the same situation quite differently both from the aging person and from the health care professionals and others who are in the context.

Literature also sensitizes us to language and makes us more conscious of the effects of what we say, especially of our "naming" of the problems (diagnosing as well as stereotyping). As this anthology shows, a good poem or play helps us realize that our thinking is strongly shaped and limited by our language. Do we see "old" first before we see an individual? What does "old" mean to us? Do we appreciate it or fear it or feel disgusted by it or honored by it? Literature helps us be much more aware of how our interactions with others tell them how we see them and, therefore, strongly affect their self-image.

When Casals said he wanted us all to be young, he was referring not to chronological age but to orientation and self-image. Someone of any age with a young attitude looks with interest and energy towards tomorrow. The opposite image portrays someone who is apathetic and weak, who always looks backward to better times in the past. As William May writes in *The Physician's Covenant:* "An image provides a compelling picture of the world and one's role in it. What one does appears to be what the world compels. The image renders another kind of behavior unthinkable." That insight helps explain the behavior of those doctors who see themselves as authoritative parents, perhaps in conflict with those aging patients who see themselves as autonomous, independent individuals. In such a situation, family members may see themselves as martyrs putting up with willful, unreasonable parents. On the other hand, if people see themselves as collaborative and mutually caring, a very different scene develops. Images of aging range from Yeats' old scarecrow and Shakespeare's infirm and choleric old hags to Donne's "No Spring nor Summer Beauty hath such grace / As I have seen in one Autumnal face" or Robinson Jeffers's "The heads of strong old age are beautiful / Beyond all grace of youth." The literature about aging in this collection lets us examine the images people have for themselves and their corresponding world views that so affect their thinking and action.

And a final, and in some ways most important, purpose for this anthology is to gather together works of art that address the themes of aging. Good stories, poems, and plays enrich us because they have intrinsic worth, like fine concertos or exquisite paintings. The works in this anthology of literature and aging all have artistic value and are worth our attention for their craftsmanship in shaping plot and character, for their masterful handling of imagery and metaphor, for their creation of fictional worlds which we can live in and learn from whether we are reading for our own pleasure or for use in an educational or clinical setting.

DELESE WEAR

As I began reading through the typeset pages of this volume for the final time, I kept thinking of something Salman Rushdie recently wrote: "Literature is the one place in any society where, within the secrecy of our own heads, we can hear *voices talking about everything in every possible way.*" I was struck time and again by this notion of multiplicity as I heard those literary voices portraying an individual's lived experience of growing older. I found, too, that there were no formulas, no models, no prototypes of "how to age," affirming Rushdie's observation that literature "tells us there are no answers; or, rather, it tells us that answers are easier to come by, and less reliable, than questions. . . . great literature, by asking extraordinary questions, opens new doors in our minds."

I think of the literature and medicine classes I teach and the doors opened for my students and me by the fiction we read. These doors seem to be rather magical (for those of us willing to entertain such thoughts); once we walk through, we are suddenly able to experience other people, other happenings more vicariously. And—the true magic—we are rendered vulnerable ourselves to the same joys and sorrows and doubts of these fictionalized others. Through the voices of Eva in Olsen's *Tell Me a Riddle* or Sylvia in Vonnegut's *Fortitude* or Frank in Canin's "We Are Nighttime Travelers," we may feel in some deeper sense what it may feel like to be someone else— here, in this volume, someone who is aging and facing changes in family, identity, health, and love relationships. Here in the private safety of reading we come to question or rethink our beliefs about aging, and to reflect more critically on our relationships, personal and professional, to those who are aging. And to the extent that we allow ourselves to become more vulnerable, we are better able to personalize to our *own* lives the human stories found in our reading, not as caregivers, or the sons and daughters of these older Others, but as individuals facing aging ourselves, sometimes fearfully, always most assuredly. Here, in what Maxine Greene calls a state of wide-awakeness, readers can be

> provoked to reach beyond themselves in their intersubjective space . . . to think about what they are doing, to become mindful, to share meanings, to conceptualize, to make varied sense of their lived worlds . . . [where] preferences may be released, languages learned, intelligences developed, perspectives opened, possibilities disclosed . . . how seldom this occurs today in our technicized, privatized, consumerist time.[1]

These stories, then, with roots in the earthy richness of a domain so different from clinical perspectives on aging, may provoke us to reflect widely and variously on one of the most mysterious and inevitable shared human experiences. I was aware of this at the initial stages of sifting and sorting for this book, and I was struck with the same mystery again as I proofread. Now, I am hopeful that other readers of these stories and poems may be as provoked and nourished as I was, and continue to be.

---

[1] Maxine Green, "Sense-Making through Story: An Autobiographical Inquiry," *Teaching Education* 2 (Autumn 1987): 12.

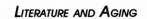

LITERATURE AND AGING

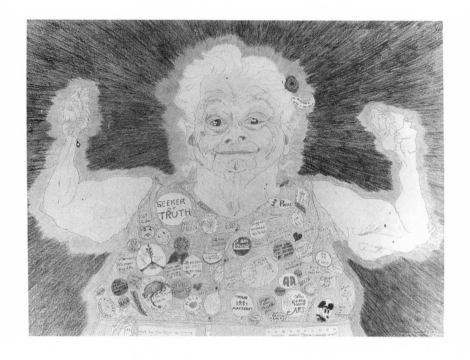

Aging and Identity

Introduction

"Who are you?" said the Caterpillar, as he began his interrogation of Alice. And her response was: "I hardly know, sir, just at present—at least I know who I was when I got up this morning, but I think I must have changed several times since then." And when the Caterpillar demanded that she explain herself, Alice replied, "I can't explain myself, I'm afraid, sir, because I'm not myself, you see."

This little excerpt from *Alice's Adventures in Wonderland* captures several of the essentials of self-recognition. One's identity requires some consistency over time; without it, the self loses itself.

When a person asks, "Who are you?" we almost always answer with our name; that name helps identify us as unique but it also places us in a family which has a history, and it may even indicate something of our ethnic and religious background. Naming has considerable bearing on identity. Note the Genesis and Exodus emphasis on the power of names, whether it be the change of name that comes with the covenant, as in Abram's name change to Abraham; or whether it be God's answer to Moses when he asked for God's name—"I am who I am." The name asserts identity. Someone who feels uncertain about selfhood can be very threatened by name calling and labeling, for such words are verbal attacks on one's identity. Consider, for example, the variety of labels for the elderly—"golden agers," "senior citizens," "old folks," "old fogies," "over the hill gang," etc.

After we have given our name, we continue to answer the question about who we are by mentioning where we live or come from, giving an environmental context. Our sense of self is closely connected to the places we inhabit; it is often very hard for us to move away from a place where we have done a lot of living, because our awareness of continuity and sameness of self has a home there—we are comfortable in this familiar space; it is full of things (furniture, pictures, doorways, trees) that carry memories for us of events in our histories associated with those things. The tenacity with which some elderly people hang onto their homes, the resistance they feel to moving into retirement centers or nursing homes, has much to do with their sense of identity—who they are is imbedded in their home place.

We may also answer the question about who we are by mentioning our jobs and roles (who we are in the context of work, of family, of community). The identification of a person with his or her career (I am a professor, I am a doctor) may make retirement extremely difficult, because the career no longer supplies a measure of one's worth. Similarly, as roles change—from mother to grandmother, for instance—a person may struggle with who she is now, when she is not needed in the same ways she used to be.

Our answers to the question of who we are all presuppose a continuity—our names, our environments, our careers and roles will not be changing every other day. We can assume that while some things may change, most of our "identifiers" will remain reasonably consistent. If they don't, we're in trouble.

During the Second World War, Eric Erikson coined the term "identity crisis" to describe the condition of shell-shocked soldiers who had lost a sense of sameness and continuity of the self. Similar identity crises also occur for some elderly people who may forget their family and friends, may lose their orientation in space and time, and finally lose "themselves."

Our sense of who we are as individuals depends on our ability to remember our own personal history and the people and places that contributed to that history. When writers create lifelike characters, they build fictional histories and contexts for them, and the characters seem alive to us in proportion to the realism of those histories. We can get quite angry and frustrated when a character suddenly does something "out of character"—our sense of who that person is gets challenged. We may be irritated with the author for not keeping the character consistent with what we remember about him or her.

The same happens in real life. A grandfather who forgets his children and grandchildren, who cannot get oriented in once-familiar places, necessarily loses continuity with his own sense of self. He may, like Alice, say, "I'm not myself." He may experience real alarm as memory fails, feeling the distress of looking at himself in the mirror and not recognizing his own face; and his family and friends may feel anger and frustration as he changes into someone other than the person they knew. For many people Alzheimer's disease and similar dementia are much harder to bear than heart disease or cancer, mainly because the patient loses identity—the person has no continuity of selfhood.

Literature can help us understand some of the problems of aging and identity by placing us in the perspectives of the elderly person experiencing the ambiguities of self and in the perspectives of friends and family around that person. Sometimes the outsiders do not recognize how much personhood is still active—as in Welty's wonderful character, Phoenix, whom everyone dismisses as mindless.

Monet Refuses the Operation

Doctor, you say there are no haloes
around the streetlights in Paris
and what I see is an aberration
caused by old age, an affliction.
I tell you it has taken me all my life
to arrive at the vision of gas lamps as angels,
to soften and blur and finally banish
the edges you regret I don't see,
to learn that the line I called the horizon
does not exist and sky and water,
so long apart, are the same state of being.
Fifty-four years before I could see
Rouen cathedral is built
of parallel shafts of sun,
and now you want to restore
my youthful errors: fixed
notions of top and bottom,
the illusion of three-dimensional space,
wisteria separate
from the bridge it covers.
What can I say to convince you
the Houses of Parliament dissolve
night after night to become
the fluid dream of the Thames?
I will not return to a universe
of objects that don't know each other,
as if islands were not the lost children
of one great continent. The world
is flux, and light becomes what it touches,
becomes water, lilies on water,
above and below water,
becomes lilac and mauve and yellow
and white and cerulean lamps,
small fists passing sunlight
so quickly to one another

that it would take long, streaming hair
inside my brush to catch it.
To paint the speed of light!
Our weighted shapes, these verticals,
burn to mix with air
and change our bones, skin, clothes
to gases. Doctor,
if only you could see
how heaven pulls earth into its arms
and how infinitely the heart expands
to claim this world, blue vapor without end.

Next Day

Moving from Cheer to Joy, from Joy to All,
I take a box
And add it to my wild rice, my Cornish game hens.
The slacked or shorted, basketed, identical
Food-gathering flocks
Are selves I overlook. Wisdom, said William James,

Is learning what to overlook. And I am wise
If that is wisdom.
Yet somehow, as I buy All from these shelves
And the boy takes it to my station wagon,
What I've become
Troubles me even if I shut my eyes.

When I was young and miserable and pretty
And poor, I'd wish
What all girls wish: to have a husband,
A house and children. Now that I'm old, my wish
Is womanish:
That the boy putting groceries in my car

See me. It bewilders me he doesn't see me.
For so many years
I was good enough to eat: the world looked at me
And its mouth watered. How often they have
    undressed me,
The eyes of strangers!
And, holding their flesh within my flesh, their vile

Imaginings within my imagining,
I too have taken
The chance of life. Now the boy pats my dog
And we start home. Now I am good.
The last mistaken,
Ecstatic, accidental bliss, the blind

Happiness that, bursting, leaves upon the palm
Some soap and water—
It was so long ago, back in some Gay
Twenties, Nineties, I don't know . . . Today I miss
My lovely daughter
Away at school, my sons away at school,

My husband away at work—I wish for them.
The dog, the maid,
And I go through the sure unvarying days
At home in them. As I look at my life,
I am afraid
Only that it will change, as I am changing:

I am afraid, this morning, of my face.
It looks at me
From the rear-view mirror, with the eyes I hate,
The smile I hate. Its plain, lined look
Of gray discovery
Repeats to me: "You're old." That's all, I'm old.

And yet I'm afraid, as I was at the funeral
I went to yesterday.
My friend's cold made-up face, granite among its
        flowers,
Her undressed, operated-on, dressed body
Were my face and body.
As I think of her I hear her telling me

How young I seem; I *am* exceptional;
I think of all I have.
But really no one is exceptional,
No one has anything, I'm anybody,
I stand beside my grave
Confused with my life, that is commonplace and
        solitary.

A Worn Path

It was December—a bright frozen day in the early morning. Far out in the country there was an old Negro woman with her head tied in a red rag, coming along a path through the pinewoods. Her name was Phoenix Jackson. She was very old and small and she walked slowly in the dark pine shadows, moving a little from side to side in her steps, with the balanced heaviness and lightness of a pendulum in a grandfather clock. She carried a thin, small cane made from an umbrella, and with this she kept tapping the frozen earth in front of her. This made a grave and persistent noise in the still air, that seemed meditative like the chirping of a solitary little bird.

She wore a dark striped dress reaching down to her shoe tops, and an equally long apron of bleached sugar sacks, with a full pocket: all neat and tidy, but every time she took a step she might have fallen over her shoelaces, which dragged from her unlaced shoes. She looked straight ahead. Her eyes were blue with age. Her skin had a pattern all its own of numberless branching wrinkles and as though a whole little tree stood in the middle of her forehead, but a golden color ran underneath, and the two knobs of her cheeks were illumined by a yellow burning under the dark. Under the red rag her hair came down on her neck in the frailest of ringlets, still black, and with an odor like copper.

Now and then there was a quivering in the thicket. Old Phoenix said, "Out of my way, all you foxes, owls, beetles, jack rabbits, coons and wild animals! . . . Keep out from under these feet, little bob-whites. . . Keep the big wild hogs out of my path. Don't let none of those come running my direction. I got a long way." Under her small black-freckled hand her cane, limber as a buggy whip, would switch at the brush as if to rouse up any hiding things.

On she went. The woods were deep and still. The sun made the pine needles almost too bright to look at, up where the wind rocked. The cones dropped as light as feathers. Down in the hollow was the mourning dove—it was not too late for him.

The path ran up a hill. "Seem like there is chains about my feet, time I get this far," she said, in the voice of argument old people keep to use with themselves. "Something always take a hold of me on this hill—pleads I should stay."

After she got to the top she turned and gave a full, severe look behind her where she had come. "Up through pines," she said at length. "Now down through oaks."

Her eyes opened their widest, and she started down gently. But before she got to the bottom of the hill a bush caught her dress.

Her fingers were busy and intent, but her skirts were full and long, so that before she could pull them free in one place they were caught in another. It was not possible to allow the dress to tear. "I in the thorny bush," she said. "Thorns, you doing your appointed work. Never want to let folks pass, no sir. Old eyes thought you was a pretty little *green* bush."

Finally, trembling all over, she stood free, and after a moment dared to stoop for her cane.

"Sun so high!" she cried, leaning back and looking, while the thick tears went over her eyes. "The time getting all gone here."

At the foot of this hill was a place where a log was laid across the creek.

"Now comes the trial," said Phoenix.

Putting her right foot out, she mounted the log and shut her eyes. Lifting her skirt, leveling her cane fiercely before her, like a festival figure in some parade, she began to march across. Then she opened her eyes and she was safe on the other side.

"I wasn't as old as I thought," she said.

But she sat down to rest. She spread her skirts on the bank around her and folded her hands over her knees. Up above her was a tree in a pearly cloud of mistletoe. She did not dare to close her eyes, and when a little boy brought her a plate with a slice of marble-cake on it she spoke to him. "That would be acceptable," she said. But when she went to take it there was just her own hand in the air.

So she left that tree, and had to go through a barbed-wire fence. There she had to creep and crawl, spreading her knees and stretching her fingers like a baby trying to climb the steps. But she talked loudly to herself: she could not let her dress be torn now, so late in the day, and she could not pay for having her arm or her leg sawed off if she got caught fast where she was.

At last she was safe through the fence and risen up out in the clearing. Big dead trees, like black men with one arm, were standing in the purple stalks of the withered cotton field. There sat a buzzard.

"Who you watching?"

In the furrows she made her way along.

"Glad this not the season for bulls," she said, looking sideways, "and the good Lord made his snakes to curl up and sleep in the winter. A pleasure I don't see no two-headed snake coming around that tree, where it come once. It took a while to get by him, back in the summer."

She passed through the old cotton and went into a field of dead corn. It whispered and shook and was taller than her head. "Through the maze now," she said, for there was no path.

Then there was something tall, black, and skinny there, moving before her.

At first she took it for a man. It could have been a man dancing in the field. But she stood still and listened, and it did not make a sound. It was as silent as a ghost.

"Ghost," she said sharply, "who be you the ghost of? For I have heard of nary death close by."

But there was no answer—only the ragged dancing in the wind.

She shut her eyes, reached out her hand, and touched a sleeve. She found a coat and inside that an emptiness, cold as ice.

"You scarecrow," she said. Her face lighted. "I ought to be shut up for good," she said with laughter. "My senses is gone. I too old. I the oldest people I ever know. Dance, old scarecrow," she said, "while I dancing with you."

She kicked her foot over the furrow, and with mouth drawn down, shook her head once or twice in a little strutting way. Some husks blew down and whirled in streamers about her skirts.

Then she went on, parting her way from side to side with the cane, through the whispering field. At last she came to the end, to a wagon track where the silver grass blew between the red ruts. The quail were walking around like pullets, seeming all dainty and unseen.

"Walk pretty," she said. "This the easy place. This the easy going."

She followed the track, swaying through the quiet bare fields, through the little strings of trees silver in their dead leaves, past cabins silver from weather, with the doors and windows boarded shut, all like old women under a spell sitting there. "I walking in their sleep," she said, nodding her head vigorously.

In a ravine she went where a spring was silently flowing through a hollow log. Old Phoenix bent and drank. "Sweet-gum makes the water sweet," she said, and drank more. "Nobody know who made this well, for it was here when I was born."

The track crossed a swampy part where the moss hung as white as lace from every limb. "Sleep on, alligators, and blow your bubbles." Then the track went into the road.

Deep, deep the road went down between the high green-colored banks. Overhead the live-oaks met, and it was as dark as a cave.

A black dog with a lolling tongue came up out of the weeds by the ditch. She was meditating, and not ready, and when he came at her she only hit him a little with her cane. Over she went in the ditch, like a little puff of milkweed.

Down there, her senses drifted away. A dream visited her, and she reached her hand up, but nothing reached down and gave her a pull. So she lay there and presently went to talking. "Old woman," she said to herself, "that black dog come up out of the weeds to stall you off, and now there he sitting on his fine tail, smiling at you."

A white man finally came along and found her—a hunter, a young man, with his dog on a chain.

"Well, Granny!" he laughed. "What are you doing there?"

"Lying on my back like a June-bug waiting to be turned over, mister," she said, reaching up her hand.

He lifted her up, gave her a swing in the air, and set her down. "Anything broken, Granny?"

"No sir, them old dead weeds is springy enough," said Phoenix, when she had got her breath. "I thank you for your trouble."

"Where do you live, Granny?" he asked, while the two dogs were growling at each other.

"Away back yonder, sir, behind the ridge. You can't even see it from here."

"On your way home?"

"No sir, I going to town."

"Why, that's too far! That's as far as I walk when I come out myself, and I get something for my trouble." He patted the stuffed bag he carried, and there hung down a little closed claw. It was one of the bob-whites, with its beak hooked bitterly to show it was dead. "Now you go on home, Granny!"

"I bound to go to town, mister," said Phoenix. "The time come around."

He gave another laugh, filling the whole landscape. "I know you old colored people! Wouldn't miss going to town to see Santa Claus!"

But something held old Phoenix very still. The deep lines in her face went into a fierce and different radiation. Without warning, she had seen with her own eyes a flashing nickel fall out of the man's pocket onto the ground.

"How old are you, Granny?" he was saying.

"There's no telling, mister," she said, "no telling."

Then she gave a little cry and clapped her hands and said, "Git on away from here, dog! Look! Look at that dog!" She laughed as if in admiration. "He ain't scared of nobody. He a big black dog." She whispered, "Sic him!"

"Watch me get rid of that cur," said the man. "Sic him, Pete! Sic him!"

Phoenix heard the dogs fighting, and heard the man running and throwing sticks. She even heard a gunshot. But she was slowly bending forward by that time, further and further forward, the lid stretched down over her eyes, as if she were doing this in her sleep. Her chin was lowered almost to her knees. The yellow palm of her hand came out from the fold of her apron.

Her fingers slid down and along the ground under the piece of money with the grace and care they would have in lifting an egg from under a setting hen. Then she slowly straightened up, she stood erect, and the nickel was in her apron pocket. A bird flew by. Her lips moved. "God watching me the whole time. I come to stealing."

The man came back, and his own dog panted about them. "Well, I scared him off that time," he said, and then he laughed and lifted his gun and pointed it at Phoenix.

She stood straight and faced him.

"Doesn't the gun scare you?" he said, still pointing it.

"No, sir, I seen plenty go off closer by, in my day, and for less than what I done," she said, holding utterly still.

He smiled, and shouldered the gun. "Well, Granny," he said, "you must be a hundred years old, and scared of nothing. I'd give you a dime if I had any money with me. But you take my advice and stay home, and nothing will happen to you."

"I bound to go on my way, mister," said Phoenix. She inclined her head in the red rag. Then they went in different directions, but she could hear the gun shooting again and again over the hill.

She walked on. The shadows hung from the oak trees to the road like curtains. Then she smelled wood-smoke, and smelled the river, and she saw a steeple and the cabins on their steep steps. Dozens of little black children whirled around her. There ahead was Natchez shining. Bells were ringing. She walked on.

In the paved city it was Christmas time. There were red and green electric lights strung and crisscrossed everywhere, and all turned on in the daytime. Old Phoenix would have been lost if she had not distrusted her eyesight and depended on her feet to know where to take her.

She paused quietly on the sidewalk where people were passing by. A lady came along in the crowd, carrying an armful of red-, green- and silver-wrapped presents; she gave off perfume like the red roses in hot summer, and Phoenix stopped her.

"Please, missy, will you lace up my shoe?" She held up her foot.

"What do you want, Grandma?"

"See my shoe," said Phoenix. "Do all right for out in the country, but wouldn't look right to go in a big building."

"Stand still then, Grandma," said the lady. She put her packages down on the sidewalk beside her and laced and tied both shoes tightly.

"Can't lace 'em with a cane," said Phoenix. "Thank you, missy. I doesn't mind asking a nice lady to tie up my shoe, when I gets out on the street."

Moving slowly and from side to side, she went into the big building, and into the tower of steps, where she walked up and around and around until her feet knew to stop.

She entered a door, and there she saw nailed up on the wall the document that had been stamped with the gold seal and framed in the gold frame, which matched the dream that was hung up in her head.

"Here I be," she said. There was a fixed and ceremonial stiffness over her body.

"A charity case, I suppose," said an attendant who sat at the desk before her.

But Phoenix only looked above her head. There was sweat on her face, the wrinkles in her skin shone like a bright net.

"Speak up, Grandma," the woman said. "What's your name? We must have your history, you know. Have you been here before? What seems to be the trouble with you?"

Old Phoenix only gave a twitch to her face as if a fly were bothering her.

"Are you deaf?" cried the attendant.

But then the nurse came in.

"Oh, that's just old Aunt Phoenix," she said. "She doesn't come for her-self—she has a little grandson. She makes these trips just as regular as clock-work. She lives away back off the Old Natchez Trace." She bent down. "Well, Aunt Phoenix, why don't you just take a seat? We won't keep you standing after your long trip." She pointed.

The old woman sat down, bolt upright in the chair.

"Now, how is the boy?" asked the nurse.

Old Phoenix did not speak.

"I said, how is the boy?"

But Phoenix only waited and stared straight ahead, her face very solemn and withdrawn into rigidity.

"Is his throat any better?" asked the nurse. "Aunt Phoenix, don't you hear me? Is your grandson's throat any better since the last time you came for the medicine?"

With her hands on her knees, the old woman waited, silent, erect and motionless, just as if she were in armor.

"You mustn't take up our time this way, Aunt Phoenix," the nurse said. "Tell us quickly about your grandson, and get it over. He isn't dead, is he?"

At last there came a flicker and then a flame of comprehension across her face, and she spoke.

"My grandson. It was my memory had left me. There I sat and forgot why I made my long trip."

"Forgot?" The nurse frowned. "After you came so far?"

Then Phoenix was like an old woman begging a dignified forgiveness for waking up frightened in the night. "I never did go to school, I was too old at the Surrender," she said in a soft voice. "I'm an old woman without an ed-ucation. It was my memory fail me. My little grandson, he is just the same, and I forgot it in the coming."

"Throat never heals, does it?" said the nurse, speaking in a loud, sure voice to old Phoenix. By now she had a card with something written on it, a little list. "Yes. Swallowed lye. When was it?—January—two-three years ago—"

Phoenix spoke unmasked now. "No, missy, he not dead, he just the same. Every little while his throat begin to close up again, and he not able to swallow. He not get his breath. He not able to help himself. So the time come around, and I go on another trip for the soothing medicine."

"All right. The doctor said as long as you came to get it, you could have it," said the nurse. "But it's an obstinate case."

"My little grandson, he sit up there in the house all wrapped up, waiting by himself," Phoenix went on. "We is the only two left in the world. He suffer and it don't seem to put him back at all. He got a sweet look. He going to last. He wear a little patch quilt and peep out holding his mouth open like a little bird. I remembers so plain now. I not going to forget him again, no, the whole enduring time. I could tell him from all the others in creation."

"All right." The nurse was trying to hush her now. She brought her a bottle of medicine. "Charity," she said, making a check mark in a book.

Old Phoenix held the bottle close to her eyes, and then carefully put it into her pocket.

"I thank you," she said.

"It's Christmas time, Grandma," said the attendant. "Could I give you a few pennies out of my purse?"

"Five pennies is a nickel," said Phoenix stiffly.

"Here's a nickel," said the attendant.

Phoenix rose carefully and held out her hand. She received the nickel and then fished the other nickel out of her pocket and laid it beside the new one. She stared at her palm closely, with her head on one side.

Then she gave a tap with her cane on the floor.

"This is what come to me to do," she said. "I going to the store and buy my child a little windmill they sells, made out of paper. He going to find it hard to believe there such a thing in the world. I'll march myself back where he waiting, holding it straight up in this hand."

She lifted her free hand, gave a little nod, turned around, and walked out of the doctor's office. Then her slow step began on the stairs, going down.

A Clean,
Well-Lighted Place

It was late and every one had left the café except an old man who sat in the shadow the leaves of the tree made against the electric light. In the daytime the street was dusty, but at night the dew settled the dust and the old man liked to sit late because he was deaf and now at night it was quiet and he felt the difference. The two waiters inside the café knew that the old man was a little drunk, and while he was a good client they knew that if he became too drunk he would leave without paying, so they kept watch on him.

"Last week he tried to commit suicide," one waiter said.

"Why?"

"He was in despair."

"What about?"

"Nothing."

"How do you know it was nothing?"

"He has plenty of money."

They sat together at a table that was close against the wall near the door of the café and looked at the terrace where the tables were all empty except where the old man sat in the shadow of the leaves of the tree that moved slightly in the wind. A girl and a soldier went by in the street. The street light shone on the brass number on his collar. The girl wore no head covering and hurried beside him.

"The guard will pick him up," one waiter said.

"What does it matter if he gets what he's after?"

"He had better get off the street now. The guard will get him. They went by five minutes ago."

The old man sitting in the shadow rapped on his saucer with his glass. The younger waiter went over to him.

"What do you want?"

The old man looked at him. "Another brandy," he said.

"You'll be drunk," the waiter said. The old man looked at him. The waiter went away.

"He'll stay all night," he said to his colleague. "I'm sleepy now. I never get into bed before three o'clock. He should have killed himself last week."

The waiter took the brandy bottle and another saucer from the counter inside the café and marched out to the old man's table. He put down the saucer and poured the glass full of brandy.

"You should have killed yourself last week," he said to the deaf man. The old man motioned with his finger. "A little more," he said. The waiter poured on into the glass so that the brandy slopped over and ran down the stem into the top saucer of the pile. "Thank you," the old man said. The waiter took the bottle back inside the café. He sat down at the table with his colleague again.

"He's drunk now," he said.

"He's drunk every night."

"What did he want to kill himself for?"

"How should I know."

"How did he do it?"

"He hung himself with a rope."

"Who cut him down?"

"His niece."

"Why did they do it?"

"Fear for his soul."

"How much money has he got?"

"He's got plenty."

"He must be eighty years old."

"Anyway I should say he was eighty."

"I wish he would go home. I never get to bed before three o'clock. What kind of hour is that to go to bed?"

"He stays up because he likes it."

"He's lonely. I'm not lonely. I have a wife waiting in bed for me."

"He had a wife once too."

"A wife would be no good to him now."

"You can't tell. He might be better with a wife."

"His niece looks after him. You said she cut him down."

"I know."

"I wouldn't want to be that old. An old man is a nasty thing."

"Not always. This old man is clean. He drinks without spilling. Even now, drunk. Look at him."

"I don't want to look at him. I wish he would go home. He has no regard for those who must work."

The old man looked from his glass across the square, then over at the waiters.

"Another brandy," he said, pointing to his glass. The waiter who was in a hurry came over.

"Finished," he said, speaking with that omission of syntax stupid people employ when talking to drunken people or foreigners. "No more tonight. Close now."

"Another," said the old man.

"No. Finished." The waiter wiped the edge of the table with a towel and shook his head.

The old man stood up, slowly counted the saucers, took a leather coin purse from his pocket and paid for the drinks, leaving half a peseta tip.

The waiter watched him go down the street, a very old man walking unsteadily but with dignity.

"Why didn't you let him stay and drink?" the unhurried waiter asked. They were putting up the shutters. "It is not half-past two."

"I want to go home to bed."

"What is an hour?"

"More to me than to him."

"An hour is the same."

"You talk like an old man yourself. He can buy a bottle and drink at home."

"It's not the same."

"No, it is not," agreed the waiter with a wife. He did not wish to be unjust. He was only in a hurry.

"And you? You have no fear of going home before your usual hour?"

"Are you trying to insult me?"

"No, hombre, only to make a joke."

"No," the waiter who was in a hurry said, rising from pulling down the metal shutters. "I have confidence. I am all confidence."

"You have youth, confidence, and a job," the older waiter said. "You have everything."

"And what do you lack?"

"Everything but work."

"You have everything I have."

"No. I have never had confidence and I am not young."

"Come on. Stop talking nonsense and lock up."

"I am of those who like to stay late at the café," the older waiter said. "With all those who do not want to go to bed. With all those who need a light for the night."

"I want to go home and into bed."

"We are of two different kinds," the older waiter said. He was now dressed to go home. "It is not only a question of youth and confidence although those things are very beautiful. Each night I am reluctant to close up because there may be some one who needs the café."

"Hombre, there are bodegas open all night long."

"You do not understand. This is a clean and pleasant café. It is well lighted. The light is very good and also, now, there are shadows of the leaves."

"Good night," said the younger waiter.

"Good night," the other said. Turning off the electric light he continued the conversation with himself. It is the light of course but it is necessary that the place be clean and pleasant. You do not want music. Certainly you do not want music. Nor can you stand before a bar with dignity although that is all that is provided for these hours. What did he fear? It was not fear or dread. It was a nothing that he knew too well. It was all a nothing and a man was nothing too. It was only that and light was all it needed and a certain cleanness and order. Some lived in it and never felt it but he knew it all was nada y pues nada y nada y pues nada. Our nada who art in nada, nada be thy name thy kingdom nada thy will be nada in nada as it is in nada. Give us this nada our daily nada and nada us our nada as we nada our nadas and nada us not into nada but deliver us from nada; pues nada. Hail nothing full of nothing, nothing is with thee. He smiled and stood before a bar with a shining steam pressure coffee machine.

"What's yours?" asked the barman.

"Nada."

"Otro loco mas," said the barman and turned away.

"A little cup," said the waiter.

The barman poured it for him.

"The light is very bright and pleasant but the bar is unpolished," the waiter said.

The barman looked at him but did not answer. It was too late at night for conversation.

"You want another copita?" the barman asked.

"No, thank you," said the waiter and went out. He disliked bars and bodegas. A clean, well-lighted café was a very different thing. Now, without thinking further, he would go home to his room. He would lie in the bed and finally, with daylight, he would go to sleep. After all, he said to himself, it is probably only insomnia. Many must have it.

The Workhouse Ward

Persons

Mike McInerney }paupers
Michael Miskell }
Mrs. Donohoe, a countrywoman

Scene:
    A ward in Cloon Workhouse. The two old men in their beds.

MICHAEL MISKELL
Isn't it a hard case, Mike McInerney, myself and yourself to be left here in the bed, and it the feast day of Saint Colman, and the rest of the ward attending on the Mass.

MIKE McINERNEY
Is it sitting up by the hearth you are wishful to be, Michael Miskell, with cold in the shoulders and with speckled shins? Let you rise up so, and you well able to do it, not like myself that has pains the same as tin-tacks within in my inside.

MICHAEL MISKELL
If you have pains within in your inside there is no one can see it or know of it the way they can see my own knees that are swelled up with the rheumatism, and my hands that are twisted in ridges the same as an old cabbage stalk. It is easy to be talking about soreness and about pains, and they maybe not to be in it at all.

MIKE McINERNEY
To open me and to analyze me you would know what sort of a pain and a soreness I have in my heart and in my chest. But I'm not one like yourself to be cursing and praying and tormenting the time the nuns are at hand, thinking to get a bigger share than myself of the nourishment and of the milk.

MICHAEL MISKELL

That's the way you do be picking at me and faulting me. I had a share and a good share in my early time, and it's well you know that, and the both of us reared in Skehanagh.

MIKE McINERNEY

You may say that, indeed, we are both of us reared in Skehanagh. Little wonder you to have good nourishment the time we were both rising, and you bringing away my rabbits out of the snare.

MICHAEL MISKELL

And you didn't bring away my own eels, I suppose, I was after spearing in the Turlough? Selling them to the nuns in the convent you did, and letting on they to be your own. For you were always a cheater and a schemer, grabbing every earthly thing for your own profit.

MIKE McINERNEY

And you were no grabber yourself, I suppose, till your land and all you had grabbed wore away from you!

MICHAEL MISKELL

If I lost it itself, it was through the crosses I met with and I going through the world. I never was a rambler and a card-player like yourself, Mike McInerney, that ran through all and lavished it unknown to your mother!

MIKE McINERNEY

Lavished it, is it? And if I did was it you yourself led me to lavish it or some other one? It is on my own floor I would be today and in the face of my family, but for the misfortune I had to be put with a bad next door neighbor that was yourself. What way did my means go from me is it? Spending on fencing, spending on walls, making up gates, putting up doors, that would keep your hens and your ducks from coming in through starvation on my floor, and every four-footed beast you had from preying and trespassing on my oats and my mangolds and my little lock of hay!

MICHAEL MISKELL

O to listen to you! And I striving to please you and to be kind to you and to close my ears to the abuse you would be calling and letting out of your mouth. To trespass on your crops is it? It's little temptation there was for my poor beasts to ask to cross the mering. My God Almighty! What had you but a little corner of a field!

MIKE McINERNEY

And what do you say to my garden that your two pigs had destroyed on me the year of the big tree being knocked, and they making gaps in the wall.

MICHAEL MISKELL

Ah, there does be a great deal of gaps knocked in a twelve-month. Why wouldn't they be knocked by thunder, the same as the tree, or some storm that came up from the west?

MIKE MCINERNEY

It was the west wind, I suppose, that devoured my green cabbage? And that rooted up my Champion potatoes? And that ate the gooseberries themselves from off the bush?

MICHAEL MISKELL

What are you saying? The two quietest pigs ever I had, no way wicked and well ringed. They were not ten minutes in it. It would be hard for them eat strawberries in that time, let alone gooseberries that's full of thorns.

MIKE MCINERNEY

They were not quiet, but very ravenous pigs you had that time, as active as a fox they were, killing my young ducks. Once they had blood tasted you couldn't stop them.

MICHAEL MISKELL

And what happened myself the fair day of Esserkelly, the time I was passing your door? Two brazened dogs that rushed out and took a piece of me. I never was the better of it or of the start I got, but wasting from then till now!

MIKE MCINERNEY

Thinking you were a wild beast they did, that had made his escape out of the travelling show, with the red eyes of you and the ugly face of you, and the two crooked legs of you that wouldn't hardly stop a pig in a gap. Sure any dog that had any life in it at all would be roused and stirred seeing the like of you going the road!

MICHAEL MISKELL

I did well taking out a summons against you that time. It is a great wonder you not to have been bound over through your lifetime, but the laws of England is queer.

MIKE MCINERNEY

What ailed me that I did not summons yourself after you stealing away the clutch of eggs I had in the barrel, and I away in Ardrahan searching out a clocking hen.

MICHAEL MISKELL

To steal your eggs is it? Is that what you are saying now? (*Holds up his hands.*) The Lord is in heaven, and Peter and the saints, and yourself that was in Ardrahan that day put a hand on them as soon as myself! Isn't it a bad story for me to wearing out my days beside you the same as a spancelled goat. Chained I am and tethered I am to a man that is ramsacking his mind for lies!

MIKE MCINERNEY

If it is a bad story for you, Michael Miskell, it is a worse story again for my-self. A Miskell to be next and near me through the whole of the four quarters of the year. I never heard there to be any great name on the Miskells as there was on my own race and name.

MICHAEL MISKELL

You didn't, is it? Well, you could hear it if you had but ears to hear it. Go across to Lisheen Crannagh and down to the sea and to Newtown Lynch and the mills of Duras and you'll find a Miskell, and as far as Dublin!

MIKE MCINERNEY

What signifies Crannagh and the mills of Duras? Look at all my own gen-erations that are buried at the Seven Churches. And how many generations of the Miskells are buried in it? Answer me that!

MICHAEL MISKELL

I tell you but for the wheat that was to be sowed there would be more side cars and more common cars at my father's funeral (God rest his soul!) than at any funeral ever left your own door. And as to my mother, she was a Cuffe from Claregalway, and it's she had the purer blood!

MIKE MCINERNEY

And what do you say to the banshee? Isn't she apt to have knowledge of the ancient race? Was ever she heard to screech or to cry for the Miskells? Or the Cuffes from Claregalway? She was not, but for the six families, the Hyneses, the Foxes, the Faheys, the Dooleys, the McInerneys. It is of the nature of the McInerneys she is I am thinking, crying them the same as a king's children.

MICHAEL MISKELL

It is a pity the banshee not to be crying for yourself at this minute, and giv-ing you a warning to quit your lies and your chat and your arguing and your contrary ways; for there is no one under the rising sun could stand you. I tell you you are not behaving as in the presence of the Lord!

23

MIKE MCINERNEY

Is it wishful for my death you are? Let it come and meet me now and welcome so long as it will part me from yourself! And I say, and I would kiss the book on it, I to have one request only to be granted, and I leaving it in my will, it is what I would request, nine furrows of the field, nine ridges of the hills, nine waves of the ocean to be put between your grave and my own grave the time we will be laid in the ground!

MICHAEL MISKELL

Amen to that! Nine ridges, is it? No, but let the whole ridge of the world separate us till the Day of Judgment! I would not be laid anear you at the Seven Churches, I to get Ireland without a divide!

MIKE MCINERNEY

And after that again! I'd sooner than ten pound in my hand, I to know that my shadow and my ghost will not be knocking about with your shadow and your ghost, and the both of us waiting our time. I'd sooner be delayed in Purgatory! Now, have you anything to say?

MICHAEL MISKELL

I have everything to say, if I had but the time to say it!

MIKE MCINERNEY

(sitting up): Let me up out of this till I'll choke you!

MICHAEL MISKELL

You scolding pauper you!

MIKE MCINERNEY

(shaking his fist at him): Wait a while!

MICHAEL MISKELL

(shaking his fist): Wait a while yourself!
  MRS. DONOHOE comes in with a parcel. She is a countrywoman
  with a frilled cap and a shawl. She stands still a minute. The two old
  men lie down and compose themselves.

MRS. DONOHOE

They bade me come up here by the stair. I never was in this place at all. I don't know am I right. Which now of the two of ye is Mike McInerney?

MIKE MCINERNEY

Who is it is calling me by my name?

MRS. DONOHOE

Sure amn't I your sister, Honor McInerney that was, that is now Honor Donohoe.

MIKE McINERNEY

So you are, I believe. I didn't know you till you pushed anear me. It is time indeed for you to come see me, and I in this place five year or more. Thinking me to be no credit to you, I suppose, among that tribe of the Donohoes. I wonder they to give you leave to come ask am I living yet or dead?

MRS. DONOHOE

Ah, sure, I buried the whole string of them. Himself was the last to go. (*Wipes her eyes.*) The Lord be praised he got a fine natural death. Sure we must go through our crosses. And he got a lovely funeral; it would delight you to hear the priest reading the Mass. My poor John Donohoe! A nice clean man, you couldn't but be fond of him. Very severe on the tobacco he was, but he wouldn't touch the drink.

MIKE McINERNEY

And is it in Curranroe you are living yet?

MRS. DONOHOE

It is so. He left all to myself. But it is a lonesome thing the head of a house to have died!

MIKE McINERNEY

I hope that he has left you a nice way of living?

MRS. DONOHOE

Fair enough, fair enough. A wide lovely house I have; a few acres of grass land . . . the grass does be very sweet that grows among the stones. And as to the sea, there is something from it every day of the year, a handful of periwinkles to make kitchen, or cockles maybe. There is many a thing in the sea is not decent, but cockles is fit to put before the Lord!

MIKE McINERNEY

You have all that! And you without ere a man in the house?

MRS. DONOHOE

It is what I am thinking, yourself might come and keep me company. It is no credit to me a brother of my own to be in this place at all.

25

MIKE MCINERNEY

I'll go with you! Let me out of this! It is the name of the McInerneys will be rising on every side!

MRS. DONOHOE

I don't know. I was ignorant of you being kept to the bed.

MIKE MCINERNEY

I am not kept to it, but maybe an odd time when there is a colic rises up within me. My stomach always gets better the time there is a change in the moon. I'd like well to draw anear you. My heavy blessing on you, Honor Donohoe, for the hand you have held out to me this day.

MRS. DONOHOE

Sure you could be keeping the fire in, and stirring the pot with the bit of Indian meal for the hens, and milking the goat and taking the tacklings off the donkey at the door; and maybe putting out the cabbage plants in their time. For when the old man died the garden died.

MIKE MCINERNEY

I could to be sure, and be cutting the potatoes for seed. What luck could there be in a place and a man not to be in it? Is that now a suit of clothes you have brought with you?

MRS. DONOHOE

It is so, the way you will be tasty coming in among the neighbors at Curranroe.

MIKE MCINERNEY

My joy you are! It is well you earned me! Let me up out of this! (*He sits up and spreads out the clothes and tries on the coat.*) That now is a good frieze coat . . . and a hat in the fashion. . . . (*He puts on hat.*)

MICHAEL MISKELL

(*alarmed*): And is it going out of this you are, Mike McInerney?

MIKE MCINERNEY

Don't you hear I am going? To Curranroe I am going. Going I am to a place where I will get every good thing!

MICHAEL MISKELL

And is it to leave me here after you, you will?

MIKE MCINERNEY

(*in a rising chant*): Every good thing! The goat and the kid are there, the sheep and the lamb are there, the cow does be running and she coming to be milked! Ploughing and seed sowing, blossom at Christmas time, the cuckoo speaking through the dark days of the year! Ah, what are you talking about? Wheat high in the hedges, no talk about the rent! Salmon in the rivers as plenty as turf! Spending and getting and nothing scarce! Sport and pleasure, and music on the strings! Age will go from me and I will be young again. Geese and turkeys for the hundreds and drinks for the whole world!

MICHAEL MISKELL

Ah, Mike, is it truth you are saying, you to go from me and to leave me with rude people and with townspeople, and with people of every parish in the union, and they having no respect for me or no wish for me at all!

MIKE MCINERNEY

Whist now and I'll leave you . . . my pipe (*hands it over*); and I'll engage it is Honor Donohoe won't refuse to be sending you a few ounces of tobacco an odd time, and neighbors coming to the fair in November or in the month of May.

MICHAEL MISKELL

Ah, what signifies tobacco? All that I am craving is the talk. There to be no one at all to say out to whatever thought might be rising in my innate mind! To be lying here and no conversible person in it would be the abomination of misery!

MIKE MCINERNEY

Look now, Honor. . . . It is what I often heard said, two to be better than one. . . . Sure if you had an old trouser was full of holes . . . or a skirt . . . wouldn't you put another in under it that might be as tattered as itself, and the two of them together would make some sort of a decent show?

MRS. DONOHOE

Ah, what are you saying? There is no holes in that suit I brought you now, but as sound it is as the day I spun it for himself.

MIKE MCINERNEY

It is what I am thinking, Honor . . . I do be weak an odd time . . . any load I would carry, it preys upon my side . . . and this man does be weak an odd time with the swelling in his knees . . . but the two of us together it's not likely it is at the one time we would fail. Bring the both of us with you,

Honor, and the height of the castle of luck on you and the both of us together will make one good hardy man!

MRS. DONOHOE

I'd like my job! Is it queer in the head you are grown asking me to bring in a stranger off the road?

MICHAEL MISKELL

I am not, ma'am, but an old neighbor I am. If I had forecasted this asking I would have asked it myself. Michael Miskell I am, that was in the next house to you in Skehanagh!

MRS. DONOHOE

For pity's sake! Michael Miskell is it? That's worse again. Yourself and Mike that never left fighting and scolding and attacking one another like two young pups you were, and threatening one another after like two grown dogs!

MIKE MCINERNEY

All the quarreling was ever in the place it was myself did it. Sure his anger rises fast and goes away like the wind. Bring him out with myself now, Honor Donohoe, and God bless you.

MRS. DONOHOE

Well, then, I will not bring him out, and I will not bring yourself out, and you not to learn better sense. Are you making yourself ready to come?

MIKE MCINERNEY

I am thinking, maybe . . . it is a mean thing for a man that is shivering into seventy years to go changing from place to place.

MRS. DONOHOE

Well, take your luck or leave it. All I asked was to save you from the hurt and the harm of the year.

MIKE MCINERNEY

Bring the both of us with you or I will not stir out of this.

MRS. DONOHOE

Give me back my fine suit so (*begins gathering up the clothes*), till I'll go look for a man of my own!

MIKE MCINERNEY

Let you go so, as you are so unnatural and so disobliging, and look for some man of your own, God help him! For I will not go with you at all!

MRS. DONOHOE

It is too much time I lost with you, and dark night waiting to overtake me on the road. Let the two of you stop together, and the back of my hand to you. It is I will leave you there the same as God left the Jews!

She goes out. The old men lie down and are silent for a moment.

MICHAEL MISKELL

Maybe the house is not so wide as what she says.

MIKE MCINERNEY

Why wouldn't it be wide?

MICHAEL MISKELL

Ah, there does be a good deal of middling poor houses down by the sea.

MIKE MCINERNEY

What would you know about wide houses? Whatever sort of a house you had yourself it was too wide for the provision you had into it.

MICHAEL MISKELL

Whatever provision I had in my house it was wholesome provision and natural provision. Herself and her periwinkles! Periwinkles is a hungry sort of food.

MIKE MCINERNEY

Stop your impudence and your chat or it will be the worse for you. I'd bear with my own father and mother as long as any man would, but if they'd vex me I would give them the length of a rope as soon as another!

MICHAEL MISKELL

I would never ask at all to go eating periwinkles.

MIKE MCINERNEY

(*sitting up*): Have you anyone to fight me?

MICHAEL MISKELL

(*whimpering*): I have not, only the Lord!

MIKE MCINERNEY

Let you leave putting insults on me so, and death picking at you!

MICHAEL MISKELL

Sure I am saying nothing at all to displease you. It is why I wouldn't go eating periwinkles, I'm in dread I might swallow the pin.

MIKE MCINERNEY

Who in the world wide is asking you to eat them? You're as tricky as a fish in the full tide!

MICHAEL MISKELL

Tricky is it! Oh, my curse and the curse of the four and twenty men upon you!

MIKE MCINERNEY

That the worm may chew you from skin to marrow bone! (*Seizes his pillow.*)

MICHAEL MISKELL

(*seizing his own pillow*): I'll leave my death on you, you scheming vagabond!

MIKE MCINERNEY

By cripes! I'll pull out your pin feathers! (*Throwing pillow.*)

MICHAEL MISKELL

(*throwing pillow*): You tyrant! You big bully you!

MIKE MCINERNEY

(*throwing pillow and seizing mug*): Take this so, you stobbing ruffian you!
They throw all within their reach at one another, mugs, prayer books, pipes, etc.

Curtain

The Space Crone

The menopause is probably the least glamorous topic imaginable; and this is interesting, because it is one of the very few topics to which cling some shreds and remnants of taboo. A serious mention of menopause is usually met with uneasy silence; a sneering reference to it is usually met with relieved sniggers. Both the silence and the sniggering are pretty sure indications of taboo.

Most people would consider the old phrase "change of life" a euphemism for the medical term "menopause," but I, who am now going through the change, begin to wonder if it isn't the other way round. "Change of life" is too blunt a phrase, too factual. "Menopause," with its chime-suggestion of a mere pause after which things go on as before, is reassuringly trivial.

But the change is not trivial, and I wonder how many women are brave enough to carry it out wholeheartedly. They give up their reproductive capacity with more or less of a struggle, and when it's gone they think that's all there is to it. Well, at least I don't get the Curse any more, they say, and the only reason I felt so depressed sometimes was hormones. Now I'm myself again. But this is to evade the real challenge, and to lose, not only the capacity to ovulate, but the opportunity to become a Crone.

In the old days women who survived long enough to attain the menopause more often accepted the challenge. They had, after all, had practice. They had already changed their life radically once before, when they ceased to be virgins and became mature women/wives/matrons/mothers/mistresses/whores/etc. This change involved not only the physiological alterations of puberty—the shift from barren childhood to fruitful maturity—but a socially recognized alteration of being: a change of condition from the sacred to the profane.

With the secularization of virginity now complete, so that the once awesome term "virgin" is now a sneer or at best a slightly dated word for a person who hasn't copulated yet, the opportunity of gaining or regaining the dangerous/sacred condition of being at the Second Change has ceased to be apparent.

Virginity is now a mere preamble or waiting room to be got out of as soon as possible; it is without significance. Old age is similarly a waiting room,

where you go after life's over and wait for cancer or a stroke. The years before and after the menstrual years are vestigial: the only meaningful condition left to women is that of fruitfulness. Curiously, this restriction of
significance coincided with the development of chemicals and instruments
that make fertility itself a meaningless or at least secondary characteristic of
female maturity. The significance of maturity now is not the capacity to con-
ceive but the mere ability to have sex. As this ability is shared by pubescents
and by postclimacterics, the blurring of distinctions and elimination of op-
portunities is almost complete. There are no rites of passage because there
is no significant change. The Triple Goddess has only one face: Marilyn
Monroe's, maybe. The entire life of a woman from ten or twelve through
seventy or eighty has become secular, uniform, changeless. As there is no
longer any virtue in virginity, so there is no longer any meaning in menopause. It requires fanatical determination now to become a Crone.

Women have thus, by imitating the life condition of men, surrendered a
very strong position of their own. Men are afraid of virgins, but they have a
cure for their own fear and the virgin's virginity: fucking. Men are afraid of
crones, so afraid of them that their cure for virginity fails them; they know it
won't work. Faced with the fulfilled Crone, all but the bravest men wilt and
retreat, crestfallen and cockadroop.

Menopause Manor is not merely a defensive stronghold, however. It is a
house or household, fully furnished with the necessities of life. In abandon-
ing it, women have narrowed their domain and impoverished their souls.
There are things the Old Woman can do, say, and think that the Woman
cannot do, say, or think. The Woman has to give up more than her menstrual
periods before she can do, say, or think them. She has got to change her life.

The nature of that change is now clearer than it used to be. Old age is not
virginity but a third and new condition; the virgin must be celibate, but the
crone need not. There was a confusion there, which the separation of female
sexuality from reproductive capacity, via modern contraceptives, has cleared
up. Loss of fertility does not mean loss of desire and fulfillment. But it does
entail a change, a change involving matters even more important—if I may
venture a heresy—than sex.

The woman who is willing to make that change must become pregnant
with herself, at last. She must bear herself, her third self, her old age, with
travail and alone. Not many will help her with that birth. Certainly no male
obstetrician will time her contractions, inject her with sedatives, stand ready
with forceps, and neatly stitch up the torn membranes. It's hard even to find
an old-fashioned midwife, these days. That pregnancy is long, that labor is
hard. Only one is harder, and that's the final one, the one that men also must
suffer and perform.

It may well be easier to die if you have already given birth to others or
yourself, at least once before. This would be an argument for going through

all the discomfort and embarrassment of becoming a Crone. Anyhow it seems a pity to have a built-in rite of passage and to dodge it, evade it, and pretend nothing has changed. That is to dodge and evade one's womanhood, to pretend one's like a man. Men, once initiated, never get the second chance. They never change again. That's their loss, not ours. Why borrow poverty?

Certainly the effort to remain unchanged, young, when the body gives so impressive a signal of change as the menopause, is gallant; but it is a stupid, self-sacrificial gallantry, better befitting a boy of twenty than a woman of forty-five or fifty. Let the athletes die young and laurel-crowned. Let the soldiers earn the Purple Hearts. Let women die old, white-crowned, with human hearts.

If a space ship came by from the friendly natives of the fourth planet of Altair, and the polite captain of the space ship said, "We have room for one passenger; will you spare us a single human being, so that we may converse at leisure during the long trip back to Altair and learn from an exemplary person the nature of the race?"—I suppose what most people would want to do is provide them with a fine, bright, brave young man, highly educated and in peak physical condition. A Russian cosmonaut would be ideal (American astronauts are mostly too old). There would surely be hundreds, thousands of volunteers, just such young men, all worthy. But I would not pick any of them. Nor would I pick any of the young women who would volunteer, some out of magnanimity and intellectual courage, others out of a profound conviction that Altair couldn't possibly be any worse for a woman than Earth is.

What I would do is go down to the local Woolworth's, or the local village marketplace, and pick an old woman, over sixty, from behind the costume jewelry counter or the betel-nut booth. Her hair would not be red or blonde or lustrous dark, her skin would not be dewy fresh, she would not have the secret of eternal youth. She might, however, show you a small snapshot of her grandson, who is working in Nairobi. She is a bit vague about where Nairobi is, but extremely proud of the grandson. She has worked hard at small, unimportant jobs all her life, jobs like cooking, cleaning, bringing up kids, selling little objects of adornment or pleasure to other people. She was a virgin once, a long time ago, and then a sexually potent fertile female, and then went through menopause. She has given birth several times and faced death several times—the same times. She is facing the final birth/death a little more nearly and clearly every day now. Sometimes her feet hurt something terrible. She never was educated to anything like her capacity, and that is a shameful waste and a crime against humanity, but so common a crime should not and cannot be hidden from Altair. And anyhow she's not dumb. She has a stock of sense, wit, patience, and experiential shrewdness, which the Altaireans might, or might not, perceive as wisdom. If they are wiser than we, then of course we don't know how they'd perceive it. But if they are wiser than we, they may know how to perceive that inmost mind and heart which we, working on mere guess and hope, proclaim to be humane. In any case, since they are curious and kindly, let's give them the best we have to give.

The trouble is, she will be very reluctant to volunteer. "What would an old woman like me do on Altair?" she'll say. "You ought to send one of those scientist men, they can talk to those funny-looking green people. Maybe Dr. Kissinger should go. What about sending the Shaman?" It will be very hard to explain to her that we want her to go because only a person who has experienced, accepted, and acted the entire human condition—the essential quality of which is Change—can fairly represent humanity. "Me?" she'll say, just a trifle slyly. "But I never did anything."

But it won't wash. She knows, though she won't admit it, that Dr. Kissinger has not gone and will never go where she has gone, that the scientists and the shamans have not done what she has done. Into the space ship, Granny.

Mr. Flood's Party

Old Eben Flood, climbing alone one night
Over the hill between the town below
And the forsaken upland hermitage
That held as much as he should ever know
On earth again of home, paused warily.
The road was his with not a native near;
And Eben, having leisure, said aloud,
For no man else in Tilbury Town to hear:

"Well, Mr. Flood, we have the harvest moon
Again, and we may not have many more;
The bird is on the wing, the poet says,
And you and I have said it here before.
Drink to the bird." He raised up to the light
The jug that he had gone so far to fill,
And answered huskily: "Well, Mr. Flood,
Since you propose it, I believe I will."

Alone, as if enduring to the end
A valiant armor of scarred hopes outworn,
He stood there in the middle of the road
Like Roland's ghost winding a silent horn.
Below him, in the town among the trees,
Where friends of other days had honored him,
A phantom salutation of the dead
Rang thinly till old Eben's eyes were dim.

Then, as a mother lays her sleeping child
Down tenderly, fearing it may awake,
He set the jug down slowly at his feet
With trembling care, knowing that most things break;
And only when assured that on firm earth
It stood, as the uncertain lives of men
Assuredly did not, he paced away,
And with his hand extended paused again:

"Well, Mr. Flood, we have not met like this
In a long time; and many a change has come
To both of us, I fear, since last it was
We had a drop together. Welcome home!"
Convivially returning with himself,
Again he raised the jug up to the light;
And with an acquiescent quaver said:
"Well, Mr. Flood, if you insist, I might.

"Only a very little, Mr. Flood—
For auld lang syne. No more, sir; that will do."
So, for the time, apparently it did,
And Eben evidently thought so too;
For soon amid the silver loneliness
Of night he lifted up his voice and sang,
Secure, with only two moons listening,
Until the whole harmonious landscape rang—

"For auld lang syne." The weary throat gave out,
The last word wavered; and the song being done,
He raised again the jug regretfully
And shook his head, and was again alone.
There was not much that was ahead of him,
And there was nothing in the town below—
Where strangers would have shut the many doors
That many friends had opened long ago.

An Old Man's Winter Night

All out-of-doors looked darkly in at him
Through the thin frost, almost in separate stars,
That gathers on the pane in empty rooms.
What kept his eyes from giving back the gaze
Was the lamp tilted near them in his hand.
What kept him from remembering what it was
That brought him to that creaking room was age.
He stood with barrels round him—at a loss.
And having scared the cellar under him
In clomping here, he scared it once again
In clomping off;—and scared the outer night,
Which has its sounds, familiar, like the roar
Of trees and crack of branches, common things,
But nothing so like beating on a box.
A light he was to no one but himself
Where now he sat, concerned with he knew what,
A quiet light, and then not even that.
He consigned to the moon, such as she was,
So late-arising, to the broken moon
As better than the sun in any case
For such a charge, his snow upon the roof,
His icicles along the wall to keep;
And slept. The log that shifted with a jolt
Once in the stove, disturbed him and he shifted,
And eased his heavy breathing, but still slept.
One aged man—one man—can't keep a house,
A farm, a countryside, or if he can,
It's thus he does it of a winter night.

Provide, Provide

The witch that came (the withered hag)
To wash the steps with pail and rag,
Was once the beauty Abishag,

The picture pride of Hollywood.
Too many fall from great and good
For you to doubt the likelihood.

Die early and avoid the fate.
Or if predestined to die late,
Make up your mind to die in state.

Make the whole stock exchange your own!
If need be occupy a throne,
Where nobody can call *you* crone.

Some have relied on what they knew;
Others on being simply true.
What worked for them might work for you.

No memory of having starred
Atones for later disregard,
Or keeps the end from being hard.

Better to go down dignified
With boughten friendship at your side
Than none at all. Provide, provide!

A Woman Alone

When she cannot be sure
which of two lovers it was with whom she felt
this or that moment of pleasure, of something fiery
streaking from head to heels, the way the white
flame of a cascade streaks a mountainside
seen from a car across a valley, the car
changing gear, skirting a precipice,
climbing . . .
When she can sit or walk for hours after a movie
talking earnestly and with bursts of laughter
with friends, without worrying
that it's late, dinner at midnight, her time
spent without counting the change . . .
When half her bed is covered with books
and no one is kept awake by the reading light
and she disconnects the phone, to sleep till noon . . .
Then
selfpity dries up, a joy
untainted by guilt lifts her.
She has fears, but not about loneliness;
fears about how to deal with the aging
of her body—how to deal
with photographs and the mirror. She feels
so much younger and more beautiful
than she looks. At her happiest
—or even in the midst of
some less than joyful hour, sweating
patiently through a heatwave in the city
or hearing the sparrows at daybreak, dully gray,
toneless, the sound of fatigue—
a kind of sober euphoria makes her believe
in her future as an old woman, a wanderer,
seamed and brown,
little luxuries of the middle of life all gone,
watching cities and rivers, people and mountains,

without being watched; not grim nor sad,
an old winedrinking woman, who knows
the old roads, grass-grown, and laughs to herself . . .
She knows it can't be:
that's Mrs. Doasyouwouldbedoneby from
                              The Water-Babies,
no one can walk the world any more,
a world of fumes and decibels.
But she thinks maybe
she could get to be tough and wise, some way,
anyway. Now at least
she is past the time of mourning,
now she can say without shame or deceit,
O blessed Solitude.

Virginia Portrait

Winter is settling on the place; the sedge
Is dry and lifeless and the woods stand bare.
The late autumnal flowers, nipped by frost,
Break from the sear stalks in the trim, neat garden,
And fall unheeded on the bleak, brown earth.

The winter of her year has come to her,
This wizened woman, spare of frame, but great
Of heart, erect, and undefeated yet.

Grief has been hers, before this wintry time.
Death has paid calls, unmannered, uninvited;
Low mounds have swollen in the fenced off corner,
Over brown children, marked by white-washed stones.
She has seen hopes that promised a fine harvest
Burnt by the drought; or bitten by the hoarfrost;
Or washed up and drowned out by unlooked for rains.
And as a warning blast of her own winter,
Death, the harsh overseer, shouted to her man,
Who answering slowly went over the hill.

She, puffing on a jagged slow-burning pipe,
By the low hearthfire, knows her winter now.
But she has strength and steadfast hardihood.
Deep-rooted is she, even as the oaks,
Hardy as perennials about her door.
The circle of the season brings no fear,
"*Folks all gits used to what dey sees so often*";
And she has helps that throng her glowing fire
Mixed with the smoke hugging her grizzled head:

Warm friends, the love of her full-blooded spouse,
Quiet companionship as age crept on him,
Laughter of babies, and their shrewd, sane raising;
These simple joys not poor to her at all;

41

The sight of smokeclouds pouring from the flue;
Her stalwart son deep busied with "book larnin',"
After the weary fields; the kettle's purr
In duet with the sleek and pampered mouser;
Twanging of dominickers; lowing of Betsey;
Old folksongs chanted underneath the stars. . . .

Even when winter settles on her heart,
She keeps a wonted, quiet nonchalance,
A courtly dignity of speech and carriage,
Unlooked for in these distant rural ways.

She has found faith sufficient for her grief,
The song of earth for bearing heavy years,
She with slow speech, and spurts of heartfelt laughter,
Illiterate, and somehow very wise.

She has been happy, and her heart is grateful.
Now she looks out, and forecasts unperturbed
Her following slowly over the lonesome hill,
Her *'layin' down her burdens, bye and bye.'*

Miss Rosie

when i watch you
wrapped up like garbage
sitting, surrounded by the smell
of too old potato peels
or
when i watch you
in your old man's shoes
with the little toe cut out
sitting, waiting for your mind
like next week's grocery
i say
when i watch you
you wet brown bag of a woman
who used to be the best looking gal in georgia
used to be called the Georgia Rose
i stand up
through your destruction
i stand up

A Lady

You are beautiful and faded
Like an old opera tune
Played upon a harpsichord;
Or like the sun-flooded silks
Of an eighteenth-century boudoir.
In your eyes
Smoulder the fallen roses of out-lived
    minutes,
And the perfume of your soul
Is vague and suffusing,
With the pungence of sealed spice-jars.
Your half-tones delight me,
And I grow mad with gazing
At your blent colours.

My vigour is a new-minted penny,
Which I cast at your feet.
Gather it up from the dust,
That its sparkle may amuse you.

On a Winter Night

On a winter night
I sat alone
In a cold room,
Feeling old, strange
At the year's change
In fire light.

Last fire of youth,
All brilliance burning
And my year turning,
One dazzling rush
Like a wild wish
Or blaze of truth.

First fire of age
And the soft snow
Of ash below—
For the clean wood
The end was good.
For me, an image.

For then I saw
That fires, not I,
Burn down and die;
That flare of gold
Turns old, turns cold.
Not I. I grow.

Nor old, nor young,
The burning sprite
Of my delight,
A salamander
In fires of wonder,
Gives tongue, gives tongue!

How to Be Old

It is easy to be young. (Everybody is,
at first.) It is not easy
to be old. It takes time.
Youth is given; age is achieved.
One must work a magic to mix with time
in order to become old.

Youth is given. One must put it away
like a doll in a closet,
take it out and play with it only
on holidays. One must have many dresses
and dress the doll impeccably
(but not to show the doll, to keep it hidden.)

It is necessary to adore the doll,
to remember it in the dark on the ordinary
days, and every day congratulate
one's aging face in the mirror.

In time one will be very old.
In time, one's life will be accomplished.
And in time, in time, the doll—
like new, though ancient—will be found.

Old

I'm afraid of needles.
I'm tired of rubber sheets and tubes.
I'm tired of faces that I don't know
and now I think that death is starting.
Death starts like a dream,
full of objects and my sister's laughter.
We are young and we are walking
and picking wild blueberries
all the way to Damariscotta.
Oh Susan, she cried,
you've stained your new waist.
Sweet taste—
my mouth so full
and the sweet blue running out
all the way to Damariscotta.
What are you doing? Leave me alone!
Can't you see I'm dreaming?
In a dream you are never eighty.

Fortitude

DR. ELBERT LITTLE   a kindly, attractive young general practitioner, is being shown around by the creator and boss of the operation, DR. NORBERT FRANKENSTEIN

FRANKENSTEIN   FRANKENSTEIN is 65, a crass medical genius.

DR. TOM SWIFT   Seated at the console, wearing headphones and watching meters and flashing lights, is FRANKENSTEIN'S enthusiastic first assistant.

The Time
> the present.

The Place
> Upstate New York, a large room filled with pulsing, writhing, panting machines that perform the functions of various organs of the human body—heart, lungs, liver, and so on. Color-coded pipes and wires swoop upward from the machines to converge and pass through a hole in the ceiling. To one side is a fantastically complicated master control console.

LITTLE

Oh, my God—oh, my God—

FRANKENSTEIN

Yeah. Those are her kidneys over there. That's her liver, of course. There you got her pancreas.

LITTLE

Amazing. Dr. Frankenstein, after seeing this, I wonder if I've even been *practicing* medicine, if I've ever even *been* to medical school. (*Pointing*) That's her *heart?*

FRANKENSTEIN

That's a Westinghouse heart. They make a damn good heart, if you ever need one. They make a kidney I wouldn't touch with a ten-foot pole.

LITTLE

That heart is probably worth more than the whole township where I practice.

FRANKENSTEIN

That pancreas is worth your whole state. *Vermont?*

LITTLE

Vermont.

FRANKENSTEIN

What we paid for the pancreas—yeah, we could have bought Vermont for that. Nobody'd ever made a pancreas before, and we had to have one in ten days or lose the patient. So we told all the big organ manufacturers, "OK, you guys got to have a crash program for a pancreas. Put every man you got on the job. We don't care what it costs, as long as we get a pancreas by next Tuesday."

LITTLE

And they succeeded.

FRANKENSTEIN

The patient's still alive, isn't she? Believe me, those are some expensive sweetbreads.

LITTLE

But the patient could afford them.

FRANKENSTEIN

You don't live like this on Blue Cross.

LITTLE

And how many operations has she had? In how many years?

FRANKENSTEIN

I gave her her first major operation thirty-six years ago. She's had seventy-eight operations since then.

LITTLE

And how old is she?

FRANKENSTEIN

One hundred.

LITTLE

What *guts* that woman must have!

FRANKENSTEIN

You're looking at 'em.

LITTLE

I mean—what *courage!* What *fortitude!*

FRANKENSTEIN

We knock her out, you know. We don't operate without anesthetics.

LITTLE

Even so . . .
    FRANKENSTEIN *taps* SWIFT *on the shoulder,* SWIFT *frees an ear
    from the headphones, divides his attention between the visitors and
    the console.*

FRANKENSTEIN

Dr. Tom Swift, this is Dr. Elbert Little. Tom here is my first assistant.

SWIFT

Howdy-doody.

FRANKENSTEIN

Dr. Little has a practice up in Vermont. He happened to be in the neighborhood. He asked for a tour.

LITTLE

What do you hear in the headphones?

SWIFT

Anything that's going on in the patient's room. (*He offers the headphones*) Be my guest.

LITTLE

(*listening to headphones*): Nothing.

SWIFT

She's having her hair brushed now. The beautician's up there. She's always quiet when her hair's being brushed. (*He takes the headphones back*)

FRANKENSTEIN

(*to* SWIFT): We should *congratulate* our young visitor here.

SWIFT

What for?

LITTLE

Good question. What for?

FRANKENSTEIN

Oh, I know about the great honor that has come your way.

LITTLE

I'm not sure *I* do.

FRANKENSTEIN

You are *the* Dr. Little, aren't you, who was named the Family Doctor of the Year by the *Ladies' Home Journal* last month?

LITTLE

Yes—that's right. I don't know how in the hell they decided. And I'm even more flabbergasted that a man of *your* caliber would know about it.

FRANKENSTEIN

I read the *Ladies' Home Journal* from cover to cover every month.

LITTLE

You *do?*

FRANKENSTEIN

I only got one patient, Mrs. Lovejoy. And Mrs. Lovejoy reads the *Ladies' Home Journal*, so I read it, too. That's what we talk about—what's in the *Ladies' Home Journal*. We read all about you last month. Mrs. Lovejoy kept saying, "Oh, what a nice young man he must be. *So understanding.*"

LITTLE

Um.

FRANKENSTEIN

Now here you are in the flesh. I bet she wrote you a letter.

LITTLE

Yes—she did.

FRANKENSTEIN

She writes thousands of letters a year, gets thousands of letters back. Some pen pal she is.

LITTLE

Is she—uh—generally *cheerful* most of the time?

FRANKENSTEIN

If she isn't, that's our fault down here. If she gets unhappy, that means something down *here* isn't working right. She was blue about a month ago. Turned out it was a bum transistor in the console. (*He reaches over* SWIFT's *shoulder, changes a setting on the console. The machinery subtly adjusts to the new setting.*) There—she'll be all depressed for a couple of minutes now. (*He changes the setting again*) There. Now, pretty quick, she'll be happier than she was before. She'll sing like a bird.

LITTLE *conceals his horror imperfectly.* CUT TO *patient's room, which is full of flowers and candy boxes and books. The patient is* SYLVIA LOVEJOY, *a billionaire's widow.* SYLVIA *is no longer anything but a head connected to pipes and wires coming up through the floor, but this is not immediately apparent. The first shot of her is a* CLOSE-UP, *with* GLORIA, *a gorgeous beautician, standing behind her.* SYLVIA *is a heartbreakingly good-looking old lady, once a famous beauty. She is crying now.*

SYLVIA

Gloria—

GLORIA

Ma'am?

SYLVIA

Wipe these tears away before somebody comes in and sees them.

GLORIA

(*wanting to cry herself*): Yes, ma'am. (*She wipes the tears away with Kleenex, studies the results*) There. There.

SYLVIA

I don't know what came over me. Suddenly I was so sad I couldn't stand it.

GLORIA

Everybody has to cry *sometimes.*

SYLVIA

It's passing now. Can you tell I've been crying?

GLORIA

No. No.
She is unable to control her own tears anymore. She goes to a window so SYLVIA *can't see her cry.* CAMERA BACKS AWAY *to reveal the tidy, clinical abomination of the head and wires and pipes. The head is on a tripod. There is a black box with winking colored lights hanging under the head, where the chest would normally be. Mechanical arms come out of the box where arms would normally be. There is a table within easy reach of the arms. On it are a pen and paper, a partially solved jigsaw puzzle and a bulky knitting bag. Sticking out of the bag are needles and a sweater in progress. Hanging over* SYLVIA's *head is a microphone on a boom.*

SYLVIA

(*sighing*): Oh, what a *foolish* old woman you must think I am. (GLORIA *shakes her head in denial, is unable to reply*) Gloria? Are you still there?

GLORIA

Yes.

SYLVIA

Is anything the matter?

GLORIA

No.

SYLVIA

You're *such* a good friend, Gloria. I want you to know I feel that with all my heart.

GLORIA

I like you, too.

SYLVIA

If you ever have any problems I can help you with, I hope you'll ask me.

GLORIA

I will, I *will*.
HOWARD DERBY, *the hospital mail clerk, dances in with an armload of letters. He is a merry old fool.*

53

DERBY

Mailman! Mailman!

SYLVIA

(*brightening*): Mailman! God *bless* the mailman!

DERBY

How's the patient today?

SYLVIA

Very sad a moment ago. But now that I see you, I want to sing like a bird.

DERBY

Fifty-three letters today. There's even one from Leningrad.

SYLVIA

There's a blind woman in Leningrad. Poor soul, *poor* soul.

DERBY

(*making a fan of the mail, reading postmarks*): West Virginia, Honolulu, Brisbane, Australia—
    SYLVIA *selects an envelope at random.*

SYLVIA

Wheeling, West Virginia. Now, who do I know in Wheeling? (*She opens the envelope expertly with her mechanical hands, reads*) "Dear Mrs. Lovejoy: You don't know me, but I just read about you in the *Reader's Digest*, and I'm sitting here with tears streaming down my cheeks." *Reader's Digest?* My goodness that article was printed fourteen years ago! And she just *read* it?

DERBY

Old *Reader's Digests* go on and on. I've got one at home I'll bet is ten years old. I still read it every time I need a little inspiration.

SYLVIA

(*reading on*): "I am never going to complain about anything that ever happens to me ever again. I thought I was as unfortunate as a person can get when my husband shot his girlfriend six months ago and then blew his own brains out. He left me with seven children and with eight payments still to go on a Buick Roadmaster with three flat tires and a busted transmission. After reading about you, though, I sit here and count my blessings." Isn't that a nice letter?

DERBY

Sure is.

SYLVIA

There's a P.S.: "Get well real soon, you *hear?*" (*She puts the letter on the table*) There isn't a letter from Vermont, is there?

DERBY

Vermont?

SYLVIA

Last month, when I had that low spell, I wrote what I'm afraid was a very stupid, self-centered, self-pitying letter to a young doctor I read about in the *Ladies' Home Journal.* I'm so ashamed. I live in fear and trembling of what he's going to say back to me—if he answers at all.

GLORIA

What could he say? What could he *possibly* say?

SYLVIA

He could tell me about the *real* suffering going on out there in the world, about people who don't know where the next meal is coming from, about people so poor they've never *been* to a doctor in their whole *lives.* And to think of all the help I've had—all the tender, loving care, all the latest wonders science has to offer.

    CUT TO *corridor outside* SYLVIA's *room. There is a sign on the door saying,* ALWAYS ENTER SMILING! FRANKENSTEIN *and* LITTLE *are about to enter.*

LITTLE

She's in *there?*

FRANKENSTEIN

Every part of her that isn't downstairs.

LITTLE

And everybody obeys this sign, I'm sure.

FRANKENSTEIN

Part of the therapy. We treat the *whole* patient here.

    GLORIA *comes from the room, closes the door tightly, then bursts into noisy tears.*

FRANKENSTEIN

(*to* GLORIA, *disgusted*): Oh, for crying out loud. And what is this?

GLORIA

Let her *die*, Dr. Frankenstein. For the love of God, let her *die*!

LITTLE

This is her *nurse?*

FRANKENSTEIN

She hasn't got the brains enough to be a nurse. She is a lousy beautician. A hundred bucks a week she makes—just to take care of one woman's face and hair. (*To* GLORIA) You blew it, honeybunch. You're through.

GLORIA

What?

FRANKENSTEIN

Pick up your check and scram.

GLORIA

I'm her closest friend.

FRANKENSTEIN

Some friend! You just asked me to knock her off.

GLORIA

In the name of mercy, yes, I did.

FRANKENSTEIN

You're that sure there's a heaven, eh? You want to send her right up there so she can get her wings and harp.

GLORIA

I know there's a hell. I've seen it. It's in there, and you're its great inventor.

FRANKENSTEIN

(*stung, letting a moment pass before replying*): Christ—the things people say sometimes.

GLORIA

It's time somebody who loves her spoke up.

FRANKENSTEIN

Love.

GLORIA

You wouldn't know what that is.

FRANKENSTEIN

Love. (*More to himself than to her*) Do I have a wife? No. Do I have a mistress? No. I have loved only two women in my life—my mother and that woman in there. I wasn't able to save my mother from death. I had just graduated from medical school and my mother was dying of cancer of the everything. "OK, wise guy," I said to myself, "you're such a hot-shot doctor from Heidelberg, now, let's see you save your mother from death." And everybody told me there wasn't anything I could do for her, and I said, "I don't give a damn. I'm gonna do something anyway." And they finally decided I was nuts and they put me in a crazyhouse for a little while. When I got out, she was dead—the way all the wise men said she had to be. What those wise men didn't know was all the wonderful things machinery could do—and neither did I, but I was gonna find out. So I went to the Massachusetts Institute of Technology and I studied mechanical engineering and electrical engineering and chemical engineering for six long years. I lived in an attic. I ate two-day-old bread and the kind of cheese they put in mousetraps. When I got out of MIT, I said to myself, "OK, boy—it's just barely possible now that you're the only guy on earth with the proper education to practice 20th century medicine." I went to work for the Curley Clinic in Boston. They brought in this woman who was beautiful on the outside and a mess on the inside. She was the image of my mother. She was the widow of a man who had left her five-hundred million dollars. She didn't have any relatives. The wise men said again, "This lady's gotta die." And I said to them, "Shut up and listen. I'm gonna tell you what we're gonna do."
Silence.

LITTLE

That's—that's quite a story.

FRANKENSTEIN

It's a story about *love*. (*To* GLORIA) That love story started years and years before you were born, you great lover, you. And it's still going on.

GLORIA

Last month, she asked me to bring her a pistol so she could shoot herself.

FRANKENSTEIN

You think I don't know that? (*Jerking a thumb at* LITTLE) Last month, she wrote him a letter and said, "Bring me some cyanide, doctor, if you're a doctor with any heart at all."

LITTLE

(*startled*): You *knew* that. You—you read her mail?

FRANKENSTEIN

So we'll know what she's *really* feeling. She might try to fool us sometime— just *pretend* to be happy. I told you about that bum transistor last month. We maybe wouldn't have known anything was wrong if we hadn't read her mail and listened to what she was saying to lame-brains like this one here. (*Feeling challenged*) Look—you go in there all by yourself. Stay as long as you want, ask her anything. Then you come back out and tell me the truth: Is that a happy woman in there, or is that a woman in hell?

LITTLE

(*hesitating*): I—

FRANKENSTEIN

Go on in! I got some more things to say to this young lady—to Miss Mercy Killing of the Year. I'd like to show her a body that's been in a casket for a couple of years sometime—let her see how pretty death is, this thing she wants for her friend.

LITTLE *gropes for something to say, finally mimes his wish to be fair to everyone. He enters the patient's room.* CUT TO *room.* SYLVIA *is alone, faced away from the door.*

SYLVIA

Who's that?

LITTLE

A friend—somebody you wrote a letter to.

SYLVIA

That could be anybody. Can I see you, please? (LITTLE *obliges. She looks him over with growing affection.*) Dr. Little—family doctor from Vermont.

LITTLE

(*bowing slightly*): Mrs. Lovejoy—how are you today?

SYLVIA

Did you bring me cyanide?

LITTLE

No.

SYLVIA

I wouldn't take it today. It's such a lovely day. I wouldn't want to miss it, or tomorrow, either. Did you come on a snow-white horse?

LITTLE

In a blue Oldsmobile.

SYLVIA

What about your patients, who love and need you so?

LITTLE

Another doctor is covering for me. I'm taking a week off.

SYLVIA

Not on my account.

LITTLE

No.

SYLVIA

Because I'm fine. You can see what wonderful hands I'm in.

LITTLE

Yes.

SYLVIA

One thing I don't need is another doctor.

LITTLE

Right.
      Pause.

SYLVIA

I do wish I had somebody to talk to about death, though. You've seen a lot of it, I suppose.

LITTLE

Some.

SYLVIA

And it was a blessing for some of them—when they died?

LITTLE

I've heard that said.

SYLVIA

But you don't say so yourself.

LITTLE

It's not a professional thing for a doctor to say, Mrs. Lovejoy.

SYLVIA

Why have other people said that certain deaths have been a blessing?

LITTLE

Because of the pain the patient was in, because he couldn't be cured at any price—at any price within his means. Or because the patient was a vegetable, had lost his mind and couldn't get it back.

SYLVIA

At any price.

LITTLE

As far as I know, it is not now possible to beg, borrow or steal an artificial mind for someone who's lost one. If I asked Dr. Frankenstein about it, he might tell me that it's the coming thing.
Pause.

SYLVIA

It *is* the coming thing.

LITTLE

He's told you so?

SYLVIA

I asked him yesterday what would happen if my brain started to go. He was serene. He said I wasn't to worry my pretty little head about that. "We'll cross that bridge when we come to it," he told me. (*Pause*) Oh, God, the bridges I've crossed!

CUT TO *room full of organs, as before.* SWIFT *is at the console.* FRANKENSTEIN *and* LITTLE *enter.*

FRANKENSTEIN

You've made the grand tour and now here you are back at the beginning.

LITTLE

And I still have to say what I said at the beginning: "My God—oh, my God."

FRANKENSTEIN

It's gonna be a little tough going back to the aspirin-and-laxative trade after this, eh?

LITTLE

Yes. (*Pause*) What's the cheapest thing here?

FRANKENSTEIN

The simplest thing. It's the goddamn pump.

LITTLE

What does a heart go for these days?

FRANKENSTEIN

Sixty thousand dollars. There are cheaper ones and more expensive ones. The cheap ones are junk. The expensive ones are jewelry.

LITTLE

And how many are sold a year now?

FRANKENSTEIN

Six hundred, give or take a few.

LITTLE

Give one, that's life. Take one, that's death.

FRANKENSTEIN

If the trouble is the heart. It's lucky if you have trouble that cheap. (*To* SWIFT) Hey, Tom—put her to sleep so he can see how the day ends around here.

SWIFT

It's twenty minutes ahead of time.

FRANKENSTEIN

What's the difference? We put her to sleep for twenty minutes extra, she still wakes up tomorrow feeling like a million bucks, unless we got another bum transistor.

LITTLE

Why don't you have a television camera aimed at her, so you can watch her on a screen?

FRANKENSTEIN

She didn't want one.

LITTLE

She gets what she wants?

FRANKENSTEIN

She got *that*. What the hell do we have to watch her face for? We can look at the meters down here and find out more about her than she can know about herself. (*To* SWIFT) Put her to sleep, Tom.

SWIFT

(*to* LITTLE): It's just like slowing down a car or banking a furnace.

LITTLE

Um.

FRANKENSTEIN

Tom, too, has degrees in both engineering and medicine.

LITTLE

Are you tired at the end of a day, Tom?

SWIFT

It's a good kind of tiredness—as though I'd flown a big jet from New York to Honolulu, or something like that. (*Taking hold of a lever*) And now we'll bring Mrs. Lovejoy in for a happy landing. (*He pulls the lever gradually and the machinery slows down*) There.

FRANKENSTEIN

Beautiful.

LITTLE

She's asleep?

FRANKENSTEIN

Like a baby.

SWIFT

All I have to do now is wait for the night man to come on.

LITTLE

Has anybody ever brought her a suicide weapon?

FRANKENSTEIN

No. We wouldn't worry about it if they did. The arms are designed so she can't possibly point a gun at herself or get poison to her lips, no matter how she tries. That was Tom's stroke of genius.

LITTLE

Congratulations.
Alarm bell rings. Light flashes.

FRANKENSTEIN

Who could that be? (*To* LITTLE) Somebody just went into her room. We better check! (*To* SWIFT) Lock the door up there, Tom—so whoever it is, we got 'em. (SWIFT *pushes a button that locks door upstairs. To* LITTLE) You come with me.
CUT TO *patient's room.* SYLVIA *is asleep, snoring gently.* GLORIA *has just sneaked in. She looks around furtively, takes a revolver from her purse, makes sure it's loaded, then hides it in* SYLVIA'S *knitting bag. She is barely finished when* FRANKENSTEIN *and* LITTLE *enter breathlessly,* FRANKENSTEIN *opening the door with a key.*

FRANKENSTEIN

What's this?

GLORIA

I left my watch up here. (*Pointing to watch*) I've got it now.

FRANKENSTEIN

Thought I told you never to come into this building again.

GLORIA

I won't.

FRANKENSTEIN

(*to* LITTLE): You keep her right there. I'm gonna check things over. Maybe there's been a little huggery buggery. (*To* GLORIA) How would you like to be in court for attempted murder, eh? (*Into microphone*) Tom? Can you hear me?

SWIFT

(*voice from squawk box on wall*): I hear you.

FRANKENSTEIN

Wake her up again. I gotta give her a check.

SWIFT

Cock-a-doodle-doo.
  Machinery can be heard speeding up below. SYLVIA *opens her eyes, sweetly dazed.*

SYLVIA

(*to* FRANKENSTEIN): Good morning, Norbert.

FRANKENSTEIN

How do you feel?

SYLVIA

The way I always feel when I wake up—fine—vaguely at sea. Gloria! Good morning!

GLORIA

Good morning.

SYLVIA

Dr. Little! You're staying another day?

FRANKENSTEIN

It isn't morning. We'll put you back to sleep in a minute.

SYLVIA

I'm sick again?

FRANKENSTEIN

I don't think so.

SYLVIA

I'm going to have to have another operation?

FRANKENSTEIN

Calm down, calm down. (*He takes an ophthalmoscope from his pocket*)

SYLVIA

How can I be calm when I think about another operation?

FRANKENSTEIN

(*into microphone*): Tom—give her some tranquilizers.

SWIFT

(*squawk box*): Coming up.

SYLVIA

What else do I have to lose? My ears? My hair?

FRANKENSTEIN

You'll be calm in a minute.

SYLVIA

My eyes? My eyes, Norbert—are they going next?

FRANKENSTEIN

(*to* GLORIA): Oh, boy, baby doll—will you look what you've done? (*Into microphone*) Where the hell are those tranquilizers?

SWIFT

Should be taking effect just about now.

SYLVIA

Oh, well. It doesn't matter. (*As* FRANKENSTEIN *examines her eyes*) It *is* my eyes, isn't it?

FRANKENSTEIN

It isn't your anything.

SYLVIA

Easy come, easy go.

FRANKENSTEIN

You're healthy as a horse.

SYLVIA

I'm sure somebody manufactures excellent eyes.

FRANKENSTEIN

RCA makes a damn good eye, but we aren't gonna buy one for a while yet. (*He backs away, satisfied*) Everything's all right up here. (*To* GLORIA) Lucky for you.

SYLVIA

I love it when friends of mine are lucky.

SWIFT

Put her to sleep again?

FRANKENSTEIN

Not yet. I want to check a couple of things down there.

SWIFT

Roger and out.
        CUT TO LITTLE, GLORIA *and* FRANKENSTEIN *entering the machinery room minutes later.* SWIFT *is at the console.*

SWIFT

Night man's late.

FRANKENSTEIN

He's got troubles at home. You want a good piece of advice, boy? Don't ever get married. (*He scrutinizes meter after meter*)

GLORIA

(*appalled by her surroundings*): My God—oh, my God—

LITTLE

You've never seen this before?

GLORIA

No.

FRANKENSTEIN

She was the great hair specialist. We took care of everything else—everything but the hair. (*The reading on a meter puzzles him*) What's this? (*He socks the meter, which then gives him the proper reading*) That's more like it.

GLORIA

(*emptily*): Science.

FRANKENSTEIN

What did you think it was like down here?

GLORIA

I was afraid to think. Now I can see why.

FRANKENSTEIN

You got any scientific background at all—any way of appreciating even slightly what you're seeing here?

GLORIA

I flunked earth science twice in high school.

FRANKENSTEIN

What do they teach in beauty college?

GLORIA

Dumb things for dumb people. How to paint a face. How to curl or uncurl hair. How to cut hair. How to dye hair. Fingernails. Toenails in the summertime.

FRANKENSTEIN

I suppose you're gonna crack off about this place after you get out of here—gonna tell people all the crazy stuff that goes on.

GLORIA

Maybe.

FRANKENSTEIN

Just remember this: You haven't got the brains or the education to talk about any aspect of our operation. Right?

GLORIA

Maybe.

FRANKENSTEIN

What *will* you say to the outside world?

GLORIA

Nothing very complicated—just that. . . .

FRANKENSTEIN

Yes?

GLORIA

That you have the head of a dead woman connected to a lot of machinery, and you play with it all day long, and you aren't married or anything, and that's all you do.

FREEZE SCENE *as a still photograph.* FADE TO *black.* FADE IN *same still. Figures begin to move.*

FRANKENSTEIN

(*aghast*): How can you call her dead? She reads the *Ladies' Home Journal!* She talks! She knits! She writes letters to pen pals all over the world!

GLORIA

She's like some horrible fortunetelling machine in a penny arcade.

FRANKENSTEIN

I thought you loved her.

GLORIA

Every so often, I see a tiny little spark of what she used to be. I love that spark. Most people say they love her for her courage. What's that courage worth, when it comes from down here? You could turn a few faucets and switches down here and she'd be volunteering to fly a rocket ship to the moon. But no matter what you do down here, that little spark goes on thinking, "For the love of God—somebody get me out of here!"

FRANKENSTEIN

(*glancing at the console*): Dr. Swift—is that microphone open?

SWIFT

Yeah. (*Snapping his fingers*) I'm sorry.

FRANKENSTEIN

Leave it open. (*To* GLORIA) She's heard every word you've said. How does that make you feel?

GLORIA

She can hear me now?

FRANKENSTEIN

Run off at the mouth some more. You're saving me a lot of trouble. Now I won't have to explain to her what sort of friend you really were and why I gave you the old heave-ho.

GLORIA
(*drawing nearer to the microphone*): Mrs. Lovejoy?

SWIFT
(*reporting what he has heard on the headphones*): She says, "What is it, dear?"

GLORIA
There's a loaded revolver in your knitting bag, Mrs. Lovejoy—in case you don't want to live anymore.

FRANKENSTEIN
(*not in the least worried about the pistol but filled with contempt and disgust for* GLORIA): You total imbecile. Where did you get a pistol?

GLORIA
From a mail-order house in Chicago. They had an ad in *True Romances*.

FRANKENSTEIN
They sell guns to crazy broads.

GLORIA
I could have had a bazooka if I'd wanted one. Fourteen-ninety-eight.

FRANKENSTEIN
I am going to get that pistol now and it is going to be exhibit A at your trial. (*He leaves*)

LITTLE
(*To* SWIFT): Shouldn't you put the patient to sleep?

SWIFT
There's no way she can hurt herself.

GLORIA
(*To* LITTLE): What does he mean?

LITTLE
Her arms are fixed so she can't point a gun at herself.

GLORIA
(*sickened*): They even thought of that.

CUT TO SYLVIA's *room.* FRANKENSTEIN *is entering.* SYLVIA *is holding the pistol thoughtfully.*

FRANKENSTEIN

Nice playthings you have.

SYLVIA

You mustn't get mad at Gloria, Norbert. I asked her for this. I begged her for this.

FRANKENSTEIN

Last month.

SYLVIA

Yes.

FRANKENSTEIN

But everything is better now.

SYLVIA

Everything but the spark.

FRANKENSTEIN

Spark?

SYLVIA

The spark that Gloria says she loves—the tiny spark of what I used to be. As happy as I am right now, that spark is begging me to take this gun and put it out.

FRANKENSTEIN

And what is your reply?

SYLVIA

I am going to do it, Norbert. This is goodbye. (*She tries every which way to aim the gun at herself, fails and fails, while* FRANKENSTEIN *stands calmly by*) That's no accident, is it?

FRANKENSTEIN

We very much don't want you to hurt yourself. We love you, too.

SYLVIA

And how much longer must I live like this? I've never dared ask before.

FRANKENSTEIN

I would have to pull a figure out of a hat.

SYLVIA

Maybe you'd better not. (*Pause*) Did you pull one out of a hat?

FRANKENSTEIN

At least five hundred years.
    Silence.

SYLVIA

So I will still be alive—long after you are gone?

FRANKENSTEIN

Now is the time, my dear Sylvia, to tell you something I have wanted to tell you for years. Every organ downstairs has the capacity to take care of two human beings instead of one. And the plumbing and wiring have been designed so that a second human being can be hooked up in two shakes of a lamb's tail. (*Silence*) Do you understand what I am saying to you, Sylvia? (*Silence. Passionately*) Sylvia! I will be that second human being! Talk about marriage! Talk about great love stories from the past! Your kidney will be my kidney! Your liver will be my liver! Your heart will be my heart! Your ups will be my ups and your downs will be my downs! We will live in such perfect harmony, Sylvia, that the Gods themselves will tear out their hair in envy!

SYLVIA

This is what you want!

FRANKENSTEIN

More than anything in this world.

SYLVIA

Well, then—here it is, Norbert. (*She empties the revolver into him*) CUT TO *same room almost a half hour later. A second tripod has been set up, with* FRANKENSTEIN'*s head on top.* FRANKENSTEIN *is asleep and so is* SYLVIA. SWIFT, *with* LITTLE *standing by, is feverishly making a final connection to the machinery below. There are pipe wrenches and a blowtorch and other plumber's and electrician's tools lying around.*

SWIFT

That's gotta be it. (*He straightens up, looks around*) That's gotta be it.

LITTLE
(*consulting watch*): Twenty-eight minutes since the first shot was fired.

SWIFT
Thank God you were around.

LITTLE
What you really needed was a plumber.

SWIFT
(*into microphone*): Charley—we're all set up here. You all set down there?

CHARLEY
(*squawk box*): All set.

SWIFT
Give 'em plenty of martinis.
    GLORIA *appears numbly in doorway.*

CHARLEY
They've got 'em. They'll be higher than kites.

SWIFT
Better give 'em a touch of LSD, too.

CHARLEY
Coming up.

SWIFT
Hold it! I forgot the phonograph. (*To* LITTLE) Dr. Frankenstein said that if this ever happened, he wanted a certain record playing when he came to. He said it was in with the other records—in a plain white jacket. (*To* GLORIA) See if you can find it.
    GLORIA *goes to phonograph, finds the record.*

GLORIA
This it?

SWIFT
Put it on.

GLORIA
Which side?

SWIFT

I don't know.

GLORIA

There's tape over one side.

SWIFT

The side *without* tape. (GLORIA *puts record on. Into microphone*) Stand by to wake up the patients.

CHARLEY

Standing by.
> *Record begins to play. It is a Jeanette MacDonald-Nelson Eddy duet, "Ah, Sweet Mystery of Life."*

SWIFT

(*into microphone*): Wake 'em up!
> FRANKENSTEIN *and* SYLVIA *wake up, filled with formless pleasure. They dreamily appreciate the music, eventually catch sight of each other, perceive each other as old and beloved friends.*

SYLVIA

Hi, there.

FRANKENSTEIN

Hello.

SYLVIA

How do you feel?

FRANKENSTEIN

Fine. Just fine.

The Jilting
of Granny Weatherall

She flicked her wrist neatly out of Dr. Harry's pudgy careful fingers and pulled the sheet up to her chin. The brat ought to be in knee breeches. Doctoring around the country with spectacles on his nose! "Get along now, take your schoolbooks and go. There's nothing wrong with me."

Doctor Harry spread a warm paw like a cushion on her forehead where the forked green vein danced and made her eyelids twitch. "Now, now, be a good girl, and we'll have you up in no time."

"That's no way to speak to a woman nearly eighty years old just because she's down. I'd have you respect your elders, young man."

"Well, Missy, excuse me." Doctor Harry patted her cheek. "But I've got to warn you, haven't I? You're a marvel, but you must be careful or you're going to be good and sorry."

"Don't tell me what I'm going to be. I'm on my feet now, morally speaking. It's Cornelia. I had to go to bed to get rid of her."

Her bones felt loose, and floated around in her skin, and Doctor Harry floated like a balloon around the foot of the bed. He floated and pulled down his waistcoat and swung his glasses on a cord. "Well, stay where you are, it certainly can't hurt you."

"Get along and doctor your sick," said Granny Weatherall. "Leave a well woman alone. I'll call for you when I want you. . . . Where were you forty years ago when I pulled through milk-leg and double pneumonia? You weren't even born. Don't let Cornelia lead you on," she shouted, because Doctor Harry appeared to float up to the ceiling and out. "I pay my own bills, and I don't throw my money away on nonsense!"

She meant to wave good-by, but it was too much trouble. Her eyes closed of themselves, it was like a dark curtain drawn around the bed. The pillow rose and floated under her, pleasant as a hammock in a light wind. She listened to the leaves rustling outside the window. No, somebody was swishing newspapers: no, Cornelia and Doctor Harry were whispering together. She leaped broad awake, thinking they whispered in her ear.

"She was never like this, *never* like this!" "Well, what can we expect?" "Yes, eighty years old. . . . "

Well, and what if she was? She still had ears. It was like Cornelia to whisper around doors. She always kept things secret in such a public way. She was always being tactful and kind. Cornelia was dutiful; that was the trouble with her. Dutiful and good: "So good and dutiful," said Granny, "that I'd like to spank her." She saw herself spanking Cornelia and making a fine job of it.

"What'd you say, Mother?"

Granny felt her face tying up in hard knots.

"Can't a body think, I'd like to know?"

"I thought you might want something."

"I do. I want a lot of things. First off, go away and don't whisper."

She lay and drowsed, hoping in her sleep that the children would keep out and let her rest a minute. It had been a long day. Not that she was tired. It was always pleasant to snatch a minute now and then. There was always so much to be done, let me see: tomorrow.

Tomorrow was far away and there was nothing to trouble about. Things were finished somehow when the time came; thank God there was always a little margin over for peace: then a person could spread out the plan of life and tuck in the edges orderly. It was good to have everything clean and folded away, with the hair brushes and tonic bottles sitting straight on the white embroidered linen: the day started without fuss and the pantry shelves laid out with rows of jelly glasses and brown jugs and white stone-china jars with blue whirligigs and words painted on them: coffee, tea, sugar, ginger, cinnamon, allspice: and the bronze clock with the lion on top nicely dusted off. The dust that lion could collect in twenty-four hours! The box in the attic with all those letters tied up, well, she'd have to go through that tomorrow. All those letters—George's letters and John's letters and her letters to them both—lying around for the children to find afterwards made her uneasy. Yes, that would be tomorrow's business. No use to let them know how silly she had been once.

While she was rummaging around she found death in her mind and it felt clammy and unfamiliar. She had spent so much time preparing for death there was no need for bringing it up again. Let it take care of itself now. When she was sixty she had felt very old, finished, and went around making farewell trips to see her children and grandchildren, with a secret in her mind: This is the very last of your mother, children! Then she made her will and came down with a long fever. That was all just a notion like a lot of other things, but it was lucky too, for she had once for all got over the idea of dying for a long time. Now she couldn't be worried. She hoped she had better sense now. Her father had lived to be one hundred and two years old and had drunk a noggin of strong hot toddy on his last birthday. He told the reporters it was his daily habit, and he owed his long life to that. He had made quite a scandal and was very pleased about it. She believed she'd just plague Cornelia a little.

"Cornelia! Cornelia!" No footsteps, but a sudden hand on her cheek. "Bless you, where have you been?"

"Here, mother."

"Well, Cornelia, I want a noggin of hot toddy."

"Are you cold, darling?"

"I'm chilly, Cornelia. Lying in bed stops the circulation. I must have told you that a thousand times."

Well, she could just hear Cornelia telling her husband that Mother was getting a little childish and they'd have to humor her. The thing that most annoyed her was that Cornelia thought she was deaf, dumb, and blind. Little hasty glances and tiny gestures tossed around her and over her head saying, "Don't cross her, let her have her way, she's eighty years old," and she sitting there as if she lived in a thin glass cage. Sometimes Granny almost made up her mind to pack up and move back to her own house where nobody could remind her every minute that she was old. Wait, wait, Cornelia, till your own children whisper behind your back!

In her day she had kept a better house and had got more work done. She wasn't too old yet for Lydia to be driving eighty miles for advice when one of the children jumped the track, and Jimmy still dropped in and talked things over: "Now, Mammy, you've a good business head, I want to know what you think of this? . . . " Old. Cornelia couldn't change the furniture around without asking. Little things, little things! They had been so sweet when they were little. Granny wished the old days were back again with the children young and everything to be done over. It had been a hard pull, but not too much for her. When she thought of all the food she had cooked, and all the clothes she had cut and sewed, and all the gardens she had made— well, the children showed it. There they were, made out of her, and they couldn't get away from that. Sometimes she wanted to see John again and point to them and say, Well, I didn't do so badly, did I? But that would have to wait. That was for tomorrow. She used to think of him as a man, but now all the children were older than their father, and he would be a child beside her if she saw him now. It seemed strange and there was something wrong in the idea. Why, he couldn't possibly recognize her. She had fenced in a hundred acres once, digging the post holes herself and clamping the wires with just a negro boy to help. That changed a woman. John would be looking for a young woman with the peaked Spanish comb in her hair and the painted fan. Digging post holes changed a woman. Riding country roads in the winter when women had their babies was another thing: sitting up nights with sick horses and sick negroes and sick children and hardly ever losing one. John, I hardly ever lost one of them! John would see that in a minute, that would be something he could understand, she wouldn't have to explain anything!

It made her feel like rolling up her sleeves and putting the whole place to rights again. No matter if Cornelia was determined to be everywhere at once, there were a great many things left undone on this place. She would start tomorrow and do them. It was good to be strong enough for everything, even if all you made melted and changed and slipped under your hands, so that by the time you finished you almost forgot what you were working for. What was it I set out to do? she asked herself intently, but she could not remember. A fog rose over the valley, she saw it marching across the creek swallowing the trees and moving up the hill like an army of ghosts. Soon it would be at the near edge of the orchard, and then it was time to go in and light the lamps. Come in, children, don't stay out in the night air.

Lighting the lamps had been beautiful. The children huddled up to her and breathed like little calves waiting at the bars in the twilight. Their eyes followed the match and watched the flame rise and settle in a blue curve, then they moved away from her. The lamp was lit, they didn't have to be scared and hang on to mother any more. Never, never, never more. God, for all my life I thank Thee. Without Thee, my God, I could never have done it. Hail, Mary, full of grace.

I want you to pick all the fruit this year and see that nothing is wasted. There's always someone who can use it. Don't let good things rot for want of using. You waste life when you waste good food. Don't let things get lost. It's bitter to lose things. Now, don't let me get to thinking, not when I am tired and taking a little nap before supper. . . .

The pillow rose about her shoulders and pressed against her heart and the memory was being squeezed out of it: oh, push down the pillow, somebody: it would smother her if she tried to hold it. Such a fresh breeze blowing and such a green day with no threats in it. But he had not come, just the same. What does a woman do when she has put on the white veil and set out the white cake for a man and he doesn't come? She tried to remember. No, I swear he never harmed me but in that. He never harmed me but in that . . . and what if he did? There was the day, the day, but a whirl of dark smoke rose and covered it, crept up and over into the bright field where everything was planted so carefully in orderly rows. That was hell, she knew hell when she saw it. For sixty years she had prayed against remembering him and against losing her soul in the deep pit of hell, and now the two things were mingled in one and the thought of him was a smoky cloud from hell that moved and crept in her head when she had just got rid of Doctor Harry and was trying to rest a minute. Wounded vanity, Ellen, said a sharp voice in the top of her mind. Don't let your wounded vanity get the upper hand of you. Plenty of girls get jilted. You were jilted, weren't you? Then stand up to it. Her eyelids wavered and let in streamers of blue-gray light like tissue paper over her eyes. She must get up and pull the shades down or she'd never sleep. She was in bed again and the shades were not down. How could that happen? Better turn over, hide from the light, sleeping in the light gave you nightmares. "Mother, how do you feel now?" and a stinging wetness on her forehead. But I don't like having my face washed in cold water!

Hapsy? George? Lydia? Jimmy? No, Cornelia, and her features were swollen and full of little puddles. "They're coming, darling, they'll all be here soon." Go wash your face, child, you look funny.

Instead of obeying, Cornelia knelt down and put her head on the pillow. She seemed to be talking but there was no sound. "Well, are you tongue-tied? Whose birthday is it? Are you going to give a party?"

Cornelia's mouth moved urgently in strange shapes. "Don't do that, you bother me, daughter."

"Oh, no, Mother. Oh, no. . . . "

Nonsense. It was strange about children. They disputed your every word. "No what, Cornelia?"

"Here's Doctor Harry."

"I won't see that boy again. He just left five minutes ago."

"That was this morning, Mother. It's night now. Here's the nurse."

"This is Doctor Harry, Mrs. Weatherall. I never saw you look so young and happy!"

"Ah, I'll never be young again—but I'd be happy if they'd let me lie in peace and get rested."

She thought she spoke up loudly, but no one answered. A warm weight on her forehead, a warm bracelet on her wrist, and a breeze went on whispering, trying to tell her something. A shuffle of leaves in the everlasting hand of God, He blew on them and they danced and rattled. "Mother, don't mind, we're going to give you a little hypodermic." "Look here, daughter, how do ants get in this bed? I saw sugar ants yesterday." Did you send for Hapsy too?

It was Hapsy she really wanted. She had to go a long way back through a great many rooms to find Hapsy standing with a baby on her arm. She seemed to herself to be Hapsy also, and the baby on Hapsy's arm was Hapsy and himself and herself, all at once, and there was no surprise in the meeting. Then Hapsy melted from within and turned flimsy as gray gauze and the baby was a gauzy shadow, and Hapsy came up close and said, "I thought you'd never come," and looked at her very searchingly and said, "You haven't changed a bit!" They leaned forward to kiss, when Cornelia began whispering from a long way off, "Oh, is there anything you want to tell me? Is there anything I can do for you?"

Yes, she had changed her mind after sixty years and she would like to see George. I want you to find George. Find him and be sure to tell him I forgot him. I want him to know I had my husband just the same and my children and my house like any other woman. A good house too and a good husband that I loved and fine children out of him. Better than I hoped for even. Tell him I was given back everything he took away and more. Oh, no, oh, God, no, there was something else besides the house and the man and the children. Oh, surely they were not all? What was it? Something not given back. . . . Her breath crowded down under her ribs and grew into a monstrous frightening shape with cutting edges; it bored up into her head, and the agony was unbelievable: Yes, John, get the Doctor now, no more talk, my time has come.

When this one was born it should be the last. The last. It should have been born first, for it was the one she had truly wanted. Everything came in good time. Nothing left out, left over. She was strong, in three days she would be as well as ever. Better. A woman needed milk in her to have her full health.

"Mother, do you hear me?"

"I've been telling you—"

"Mother, Father Connolly's here."

"I went to Holy Communion only last week. Tell him I'm not so sinful as all that."

"Father just wants to speak to you."

He could speak as much as he pleased. It was like him to drop in and inquire about her soul as if it were a teething baby, and then stay on for a cup of tea and a round of cards and gossip. He always had a funny story of some sort, usually about an Irishman who made his little mistakes and confessed them, and the point lay in some absurd thing he would blurt out in the confessional showing his struggles between native piety and original sin. Granny felt easy about her soul. Cornelia, where are your manners? Give Father Connolly a chair. She had her secret comfortable understanding with a few favorite saints who cleared a straight road to God for her. All as surely signed and sealed as the papers for the new Forty Acres. Forever . . . heirs and assigns forever. Since the day the wedding cake was not cut, but thrown out and wasted. The whole bottom dropped out of the world, and there she was blind and sweating with nothing under her feet and the walls falling away. His hand had caught her under the breast, she had not fallen, there was the freshly polished floor with the green rug on it, just as before. He had cursed like a sailor's parrot and said, "I'll kill him for you." Don't lay a hand on him, for my sake leave something to God. "Now, Ellen, you must believe what I tell you. . . . "

So there was nothing, nothing to worry about any more, except sometimes in the night one of the children screamed in a nightmare, and they both hustled out shaking and hunting for the matches and calling, "There, wait a minute, here we are!" John, get the doctor now, Hapsy's time has come. But there was Hapsy standing by the bed in a white cap. "Cornelia, tell Hapsy to take off her cap. I can't see her plain."

Her eyes opened very wide and the room stood out like a picture she had seen somewhere. Dark colors with the shadows rising towards the ceiling in long angles. The tall black dresser gleamed with nothing on it but John's picture, enlarged from a little one, with John's eyes very black when they should have been blue. You never saw him, so how do you know how he looked? But the man insisted the copy was perfect, it was very rich and handsome. For a picture, yes, but it's not my husband. The table by the bed had a linen cover and a candle and a crucifix. The light was blue from Cornelia's silk lampshades. No sort of light at all, just frippery. You had to live forty years with kerosene lamps to appreciate honest electricity. She felt very strong and she saw Doctor Harry with a rosy nimbus around him.

"You look like a saint, Doctor Harry, and I vow that's as near as you'll ever come to it."

"She's saying something."

"I heard you, Cornelia. What's all this carrying-on?"

"Father Connolly's saying—"

Cornelia's voice staggered and bumped like a cart in a bad road. It rounded corners and turned back again and arrived nowhere. Granny stepped up in the cart very lightly and reached for the reins, but a man sat beside her and she knew him by his hands, driving the cart. She did not look in his face, for she knew without seeing, but looked instead down the road where the trees leaned over and bowed to each other and a thousand birds were singing a Mass. She felt like singing too, but she put her hand in the bosom of her dress and pulled out a rosary, and Father Connolly murmured Latin in a very solemn voice and tickled her feet. My God, will you stop that nonsense? I'm a married woman. What if he did run away and leave me to face the priest by myself? I found another a whole world better. I wouldn't have exchanged my husband for anybody except St. Michael himself, and you may tell him that for me with a thank you in the bargain.

Light flashed on her closed eyelids, and a deep roaring shook her. Cornelia, is that lightning? I hear thunder. There's going to be a storm. Close all the windows. Call the children in. . . . "Mother, here we are, all of us." "Is that you, Hapsy?" "Oh, no, I'm Lydia. We drove as fast as we could." Their faces drifted above her, drifted away. The rosary fell out of her hands and Lydia put it back. Jimmy tried to help, their hands fumbled together, and Granny closed two fingers around Jimmy's thumb. Beads wouldn't do, it must be something alive. She was so amazed her thoughts ran round and round. So, my dear Lord, this is my death and I wasn't even thinking about it. My children have come to see me die. But I can't, it's not time. Oh, I always hated surprises. I wanted to give Cornelia the amethyst set—Cornelia, you're to have the amethyst set, but Hapsy's to wear it when she wants, and, Doctor Harry, do shut up. Nobody sent for you. Oh, my dear Lord, do wait a minute. I meant to do something about the Forty Acres, Jimmy doesn't need it and Lydia will later on, with that worthless husband of hers. I meant to finish the alter cloth and send six bottles of wine to Sister Borgia for her dyspepsia. I want to send six bottles of wine to Sister Borgia, Father Connolly, now don't let me forget.

Cornelia's voice made short turns and tilted over and crashed. "Oh, Mother, oh, Mother, oh, Mother. . . . "

"I'm not going, Cornelia. I'm taken by surprise. I can't go."

You'll see Hapsy again. What about her? "I thought you'd never come." Granny made a long journey outward, looking for Hapsy. What if I don't find her? What then? Her heart sank down and down, there was no bottom to death, she couldn't come to the end of it. The blue light from Cornelia's lampshade drew into a tiny point in the center of her brain, it flickered and winked like an eye, quietly it fluttered and dwindled. Granny lay curled down within herself, amazed and watchful, staring at the point of light that was herself; her body was now only a deeper mass of shadow in an endless darkness and this darkness would curl around the light and swallow it up. God, give a sign!

For the second time there was no sign. Again no bridegroom and the priest in the house. She could not remember any other sorrow because this grief wiped them all away. Oh, no, there's nothing more cruel than this—I'll never forgive it. She stretched herself with a deep breath and blew out the light.

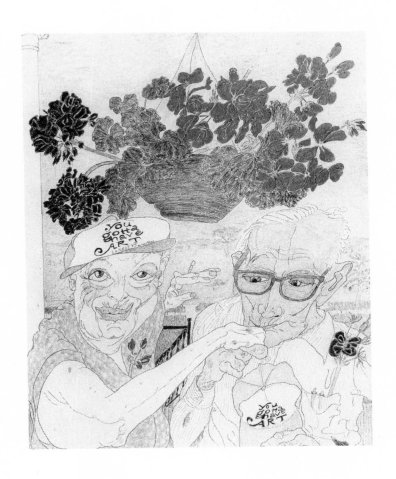

AGING AND LOVE

Introduction

The burden of proof to questions about aging and love lies with the questioner, not with those being questioned. Why shouldn't love be an integral part of an older person's life? Why should we be surprised to see that that love is evident in manifold ways? Searching more deeply we ask: What is it that binds two persons to one another in their later years? Literature provides some examples.

In Albert Camus's *The Plague* we find an elderly couple, the Castels; she is outside the quarantined city and he, a physician, is inside. When separated loved ones are given access to the closed city theirs becomes the

> one case in which natural emotions overcame the fear of death. [Yet] they weren't one of those exemplary married couples. . . . Neither partner felt quite sure the marriage was all that could have been desired. But this ruthless, protracted separation enabled them to realize that they could not live apart. . . . [1]

We may in a cynical way claim that it was merely habit that fueled this noble act. But we must be careful not to denigrate the simple, yet sometimes overwhelming, need for another and the comfort, coherence and security it brings.

We also may find that couples in their later years are bound by sensual and sexual attachments. In García Márquez's *Love in the Time of Cholera*, Florentino Ariza steadfastly waits "fifty-three years, seven months, and eleven days and nights" for *his* night with Fermina Daza. And although

> they had leapt over the arduous calvary of conjugal life and gone straight to the heart of love . . . they had lived together long enough to know that love was always love, anytime and anyplace, but it was more solid the closer it came to death.[2]

---

[1] Albert Camus, *The Plague* (New York: Vintage Books, 1972), 66.
[2] Gabriel García Márquez, *Love in the Time of Cholera* (New York: Penguin Books, 1989), 348, 345.

Between the need for the mere presence of another and total embrace, literature further offers an array of expressions of love in later life. Companionship, a comforting knowing of and sharing with another, might best characterize this state of being of older lovers (even when the loves or lovers are imagined). What do these companions share? Often remembrances, as do "The Bean Eaters" who remember "with twinklings and twinges, / As they lean over the beans in their rented back room." And remember, too, does the husband—in Williams's "Asophodel That Greeny Flower"—whose memory of a long ago wedding day is revived by the imagined scent of a flower.

Companions also share simple acts of affection, especially the holding of hands, as in the poem "Now, Before the End, I Think": "Now, wordless again, you reach to hold / my hand as if to say in silence, / it is healed, we touch, we are together." Perhaps the tactile sense rises in importance as other senses are in decline; it falls to the hands to connect two beings and serve as conduit for the soul. In "The Linden Tree" it is the holding of hands through the night, when separation threatens most, that soothes the ill Giulio and the suffering George. And what are we to make of Goldie's gesture of love to her husband Lou in Philip Roth's "Epstein"? Theirs is a marriage fed by a well-spring of bitterness and loss. Yet Goldie shares the ambulance ride with her stricken (and adulterous) husband, and while doing so, grips his hand and begins to reconstruct their life together.

What can we do to overcome the conventional wisdom that love (in all its forms) diminishes as our years increase? We must keep alert to the gestures of love that older persons share in literature and in our everyday world. We also must nourish, as well, the sources of love—imagination and touch—in their lives and in our own.

The Pleasures
of Old Age

When my grandmother Lisette turned ninety-nine,
all she could think of was men—
how they would enter her room during the night
from the vast mixer of the mind, wild
with desire, drunk with a desperate love
for only her. All day she sat, spectacle-less,
over romance magazines, until, at night,
she could dream them back into her arms,
those beautiful men, and, when morning came,
rise from her immaculate bed, pink
with the glow of the newly deflowered,
to enter the world again. All over our island
that was Manhattan, bachelors sprouted like dandelions
in the field of her hungers—Baruch Oestrich, stifled
by shyness at eighty-eight, for whom she would primp for hours;
Hugo Marx, a youthful seventy-seven, but too tired to notice;
Walter Hass, a sprightly eighty, who had sat *shivah*
for his wife for thirty years. Afternoons,
like a young girl dateless at prom time,
she would wait by the phone, sure that deliverance
would come in the voice of some stranger, resolved
that her double digitry would grow centuried
in a whirl of romance. I don't know what she was thinking
that day, when she fell from the top of the stairs
to die at the bottom, but I like to imagine
it was of who would enter her room that night,
and of her great joy in beautiful men—
how she had trembled for them once,
how she would gladly tremble for them again,
even now.

Medicine

Grandma sleeps with
my sick
grand-
pa so she
can get him
during the night
medicine
to stop
the pain

In
the morning
clumsily
I
wake
them

Her eyes
look at me
from under-
neath
his withered
arm

The
medicine
is all
in
her long
un-
braided
hair.

Now, Before the End,
I Think

Now, before the end, I think
of how it was when we began:
in holding hands before we knew
each other, in touch there was the silent
awe of what we soon would know
in knowing one another later,
as though to heal the wounds that words
would cause before they were inflicted.

Now, wordless again, you reach to hold
my hand as if to say in silence,
it is healed, we touch, we are together.
We have heard the end, drifting
to the brink of a new silence,
holding hands in awe of being
now together, this moment, now,
now before we part forever.

The Bean Eaters

They eat beans mostly, this old yellow pair.
Dinner is a casual affair.
Plain chipware on a plain and creaking wood,
Tin flatware.

Two who are Mostly Good.
Two who have lived their day,
But keep on putting on their clothes
And putting things away.

And remembering . . .
Remembering, with twinklings and twinges,
As they lean over the beans in their rented back room that
       is full of beads and receipts and dolls and cloths,
       tobacco crumbs, vases and fringes.

Crazy Jane Talks with the Bishop

I met the Bishop on the road
And much said he and I.
'Those breasts are flat and fallen now,
Those veins must soon be dry;
Live in a heavenly mansion,
Not in some foul sty.'

'Fair and foul are near of kin,
And fair needs foul,' I cried.
'My friends are gone, but that's a truth
Nor grave nor bed denied,
Learned in bodily lowliness
And in the heart's pride.

'A woman can be proud and stiff
When on love intent;
But Love has pitched his mansion in
The place of excrement;
For nothing can be sole or whole
That has not been rent.'

from Asphodel, That Greeny Flower

CODA

Inseparable from the fire
        its light
                takes precedence over it.
Then follows
        what we have dreaded—
                but it can never
overcome what has gone before.
        In the huge gap
                between the flash
and the thunderstroke
        spring has come in
                or a deep snow fallen.
Call it old age.
        In that stretch
                we have lived to see
a colt kick up his heels.
        Do not hasten
                laugh and play
in an eternity
        the heat will not overtake the light.
                That's sure.
That gelds the bomb,
        permitting
                that the mind contain it.
This is that interval,
        that sweetest interval,
                when love will blossom,
come early, come late
        and give itself to the lover.
Only the imagination is real!
        I have declared it
                time without end.

If a man die
                    it is because death
                            has first
possessed his imagination.
                    But if he refuse death—
                            no greater evil
can befall him
                    unless it be the death of love
                            meet him
in full career.
                    Then indeed
                            for him
the light has gone out.
But love and the imagination
                    are of a piece,
                            swift as the light
to avoid destruction.
                    So we come to watch time's flight
                            as we might watch
summer lightning
                    or fireflies, secure,
                            by grace of the imagination,
safe in its care.
                    For if
                            the light itself
has escaped,
                    the whole edifice opposed to it
                            goes down.
Light, the imagination
                    and love,
                            in our age,
by natural law,
                    which we worship,
                            maintain
all of a piece
                    their dominance.
So let us love
                    confident as is the light
                            in its struggle with darkness
that there is as much to say
                    and more
                            for the one side
and that not the darker

which John Donne
for instance
among many men
presents to us.
In the controversy
touching the younger
and the older Tolstoy,
Villon, St. Anthony, Kung,
Rimbaud, Buddha
and Abraham Lincoln
the palm goes
always to the light:
Who most shall advance the light—
call it what you may!
The light
for all time shall outspeed
the thunder crack.
Medieval pageantry
is human and we enjoy
the rumor of it
as in our world we enjoy
the reading of Chaucer,
likewise
a priest's raiment
(or that of a savage chieftain).
It is all
a celebration of the light.
All the pomp and ceremony
of weddings,
"Sweet Thames, run softly
till I end
my song,"—
are of an equal sort.
For our wedding, too,
the light was wakened
and shone. The light!
the light stood before us
waiting!
I thought the world
stood still.
At the altar
so intent was I
before my vows,

                    so moved by your presence
                              a girl so pale
and ready to faint
              that I pitied
                        and wanted to protect you.
As I think of it now,
              after a lifetime,
                        it is as if
a sweet-scented flower
              were poised
                        and for me did open.
Asphodel
              has no odor
                        save to the imagination
but it too
              celebrates the light.
                        It is late
but an odor
              as from our wedding
                        has revived for me
and begun again to penetrate
              into all crevices
                        of my world.

We Are Nighttime Travelers

Where are we going? Where, I might write, is this path leading us? Francine is asleep and I am standing downstairs in the kitchen with the door closed and the light on and a stack of mostly blank paper on the counter in front of me. My dentures are in a glass by the sink. I clean them with a tablet that bubbles in the water, and although they were clean already I just cleaned them again because the bubbles are agreeable and I thought their effervescence might excite me to action. By action, I mean I thought they might excite me to write. But words fail me.

This is a love story. However, its roots are tangled and involve a good bit of my life, and when I recall my life my mood turns sour and I am reminded that no man makes truly proper use of his time. We are blind and small-minded. We are dumb as snails and as frightened, full of vanity and misinformed about the importance of things. I'm an average man, without great deeds except maybe one, and that has been to love my wife.

I have been more or less faithful to Francine since I married her. There has been one transgression—leaning up against a closet wall with a red-haired purchasing agent at a sales meeting once in Minneapolis twenty years ago; but she was buying auto upholstery and I was selling it and in the eyes of judgment this may bear a key weight. Since then, though, I have ambled on this narrow path of life bound to one woman. This is a triumph and a regret. In our current state of affairs it is a regret because in life a man is either on the uphill or on the downhill, and if he isn't procreating he is on the downhill. It is a steep downhill indeed. These days I am tumbling, falling headlong among the scrub oaks and boulders, tearing my knees and abrading all the bony parts of the body. I have given myself to gravity.

Francine and I are married now forty-six years, and I would be a bamboozler to say that I have loved her for any more than half of these. Let us say that for the last year I haven't; let us say this for the last ten, even. Time has made torments of our small differences and tolerance of our passions. This is our state of affairs. Now I stand by myself in our kitchen in the middle of the night; now I lead a secret life. We wake at different hours now, sleep in different corners of the bed. We like different foods and different music, keep our clothing in different drawers, and if it can be said that either of us

96

has aspirations, I believe that they are to a different bliss. Also, she is healthy and I am ill. And as for conversation—that feast of reason, that flow of the soul—our house is silent as the bone yard.

Last week we did talk. "Frank," she said one evening at the table, "there is something I must tell you."

The New York game was on the radio, snow was falling outside, and the pot of tea she had brewed was steaming on the table between us. Her medicine and my medicine were in little paper cups at our places.

"Frank," she said, jiggling her cup, "what I must tell you is that someone was around the house last night."

I tilted my pills onto my hand. "Around the house?"

"Someone was at the window."

On my palm the pills were white, blue, beige, pink: Lasix, Diabinese, Slow-K, Lopressor. "What do you mean?"

She rolled her pills onto the tablecloth and fidgeted with them, made them into a line, then into a circle, then into a line again. I don't know her medicine so well. She's healthy, except for little things. "I mean," she said, "there was someone in the yard last night."

"How do you know?"

"Frank, will you really, please?"

"I'm asking how you know."

"I heard him," she said. She looked down. "I was sitting in the front room and I heard him outside the window."

"You heard him?"

"Yes."

"The front window?"

She got up and went to the sink. This is a trick of hers. At that distance I can't see her face.

"The front window is ten feet off the ground," I said.

"What I know is that there was a man out there last night, right outside the glass." She walked out of the kitchen.

"Let's check," I called after her. I walked into the living room, and when I got there she was looking out the window.

"What is it?"

She was peering out at an angle. All I could see was snow, blue-white.

"Footprints," she said.

I built the house we live in with my two hands. That was forty-nine years ago, when, in my foolishness and crude want of learning, everything I didn't know seemed like a promise. I learned to build a house and then I built one. There are copper fixtures on the pipes, sanded edges on the struts and queen posts. Now, a half-century later, the floors are flat as a billiard table but the man who laid them needs two hands to pick up a woodscrew. This is the diabetes. My feet are gone also. I look down at them and see two black shapes when I walk, things I can't feel. Black clubs. No connection with the ground. If I didn't look, I could go to sleep with my shoes on.

Life takes its toll, and soon the body gives up completely. But it gives up the parts first. This sugar in the blood: God says to me: "Frank Manlius— codger, man of prevarication and half-truth—I shall take your life from you, as from all men. But first—" But first! Clouds in the eyeball, a heart that makes noise, feet cold as uncooked roast. And Francine, beauty that she was—now I see not much more than the dark line of her brow and the intersections of her body: mouth and nose, neck and shoulders. Her smells have changed over the years so that I don't know what's her own anymore and what's powder.

We have two children, but they're gone now too, with children of their own. We have a house, some furniture, small savings to speak of. How Francine spends her day I don't know. This is the sad truth, my confession. I am gone past nightfall. She wakes early with me and is awake when I return, but beyond this I know almost nothing of her life.

I myself spend my days at the aquarium. I've told Francine something else, of course, that I'm part of a volunteer service of retired men, that we spend our days setting young businesses afoot: "Immigrants," I told her early on, "newcomers to the land." I said it was difficult work. In the evenings I could invent stories, but I don't, and Francine doesn't ask.

I am home by nine or ten. Ticket stubs from the aquarium fill my coat pocket. Most of the day I watch the big sea animals—porpoises, sharks, a manatee—turn their saltwater loops. I come late morning and move a chair up close. They are waiting to eat then. Their bodies skim the cool glass, full of strange magnifications. I think, if it is possible, that they are beginning to know me: this man—hunched at the shoulder, cataractic of eye, breathing through water himself—this man who sits and watches. I do not pity them. At lunchtime I buy coffee and sit in one of the hotel lobbies or in the cafeteria next door, and I read poems. Browning, Whitman, Eliot. This is my secret. It is night when I return home. Francine is at the table, four feet across from my seat, the width of two dropleaves. Our medicine is in cups. There have been three Presidents since I held her in my arms.

The cafeteria moves the men along, old or young, who come to get away from the cold. A half-hour for a cup, they let me sit. Then the manager is at my table. He is nothing but polite. I buy a pastry then, something small. He knows me—I have seen him nearly every day for months now—and by his slight limp I know he is a man of mercy. But business is business.

"What are you reading?" he asks me as he wipes the table with a wet cloth. He touches the saltshaker, nudges the napkins in their holder. I know what this means.

"I'll take a cranberry roll," I say. He flicks the cloth and turns back to the counter.

This is what:

> *Shall I say, I have gone at dusk through narrow streets*
> *And watched the smoke that rises from the pipes*
> *Of lonely men in shirt-sleeves, leaning out of windows?*

Through the magnifier glass the words come forward, huge, two by two. With spectacles, everything is twice enlarged. Still, though, I am slow to read it. In a half-hour I am finished, could not read more, even if I bought another roll. The boy at the register greets me, smiles when I reach him. "What are you reading today?" he asks, counting out the change.

The books themselves are small and fit in the inside pockets of my coat. I put one in front of each breast, then walk back to see the fish some more. These are the fish I know: the gafftopsail pompano, sixgill shark, the starry flounder with its upturned eyes, queerly migrated. He rests half-submerged in sand. His scales are platey and flat-hued. Of everything upward he is wary, of the silvery seabass and the bluefin tuna that pass above him in the region of light and open water. For a life he lies on the bottom of the tank. I look at him. His eyes are dull. They are ugly and an aberration. Above us the bony fishes wheel at the tank's corners. I lean forward to the glass. "*Platichthys stellatus*," I say to him. The caudal fin stirs. Sand moves and resettles, and I see the black and yellow stripes. "Flatfish," I whisper, "we are, you and I, observers of this life."

"A man on our lawn," I say a few nights later in bed.

"Not just that."

I breathe in, breathe out, look up at the ceiling. "What else?"

"When you were out last night he came back."

"He came back."

"Yes."

"What did he do?"

"Looked in at me."

Later, in the early night, when the lights of cars are still passing and the walked dogs still jingle their collar chains out front, I get up quickly from bed and step into the hall. I move fast because this is still possible in short bursts and with concentration. The bed sinks once, then rises. I am on the landing and then downstairs without Francine waking. I stay close to the staircase joists.

In the kitchen I take out my almost blank sheets and set them on the counter. I write standing up because I want to take more than an animal's pose. For me this is futile, but I stand anyway. The page will be blank when

I finish. This I know. The dreams I compose are the dreams of others, re-membered bits of verse. Songs of greater men than I. In months I have writ-ten few more than a hundred words. The pages are stacked, sheets of different sizes.

If I could

one says.

It has never seemed

says another. I stand and shift them in and out. They are mostly blank, sheets from months of nights. But this doesn't bother me. What I have is patience.

Francine knows nothing of the poetry. She's a simple girl, toast and but-ter. I myself am hardly the man for it: forty years selling (anything—steel piping, heater elements, dried bananas). Didn't read a book except one on sales. Think victory, the book said. Think *sale*. It's a young man's bag of ap-ples, though; young men in pants that nip at the waist. Ten years ago I left the Buick in the company lot and walked home, dye in my hair, cotton rect-angles in the shoulders of my coat. Francine was in the house that afternoon also, the way she is now. When I retired we bought a camper and went on a trip. A traveling salesman retires, so he goes on a trip. Forty miles out of town the folly appeared to me, big as a balloon. To Francine, too. "Frank," she said in the middle of a bend, a prophet turning to me, the camper push-ing sixty and rocking in the wind, trucks to our left and right big as trains— "Frank," she said, "these roads must be familiar to you."

So we sold the camper at a loss and a man who'd spent forty years at high-way speed looked around for something to do before he died. The first poem I read was in a book on a table in a waiting room. My eyeglasses made half-sense of things.

THESE
are the desolate, dark weeks

I read

when nature in its barrenness
equals the stupidity of man.

Gloom, I thought, and nothing more, but then I reread the words, and sud-denly there I was, hunched and wheezing, bald as a trout, and tears were in my eye. I don't know where they came from.

In the morning an officer visits. He has muscles, mustache, skin red from the cold. He leans against the door frame.

"Can you describe him?" he says.

"It's always dark," says Francine.

"Anything about him?"

"I'm an old woman. I can see that he wears glasses."

"What kind of glasses?"

"Black."

"Dark glasses?"

"Black glasses."

"At a particular time?"

"Always when Frank is away."

"Your husband has never been here when he's come?"

"Never."

"I see." He looks at me. This look can mean several things, perhaps that he thinks Francine is imagining. "But never at a particular time?"

"No."

"Well," he says. Outside on the porch his partner is stamping his feet. "Well," he says again. "We'll have a look." He turns, replaces his cap, heads out to the snowy steps. The door closes. I hear him say something outside.

"Last night—" Francine says. She speaks in the dark. "Last night I heard him on the side of the house."

We are in bed. Outside, on the sill, snow has been building since morning.

"You heard the wind."

"Frank." She sits up, switches on the lamp, tilts her head toward the window. Through a ceiling and two walls I can hear the ticking of our kitchen clock.

"I heard him climbing," she says. She has wrapped her arms about her own waist. "He was on the house. I heard him. He went up the drainpipe." She shivers as she says this. "There was no wind. He went up the drainpipe and then I heard him on the porch roof."

"Houses make noise."

"I heard him. There's gravel there."

I imagine the sounds, amplified by hollow walls, rubber heels on timber. I don't say anything. There is an arm's length between us, cold sheet, a space uncrossed since I can remember.

"I have made the mistake in my life of not being interested in enough people," she says then. "If I'd been interested in more people, I wouldn't be alone now."

"Nobody's alone," I say.

"I mean that if I'd made more of an effort with people I would have friends now. I would know the postman and the Giffords and the Kohlers, and we'd be together in this, all of us. We'd sit in each other's living rooms on rainy days and talk about the children. Instead we've kept to ourselves. Now I'm alone."

"You're not alone," I say.

"Yes, I am." She turns the light off and we are in the dark again. "You're alone, too."

My health has gotten worse. It's slow to set in at this age, not the violent shaking grip of death; instead—a slow leak, nothing more. A bicycle tire: rimless, thready, worn treadless already and now losing its fatness. A war of attrition. The tall camels of the spirit steering for the desert. One morning I realized I hadn't been warm in a year.

And there are other things that go, too. For instance, I recall with certainty that it was on the 23rd of April, 1945, that, despite German counteroffensives in the Ardennes, Eisenhower's men reach the Elbe; but I cannot remember whether I have visited the savings and loan this week. Also, I am unable to produce the name of my neighbor, though I greeted him yesterday in the street. And take, for example, this: I am at a loss to explain whole decades of my life. We have children and photographs, and there is an understanding between Francine and me that bears the weight of nothing less than half a century, but when I gather my memories they seem to fill no more than an hour. Where has my life gone?

It has gone partway to shoddy accumulations. In my wallet are credit cards, a license ten years expired, twenty-three dollars in cash. There is a photograph but it depresses me to look at it, and a poem, half-copied and folded into the billfold. The leather is pocked and has taken on the curve of my thigh. The poem is from Walt Whitman. I copy only what I need.

But of all things to do last, poetry is a barren choice. Deciphering other men's riddles while the world is full of procreation and war. A man should go out swinging an axe. Instead, I shall go out in a coffee shop.

But how can any man leave this world with honor? Despite anything he does, it grows corrupt around him. It fills with locks and sirens. A man walks into a store now and the microwaves announce his entry; when he leaves, they make electronic peeks into his coat pockets, his trousers. Who doesn't feel like a thief? I see a policeman now, any policeman, and I feel a fright. And the things I've done wrong in my life haven't been crimes. Crimes of the heart perhaps, but nothing against the state. My soul may turn black but I can wear white trousers at any meeting of men. Have I loved my wife? At one time, yes—in rages and torrents. I've been covered by the pimples of ecstasy and have rooted in the mud of despair; and I've lived for months, for whole years now, as mindless of Francine as a tree of its mosses.

And this is what kills us, this mindlessness. We sit across the tablecloth now with our medicines between us, little balls and oblongs. We sit, sit. This has become our view of each other, a tableboard apart. We sit.

"Again?" I say.
"Last night."
We are at the table. Francine is making a twisting motion with her fingers. She coughs, brushes her cheek with her forearm, stands suddenly so that the table bumps and my medicines move in the cup.
"Francine," I say.
The half-light of dawn is showing me things outside the window: silhouettes, our maple, the eaves of our neighbor's garage. Francine moves and stands against the glass, hugging her shoulders.
"You're not telling me something," I say.
She sits and makes her pills into a circle again, then into a line. Then she is crying.
I come around the table, but she gets up before I reach her and leaves the kitchen. I stand there. In a moment I hear a drawer open in the living room. She moves things around, then shuts it again. When she returns she sits at the other side of the table. "Sit down," she says. She puts two folded sheets of paper onto the table. "I wasn't hiding them," she says.
"What weren't you hiding?"
"These," she says. "He leaves them."
"He leaves them?"
"They say he loves me."
"Francine."
"They're inside the windows in the morning." She picks one up, unfolds it. Then she reads:

> Ah, I remember well (and how can I
> But evermore remember well) when first

She pauses, squint-eyed, working her lips. It is a pause of only faint understanding. Then she continues:

> Our flame began, when scarce we knew what was
> The flame we felt.

When she finishes she refolds the paper precisely. "That's it," she says. "That's one of them."

At the aquarium I sit, circled by glass and, behind it, the senseless eyes of fish. I have never written a word of my own poetry but can recite the verse of others. This is the culmination of a life. *Coryphaena hippurus*, says the plaque on the dolphin's tank, words more beautiful than any of my own. The dolphin circles, circles, approaches with alarming speed, but takes no notice of, if he even sees, my hands. I wave them in front of his tank. What must he think has become of the sea? He turns and his slippery proboscis nudges the glass. I am every part sore from life.

> *Ah, silver shrine, here will I take my rest*
> *After so many hours of toil and quest,*
> *A famished pilgrim—saved by miracle.*

There is nothing noble for either of us here, nothing between us, and no miracles. I am better off drinking coffee. Any fluid refills the blood. The counter boy knows me and later at the café he pours the cup, most of a dollar's worth. Refills are free but my heart hurts if I drink more than one. It hurts no different from a bone, bruised or cracked. This amazes me.

Francine is amazed by other things. She is mystified, thrown beam ends by the romance. She reads me the poems now at breakfast, one by one. I sit. I roll my pills. "Another came last night," she says, and I see her eyebrows rise. "Another this morning." She reads them as if every word is a surprise. Her tongue touches teeth, shows between lips. These lips are dry. She reads:

> *Kiss me as if you made believe*
> *You were not sure, this eve,*
> *How my face, your flower, had pursed*
> *Its petals up*

That night she shows me the windowsill, second story, rimmed with snow, where she finds the poems. We open the glass. We lean into the air. There is ice below us, sheets of it on the trellis, needles hanging from the drainwork.

"Where do you find them?"

"Outside," she says. "Folded, on the lip."

"In the morning?"

"Always in the morning."

"The police should know about this."

"What will they be able to do?"

I step away from the sill. She leans out again, surveying her lands, which are the yard's-width spit of crusted ice along our neighbor's chain link and the three maples out front, now lost their leaves. She peers as if she expects this man to appear. An icy wind comes inside. "Think," she says. "Think. He could come from anywhere."

One night in February, a month after this began, she asks me to stay awake and stand guard until the morning. It is almost spring. The earth has reappeared in patches. During the day, at the borders of yards and driveways, I see glimpses of brown—though I know I could be mistaken. I come home early that night, before dusk, and when darkness falls I move a chair by the window downstairs. I draw apart the outer curtain and raise the shade. Francine brings me a pot of tea. She turns out the light and pauses next to me, and as she does, her hand on the chair's backbrace, I am so struck by the proximity of elements—of the night, of the teapot's heat, of the sounds of water outside—that I consider speaking. I want to ask her what has become of us, what has made our breathed air so sorry now, and loveless. But the timing is wrong and in a moment she turns and climbs the stairs. I look out into the night. Later, I hear the closet shut, then our bed creak.

There is nothing to see outside, nothing to hear. This I know. I let hours pass. Behind the window I imagine fish moving down to greet me: broomtail grouper, surfperch, sturgeon with their prehistoric rows of scutes. It is almost possible to see them. The night is full of shapes and bits of light. In it the moon rises, losing the colors of the horizon, so that by early morning it is high and pale. Frost has made a ring around it.

A ringed moon above, and I am thinking back on things. What have I regretted in my life? Plenty of things, mistakes enough to fill the car showroom, then a good deal of the back lot. I've been a man of gains and losses. What gains? My marriage, certainly, though it has been no knee-buckling windfall but more like a split decision in the end, a stock risen a few points since bought. I've certainly enjoyed certain things about the world, too. These are things gone over and over again by the writers and probably enjoyed by everybody who ever lived. Most of them involve air. Early morning air, air after a rainstorm, air through a car window. Sometimes I think the cerebrum is wasted and all we really need is the lower brain, which I've been told is what makes the lungs breathe and the heart beat and what lets us smell pleasant things. What about the poetry? That's another split decision, maybe going the other way if I really made a tally. It's made me melancholy in old age, sad when if I'd stuck with motor homes and the national league standings I don't think I would have been rooting around in regret and doubt at this point. Nothing wrong with sadness, but this is not the real thing—not the death of a child but the feelings of a college student reading *Don Quixote* on a warm afternoon before going out to the lake.

Now, with Francine upstairs, I wait for a night prowler. He will not appear. This I know, but the window glass is ill-blown and makes moving shadows anyway, shapes that change in the wind's rattle. I look out and despite myself am afraid.

Before me, the night unrolls. Now the tree leaves turn yellow in moon-shine. By two or three, Francine sleeps, but I get up anyway and change into my coat and hat. The books weigh against my chest. I don gloves, scarf, ga-loshes. Then I climb the stairs and go into our bedroom, where she is sleep-ing. On the far side of the bed I see her white hair and beneath the blankets the uneven heave of her chest. I watch the bedcovers rise. She is probably dreaming at this moment. Though we have shared this bed for most of a life-time I cannot guess what her dreams are about. I step next to her and touch the sheets where they lie across her neck.

"Wake up," I whisper. I touch her cheek, and her eyes open. I know this though I cannot really see them, just the darkness of their sockets.

"Is he there?"

"No."

"Then what's the matter?"

"Nothing's the matter," I say. "But I'd like to go for a walk."

"You've been outside," she says. "You saw him, didn't you?"

"I've been at the window."

"Did you see him?"

"No. There's no one there."

"Then why do you want to walk?" In a moment she is sitting aside the bed, her feet in slippers. "We don't ever walk," she says.

I am warm in all my clothing. "I know we don't," I answer. I turn my arms out, open my hands toward her. "But I would like to. I would like to walk in air that is so new and cold."

She peers up at me. "I haven't been drinking," I say. I bend at the waist, and though my head spins, I lean forward enough so that the effect is of a bow. "Will you come with me?" I whisper. "Will you be queen of this crystal night?" I recover from my bow, and when I look up again she has risen from the bed, and in another moment she has dressed herself in her wool robe and is walking ahead of me to the stairs.

Outside, the ice is treacherous. Snow had begun to fall and our galoshes squeak and slide, but we stay on the plowed walkway long enough to leave our block and enter a part of the neighborhood where I have never been. Ice hangs from the lamps. We pass unfamiliar houses and unfamiliar trees, street signs I have never seen, and as we walk the night begins to change. It is becoming liquor. The snow is banked on either side of the walk, plowed into hillocks at the corners. My hands are warming from the exertion. They are the hands of a younger man now, someone else's fingers in my gloves. They tingle. We take ten minutes to cover a block but as we move through this neighborhood my ardor mounts. A car approaches and I wave, a boat-man's salute, because here we are together on these rare and empty seas. We are nighttime travelers. He flashes his headlamps as he passes, and this fills me to the gullet with celebration and bravery. The night sings to us. I am Bluebeard now, Lindbergh, Genghis Khan.

No, I am not.

I am an old man. My blood is dark from hypoxia, my breaths singsong from disease. It is only the frozen night that is splendid. In it we walk, stepping slowly, bent forward. We take steps the length of table forks. Francine holds my elbow.

I have mean secrets and small dreams, no plans greater than where to buy groceries and what rhymes to read next, and by the time we reach our porch again my foolishness has subsided. My knees and elbows ache. They ache with a mortal ache, tired flesh, the cartilage gone sandy with time. I don't have the heart for dreams. We undress in the hallway, ice in the ends of our hair, our coats stiff from cold. Francine turns down the thermostat. Then we go upstairs and she gets into her side of the bed and I get into mine.

It is dark. We lie there for some time, and then, before dawn, I know she is asleep. It is cold in our bedroom. As I listen to her breathing I know my life is coming to an end. I cannot warm myself. What I would like to tell my wife is this:

> *What the*
> *imagination*
> *seizes*
> *as beauty must be truth. What holds you*
> *to what you see of me is*
> *that grasp alone.*

But I do not say anything. Instead I roll in the bed, reach across, and touch her, and because she is surprised she turns to me.

When I kiss her the lips are dry, cracking against mine, unfamiliar as the ocean floor. But then the lips give. They part. I am inside her mouth, and there, still, hidden from the world, as if ruin had forgotten a part, it is wet—Lord! I have the feeling of a miracle. Her tongue comes forward. I do not know myself then, what man I am, whom I lie with in embrace. I can barely remember her beauty. She touches my chest and I bite lightly on her lip, spread moisture to her cheek and then kiss there. She makes something like a sigh. "Frank," she says. "Frank." We are lost now in seas and deserts. My hand finds her fingers and grips them, bone and tendon, fragile things.

Grandma's Got a Wig

Now I peeped in the closet
        I know why grandma's lookin so good
Yeah, think I know why's grandma's lookin so good
Grandma's got a red wig, baby
        she's swingin like I know she could

Yeah, Granny's got her wig on now
        Grandpa's give her the eye
Yeah, Granny's got her wig on
        Grandpa's give her the koochy eye
Well, I think I'm gonna buy you a wig baby,
        so I won't have to say bye-bye

Yeah, Granny's got her wig on now
        and granpa's got his shirt half off
Yeah, a pretty red wig,
        granpa's got his shirt half off
Well, I dont mind you wearin a wig baby
        but dont cut your nappy hair off

Yeah, Granny's got her wig on now
        and granpa's workin on his shoes
Yeah, a pretty red wig
        grandpa's takin off his shoes
Keep you wig on pretty baby,
        or I have to sing the nappy haired blues

In Retirement

He had lately taken to studying his old Greek grammar of fifty years ago. He read in Bulfinch and wanted to reread the *Odyssey* in Greek. His life had changed. He slept less these days and in the morning got up to stare at the sky over Gramercy Park. He watched the clouds until they took on shapes he could reflect on. He liked strange, haunted vessels and he liked to watch mythological birds and animals. He had noticed that if he contemplated these forms in the clouds, could keep his mind on them for a while, there might be a diminution of his morning depression. Dr. Morris was sixty-six, a physician, retired for two years. He had shut down his practice in Queens and moved to Manhattan. He had retired himself after a heart attack, not too serious but serious enough. It was his first attack and he hoped his last, though in the end he hoped to go quickly. His wife was dead and his daughter lived in Scotland. He wrote her twice a month and heard from her twice a month. And though he had a few friends he visited, and kept up with medical journals, and liked museums and theater, generally he contended with loneliness. And he was concerned about the future; the future was old age possessed.

After a light breakfast he would dress warmly and go out for a walk around the Square. That was the easy part of the walk. He took this walk even when it was very cold, or nasty rainy, or had snowed several inches and he had to proceed very slowly. After the Square he crossed the street and went down Irving Place, a tall figure with a cape and cane, and picked up his *Times.* If the weather was not too bad he continued on to Fourteenth Street, around to Park Avenue South, up Park and along East Twentieth back to the narrow, tall, white stone apartment building he lived in. Rarely, lately, had he gone in another direction, though when on the long walk, he stopped at least once on the way, perhaps in front of a mid-block store, perhaps at a street corner, and asked himself where else he might go. This was the difficult part of the walk. What was difficult was that it made no difference where he went. He now wished he had not retired. He had become more conscious of his age since his retirement, although sixty-six was not eighty. Still it was old. He experienced moments of anguish.

One morning after his rectangular long walk in the rain, Dr. Morris found a letter on the rubber mat under the line of mailboxes in the lobby. It was a narrow, deep lobby with false green marble columns and several bulky chairs where few people ever sat. Dr. Morris had seen a young woman with long hair, in a white raincoat and maroon shoulder bag, carrying a cellophane bubble umbrella, hurry down the vestibule steps and leave the house as he was about to enter. In fact he held the door open for her and got a breath of her bold perfume. He did not remember seeing her before and felt a momentary confusion as to who she might be. He later imagined her taking the letter out of her box, reading it hastily, then stuffing it into the maroon cloth purse she carried over her shoulder; but she had stuffed in the envelope and not the letter. That had fallen to the floor. He imagined this as he bent to retrieve it. It was a folded sheet of heavy white writing paper, written on in black in a masculine hand. The doctor unfolded and glanced at it without making out the salutation or any of its contents. He would have to put on his reading glasses, and he thought Flaherty, the doorman and elevator man, might see him if the elevator should suddenly descend. Of course Flaherty might think the doctor was reading his own mail, except that he never read it, such as it was, in the lobby. He did not want the man thinking he was reading someone else's letter. He also thought of handing him the letter and describing the young woman who had dropped it. Perhaps he could return it to her? But for some reason not at once clear to him the doctor slipped it into his pocket to take upstairs to read. His arm began to tremble and he felt his heart racing at a rate that bothered him.

After the doctor had got his own mail out of the box—nothing more than the few circulars he held in his hand—Flaherty took him up to the fifteenth floor. Flaherty spelled the night man at 8 a.m. and was himself relieved at 4 p.m. He was a slender man of sixty with sparse white hair on his half-bald head, who had lost part of his jaw under the left ear after two bone operations. He would be out for a few months; then return, the lower part of the left side of his face caved in; still it was not a bad face to look at. Although the doorman never spoke about his ailment, the doctor knew he was not done with cancer of the jaw, but of course he kept this to himself; and he sensed when the man was concealing pain.

This morning, though preoccupied, he asked, "How is it going, Mr. Flaherty?"

"Not too tough."

"Not a bad day." He said this, thinking not of the rain but of the letter in his pocket.

"Fine and dandy," Flaherty quipped. On the whole he moved and talked animatedly and was careful to align the elevator with the floor before letting passengers off. Sometimes the doctor wished he could say more to him than he did; but not this morning.

He stood by the large double window of his living room overlooking the Square, in the dull rainy-day February light, in pleasurable excitement reading the letter he had found, the kind he had anticipated it might be. It was a letter written by a father to his daughter, addressed to "Dear Evelyn." What it expressed after an irresolute start was the father's dissatisfaction with his daughter's way of life. And it ended with an exhortatory paragraph of advice: "You have slept around long enough. I don't understand what you get out of that type of behavior any more. I think you have tried everything there is to try. You claim you are a serious person but let men use you for what they can get. There is no true payoff to you unless it is very temporary, and the real payoff to them is that they have got themselves an easy lay. I know how they think about this and how they talk about it in the lavatory the next day. Now I want to urge you once and for all that you ought to be more serious about your life. You have experimented long enough. I honestly and sincerely and urgently advise you to look around for a man of steady habits and good character who will marry you and treat you like the person I believe you want to be. I don't want to think of you any more as a drifting semi-prostitute. Please follow this advice, the age of twenty-nine is no longer sixteen." The letter was signed, "Your Father," and under his signature, another sentence, in neat small handwriting, was appended: "Your sex life fills me full of fear." "Mother."

The doctor put the letter away in a drawer. His excitement had left him and he felt ashamed of having read it. He was sympathetic to the father and at the same time sympathetic to the young woman, though perhaps less so to her. After a while he tried to study his Greek grammar but could not concentrate. The letter remained in his mind like a billboard sign as he was reading *The Times* and he was conscious of it throughout the day, as though it had aroused in him some sort of expectation he could not define. Sentences from it would replay themselves in his thoughts. He reveried the young woman as he had imagined her after reading what the father had written, and as the woman—was she Evelyn?—he had seen coming out of the house. He could not be certain the letter was hers. Perhaps it was not; still he thought of the letter as though belonging to her, the woman he had held the door for, whose perfume still lingered in his senses. That night thoughts of her kept him from falling asleep. "I'm too old for this nonsense." He got up to read and was able to concentrate, but when his head lay once more on the pillow, a long freight train of thoughts of her rumbled by drawn by a black locomotive. He pictured Evelyn, the drifting semi-prostitute, in bed with various lovers, engaged in various acts of sex. Once she lay alone, erotically naked in bed, her maroon cloth purse drawn close to her nude body. He also thought of her as an ordinary girl with many fewer lovers than her father seemed to think. This was probably closer to the truth. He wondered if he could be useful to her in some way. He then felt a fright he could not explain but managed to dispel it by promising himself to burn the letter in the morning. The freight train, with its many cars, disappeared in the foggy distance. When the doctor awoke at 10 a.m. on a sunny winter's morning, there was no sense, light or heavy, of his usual depression.

But he did not burn the letter. He reread it several times during the day, each time returning it to his desk drawer and locking it there. Then he unlocked the drawer to read it again. As the day passed he was aware of an unappeased insistent hunger in himself. He recalled memories, experienced intense longing, desires he had not felt in years. The doctor was worried, alarmed by this change in him, this disturbance. He tried to blot the letter out of his mind but could not. Yet he would still not burn it, as though if he did he had shut the door on certain possibilities in his life, other ways to go, whatever that might mean. He was astonished—even thought of it as affronted, that this should be happening to him at his age. He had seen it in others, in former patients, but had not expected it in himself. The hunger he felt, a hunger for pleasure, disruption of habit, renewal of feeling, yet a fear of it, continued to grow in him like a dead tree come to life and spreading its branches. He felt as though he were hungry for exotic experience, which, if he were to have it, might make him forever ravenously hungry. He did not want that to happen to him. He recalled mythological figures: Sisyphus, Midas, who for one reason or another had been eternally cursed. He thought of Tithonus, his youth gone, become a grasshopper living forever. The doctor felt he was caught in an overwhelming emotion, a fearful dark wind.

When Flaherty left for the day at 4 p.m. and Silvio, who had tight curly black hair, was on duty, Dr. Morris came down and sat in the lobby, pretending to read his newspaper. As soon as the elevator ascended he approached the letter boxes and quickly scanned the name plates for an Evelyn, whoever she might be. He found no Evelyns though there was an E. Gordon and E. Cummings. He suspected one of them might be she. He knew that single women often preferred not to reveal their first names in order to keep cranks at a distance, conceal themselves from potential annoyers. He casually asked Silvio if Miss Gordon or Miss Cummings was named Evelyn, but Silvio said he didn't know although probably Mr. Flaherty would because he distributed the mail. "Too many peoples in this house," Silvio shrugged. Embarrassed, the doctor remarked he was just curious, a lame remark but all he could think of. He went out for an aimless short walk and when he returned said nothing more to Silvio. They rode silently up in the elevator, the doctor standing tall, almost stiff. That night he again slept badly. When he fell deeply asleep a moment his dreams were erotic. He woke with desire mixed with repulsion and lay quietly mourning himself. He felt powerless to be other than he was.

He was up before five and though he tried to kill time was uselessly in the lobby before seven. He felt he must find out, settle in his mind, who she was. In the lobby, Richard, the night man who had brought him down, returned to a pornographic paperback he was reading; the mail, as Dr. Morris knew, hadn't come. He knew it would not arrive until shortly after eight but hadn't the patience to wait in his apartment. So he left the building, bought *The Times* on Irving Place, continued on his walk, and because it was a pleasant morning, not too cold, sat on a bench in Union Square Park. He stared at the paper but could not read it. He watched some sparrows pecking at dead grass. He was an old man, true enough; but he had lived long enough to know that age often meant little in man-woman relationships. He was still vigorous and bodies are bodies. He was back in the lobby at eight-thirty, an act of great restraint. Flaherty had received the mail sack and was alphabetizing the first-class letters on a long large table before distributing them into the boxes. He did not look well today. He moved slowly. His misshapen face was gray; the mouth slack, one heard his breathing; his eyes harbored pain.

"Nothin for you yet," he said to the doctor without looking up.

"I'll wait this morning," said Dr. Morris. "I ought to be hearing from my daughter."

"Nothin yet but you might hit the lucky number in this last bundle." He removed the string.

As he was alphabetizing the last bundle of letters the elevator buzzed and Flaherty had to go up for a call.

The doctor pretended to be absorbed in his *Times*. When he heard the elevator door shut he sat momentarily still, then went to the table and hastily rifled through the C pile of letters. E. Cummings was Ernest Cummings. He shuffled through the G's, watching the metal arrow as it showed the elevator beginning to descend. In the G pile there were two letters addressed to Evelyn Gordon. One was from her mother. The other, also handwritten, was from a Lee Bradley. Almost against his will the doctor removed this letter and slipped it into his suit pocket. His body was sweaty hot. This is an aberration, he thought. He was sitting in the chair turning the page of his newspaper when the elevator door opened.

"Nothin at all for you," Flaherty said after a moment.

"Thank you," said Dr. Morris. "I think I'll go up now."

In his apartment the doctor, conscious of his whisperous breathing, placed the letter on the kitchen table and sat looking at it, waiting for a tea kettle of water to boil. The kettle whistled as it boiled but still he sat with the unopened letter before him. For a while he sat there with dulled thoughts. Soon he fantasied what the letter said. He fantasied Lee Bradley describing the sexual pleasure he had had with Evelyn Gordon, and telling her what else they might try. He fantasied the lovers' acts they engaged in. Then though he audibly told himself not to, he steamed open the flap of the envelope. His hands trembled as he held the letter. He had to place it down flat on the table so he could read it. His heart beat heavily in anticipation of what he might read. But to his surprise the letter was a bore, an egoistic account of some stupid business deal this Bradley was concocting. Only the last sentences came surprisingly to life. "Be in your bed when I get there tonight. Be wearing only your white panties. I don't like to waste time once we are together." The doctor didn't know whom he was more disgusted with, this fool or himself. In truth, himself. Slipping the sheet of paper into the envelope, he resealed it with a thin layer of paste he had rubbed carefully on the flap with his fingertip. Later in the day he tucked the letter into his inside pocket and pressed the elevator button for Silvio. The doctor left the building and soon returned with a copy of the afternoon *Post* he seemed to be involved with until Silvio had to take up two women who had come into the lobby; then the doctor thrust the letter into Evelyn Gordon's box and went out for a breath of air.

He was sitting near the table in the lobby when the young woman he had held the door open for came in shortly after 6 p.m. He was aware of her cool perfume almost at once. Silvio was not around at that moment; he had gone down to the basement to eat a sandwich. She inserted a small key into Evelyn Gordon's mailbox and stood before the open box, smoking, as she read Bradley's letter. She was wearing a light-blue pants suit with a brown knit sweater-coat. Her tail of black hair was tied with a brown silk scarf. Her face, though a little heavy, was pretty, her intense eyes blue, the lids lightly eyeshadowed. Her body, he thought, was finely proportioned. She had not noticed him but he was more than half in love with her.

He observed her many mornings. He would come down later now, at nine, and spend some time going through the medical circulars he had got out of his box, sitting on a thronelike wooden chair near a tall unlit lamp in the rear of the lobby. He would watch people as they left for work or shopping in the morning. Evelyn appeared at about half-past nine and stood smoking in front of her box, absorbed in the morning's mail. When spring came she wore brightly colored skirts with pastel blouses, or light slim pants suits. Sometimes she wore very short minidresses. Her figure was exquisite. She received many letters and read most of them with apparent pleasure, some with what seemed suppressed excitement. A few she gave short shrift to, scanned these quickly and stuffed them into her bag. He imagined they were from her father, or mother. He thought that most of her letters came from lovers, past and present, and he felt a curious anguish that there was none from him in her box. He would write to her.

He thought it through carefully. Some women needed an older man; it stabilized their lives. Sometimes a difference of as many as thirty or even thirty-five years offered no serious disadvantages, granted differences in metabolism, energy. There would of course be less sex, but there would be sex. His would go on for a long time; he knew that from the experience of friends and former patients, not to speak of medical literature. A younger woman inspired an older man to remain virile. And despite the heart incident his health was good, in some ways better than before. A girl like Evelyn, probably at odds with herself, could benefit from a steadying relationship with an older man, someone who would respect and love her and help her to respect and love herself more than she perhaps presently did; who would demand less from her in certain ways than some young men awash in their egoism; who would awake in her a stronger sense of well-being, and if things went quite well, perhaps even love for one particular man.

"I am a retired physician, a widower," he wrote to Evelyn Gordon. "I write to you with some hesitation and circumspection, although needless to say with high regard, because I am old enough to be your father. I have observed you often in this building and sometimes as we passed by each other in nearby streets, and I have grown to admire you deeply. I wonder if you will permit me to make your acquaintance? I wonder if you would care to have dinner with me and perhaps enjoy a film or performance of a play? My intentions, as used to be said when I was a young man, are 'ancient and honorable.' I do not think my company will disappoint you. If you are so inclined—so kind, certainly—to consider this request tolerantly, I will be obliged if you will place a note to that effect in my mailbox. I am respectfully yours, Simon Morris, M.D."

He did not go down to mail his letter at once. He thought he would keep it to the last moment. Then he had a fright about it that woke him out of momentary deep sleep. He dreamed he had written and sealed the letter and then remembered he had appended another sentence: "Be wearing only your white panties." When he woke he wanted to tear open the envelope to see whether he had included Bradley's remark. But when he was thoroughly waked up, in his senses, he knew he had not. He bathed and shaved early and for a while observed the cloud formations out the window. None of them interested him. At close to nine Dr. Morris descended to the lobby. He would wait till Flaherty answered a buzz, and when he was gone, drop his letter into her box; but Flaherty that morning seemed to have no calls to answer. The doctor had forgotten it was Saturday. He did not know it was till he got his *Times* and sat with it in the lobby, pretending to be waiting for the mail delivery. The mail sack arrived late on Saturdays. At last he heard a prolonged buzz, and Flaherty, who had been on his knees polishing the brass door knob, got up on one foot, then rose on both legs and walked slowly to the elevator. His asymmetric face was gray. Shortly before ten o'clock the doctor slipped his letter into Evelyn Gordon's mailbox. He decided to withdraw to his apartment but then thought he would rather wait where he usually waited while she collected her mail. She had never noticed him there.

The mail sack was dropped in the vestibule at ten-after, and Flaherty alphabetized the first bundle before he had to respond to another call. The doctor read his paper in the dark rear of the lobby because he was really not reading it. He was anticipating Evelyn's coming. He had on a new green suit, blue striped shirt, and a pink tie. He was wearing a new hat. He waited in anticipation and love.

When the elevator door opened Evelyn walked out in an elegant slit black skirt, sandals, her hair tied with a red scarf. A sharp-featured man with puffed sideburns and carefully combed medium-long hair, in a turn-of-the-century haircut, followed her out of the elevator. He was shorter than she by half a head. Flaherty handed her two letters, which she dropped into the black patent-leather pouch she was carrying. The doctor thought—hoped—she would walk past the mailboxes without stopping; but she saw the white of his letter through the slot and stopped to remove it. She tore open the envelope, pulled out the single sheet of handwritten paper, and read it with immediate intense concentration. The doctor raised his newspaper to his eyes, though he could still watch over the top of it. He watched in fear.

How mad I was not to anticipate she might come down with a man.

When she had finished reading the letter, she handed it to her companion—possibly Bradley—who read it, grinned broadly, and said something inaudible when he handed it back to her.

Evelyn Gordon quietly ripped the letter into small bits, and turning, flung the pieces in the doctor's direction. The fragments came at him like a blast of wind-driven snow. He thought he would sit forever on his wooden throne in the swirling snow.

The old doctor sat lifelessly in his chair, the floor around him littered with his torn-up letter.

Flaherty swept it up with his little broom into a metal container. He handed the doctor a thin envelope stamped with foreign stamps.

"Here's a letter from your daughter just came."

The doctor, trying to stand without moving, pressed the bridge of his nose. He wiped his eyes with his fingers.

"There's no setting old age aside," he said after a while.

"Not in some ways," said Flaherty.

"Or death."

"It moves up on you."

The doctor tried to say something kind to him but could not.

Flaherty took him up to the fifteenth floor in his elevator.

Epstein

Michael, the weekend guest, was to spend the night in one of the twin beds in Herbie's old room, where the baseball pictures still hung on the wall. Lou Epstein lay with his wife in the room with the bed pushed cater-corner. His daughter Sheila's bedroom was empty; she was at a meeting with her fiancé, the folk singer. In the corner of her room a childhood teddy bear balanced on its bottom, a VOTE SOCIALIST button pinned to its left ear; on her bookshelves, where volumes of Louisa May Alcott once gathered dust, were now collected the works of Howard Fast. The house was quiet. The only light burning was downstairs in the dining room where the *shabus* candles flickered in their tall golden holders and Herbie's jahrzeit candle trembled in its glass.

Epstein looked at the dark ceiling of his bedroom and let his head that had been bang-banging all day go blank for a moment. His wife Goldie breathed thickly beside him, as though she suffered from eternal bronchitis. Ten minutes before she had undressed and he had watched as she dropped her white nightdress over her head, over the breasts which had funneled down to her middle, over the behind like a bellows, the thighs and calves veined blue like a roadmap. What once could be pinched, what once was small and tight, now could be poked and pulled. Everything hung. He had shut his eyes while she had dressed for sleep and had tried to remember the Goldie of 1927, the Lou Epstein of 1927. Now he rolled his stomach against her backside, remembering, and reached around to hold her breasts. The nipples were dragged down like a cow's, long as his little finger. He rolled back to his own side.

A key turned in the front door—there was whispering, then the door gently shut. He tensed and waited for the noises—it didn't take those Socialists long. At night the noise from the zipping and the unzipping was enough to keep a man awake. "What are they doing down there?" he had screamed at his wife one Friday night, "trying on clothes?" Now, once again, he waited. It wasn't that he was against their playing. He was no puritan, he believed in young people enjoying themselves. Hadn't he been a young man himself? But in 1927 he and his wife were handsome people. Lou Epstein had never resembled that chinless, lazy smart aleck whose living was earned singing folk songs at a saloon, and who once had asked Epstein if it hadn't been "thrilling" to have lived through "a period of great social upheaval" like the thirties.

And his daughter, why couldn't she have grown up to be like—like the girl across the street whom Michael had the date with, the one whose father had died. Now there was a pretty girl. But not his Sheila. What happened, he wondered, what happened to that little pink-skinned baby? What year, what month did those skinny ankles grow thick as logs, the peaches-and-cream turn to pimples? That lovely child was now a twenty-three-year-old woman with "a social conscience"! Some conscience, he thought. She hunts all day for a picket line to march in so that at night she can come home and eat like a horse. . . . For her and that guitar plucker to touch each other's unmentionables seemed worse than sinful—it was disgusting. When Epstein tossed in bed and heard their pantings and the zipping it sounded in his ears like thunder.

Zip!

They were at it. He would ignore them, think of his other problems. The business . . . here he was a year away from the retirement he had planned but with no heir to Epstein Paper Bag Company. He had built the business from the ground, suffered and bled during the Depression and Roosevelt, only, finally, with the war and Eisenhower to see it succeed. The thought of a stranger taking it over made him sick. But what could be done? Herbie, who would have been twenty-eight, had died of polio, age eleven. And Sheila, his last hope, had chosen as her intended a lazy man. What could he do? Does a man of fifty-nine all of a sudden start producing heirs?

Zip! Pant-pant-pant! Ahh!

He shut his ears and mind, tighter. He tried to recollect things and drown himself in them. For instance, dinner . . .

He had been startled when he arrived home from the shop to find the soldier sitting at his dinner table. Surprised because the boy, whom he had not seen for ten or twelve years, had grown up with the Epstein face, as his son would have, the small bump in the nose, the strong chin, dark skin, and shock of shiny black hair that, one day, would turn gray as clouds.

"Look who's here," his wife shouted at him the moment he entered the door, the day's dirt still under his fingernails. "Sol's boy."

The soldier popped up from his chair and extended his hand. "How do you do, Uncle Louis?"

"A Gregory Peck," Epstein's wife said, "a Monty Clift your brother has. He's been here only three hours already he has a date. And a regular gentleman . . ."

Epstein did not answer.

The soldier stood at attention, square, as though he'd learned courtesy long before the Army. "I hope you don't mind my barging in, Uncle Louis.

I was shipped to Monmouth last week and Dad said I should stop off to see you people. I've got the weekend off and Aunt Goldie said I should stay—"
He waited.

"Look at him," Goldie was saying, "a Prince!"

"Of course," Epstein said at last, "stay. How is your father?" Epstein had not spoken to his brother Sol since 1945 when he had bought Sol's share of the business and his brother had moved to Detroit, with words.

"Dad's fine," Michael said. "He sends his regards."

"Sure, I send mine too. You'll tell him."

Michael sat down, and Epstein knew that the boy must think just as his father did: that Lou Epstein was a coarse man whose heart beat faster only when he was thinking of Epstein Paper Bag.

When Sheila came home they all sat down to eat, four, as in the old days. Goldie Epstein jumped up and down, up and down, slipping each course under their noses the instant they had finished the one before. "Michael," she said historically, "Michael, as a child you were a very poor eater. Your sister Ruthie, God bless her, was a nice eater. Not a good eater, but a nice eater."

For the first time Epstein remembered his little niece Ruthie, a little dark-haired beauty, a Bible Ruth. He looked at his own daughter and heard his wife go on, and on. "No, Ruthie wasn't such a good eater. But she wasn't a picky eater. Our Herbie, he should rest in peace, was a picky eater . . . "
Goldie looked towards her husband as though he would remember precisely what category of eater his beloved son had been; he stared into his pot roast.

"But," Goldie Epstein resumed, "You should live and be well, Michael, you turned out to be a good eater . . . "

Ahhh! Ahhh!

The noises snapped Epstein's recollection in two.

Aaahhhh!

Enough was enough. He got out of bed, made certain that he was tucked into his pajamas, and started down to the living room. He would give them a piece of his mind. He would tell them that—that 1927 was not 1957! No, that was what they would tell him.

But in the living room it was not Sheila and the folk singer. Epstein felt the cold from the floor rush up the loose legs of his pajamas and chill his crotch, raising goose flesh on his thighs. They did not see him. He retreated a step, back behind the archway to the dining room. His eyes, however, remained fixed on the living room floor, on Sol's boy and the girl from across the street.

The girl had been wearing shorts and a sweater. Now they were thrown over the arm of the sofa. The light from the candles was enough for Epstein to see that she was naked. Michael lay beside her, squirming and potent, wearing only his army shoes and khaki socks. The girl's breasts were like two small white cups. Michael kissed them, and more. Epstein tingled; he did not dare move, he did not want to move, until the two, like cars in a railroad yard, slammed fiercely together, coupled, shook. In their noise Epstein tiptoed, trembling, up the stairs and back to his wife's bed.

He could not force himself to sleep for what seemed like hours, not until the door had opened downstairs and the two young people had left. When, a minute or so later, he heard another key turn in the lock he did not know whether it was Michael returning to go to sleep, or—

Zip!

Now it was Sheila and the folk singer! The whole world, he thought, the whole young world, the ugly ones and the pretty ones, the fat and the skinny ones, zipping and unzipping! He grabbed his great shock of gray hair and pulled it till his scalp hurt. His wife shuffled, mumbled a noise. "Brrr . . . brrrrr . . . " She captured the blankets and pulled them over her. "Brrr . . ."

Butter! She's dreaming about butter. Recipes she dreams while the world zips. He closed his eyes and pounded himself down down into an old man's sleep.

2

How far back must you go to discover the beginning of trouble? Later, when Epstein had more time he would ask himself this question. When did it begin? That night he'd seen those two on the floor? Or the summer night seventeen years before when he had pushed the doctor away from the bed and put his lips to his Herbie's? Or, Epstein wondered, was it that night fifteen years ago when instead of smelling a woman between his sheets he smelled Bab-O? Or the time when his daughter had first called him "capitalist" as though it were a dirty name, as though it were a crime to be successful? Or was it none of these times? Maybe to look for a beginning was only to look for an excuse. Hadn't the trouble, the big trouble, begun simply when it appeared to, the morning he saw Ida Kaufman waiting for the bus?

And about Ida Kaufman, why in God's name was it a stranger, nobody he loved or ever could love, who had finally changed his life?—she, who had lived across the street for less than a year, and who (it was revealed by Mrs. Katz, the neighborhood Winchell) would probably sell her house now that Mr. Kaufman was dead and move all-year-round into their summer cottage at Barnegat? Until that morning Epstein had not more than noticed the woman: dark, good-looking, a big chest. She hardly spoke to the other housewives, but spent every moment, until a month ago, caring for her cancer-eaten husband. Once or twice Epstein had tipped his hat to her, but even then he had been more absorbed in the fate of Epstein Paper Bag than in the civility he was practicing. Actually then, on that Monday morning it would not have been unlikely for him to have driven right past the bus stop. It was a warm April day, certainly not a bad day to be waiting for a bus. Birds fussed and sang in the elm trees, and the sun glinted in the sky like a young athlete's trophy. But the woman at the bus stop wore a thin dress and no coat, and Epstein saw her waiting, and beneath the dress, the stockings, the imagined underthings he saw the body of the girl on his living room rug, for Ida Kaufman was the mother of Linda Kaufman, the girl Michael had befriended. So Epstein pulled slowly to the curb and, stopping for the daughter, picked up the mother.

"Thank you, Mr. Epstein," she said. "This is kind of you."

"It's nothing," Epstein said. "I'm going to Market Street."

"Market Street will be fine."

He pressed down too hard on the accelerator and the big Chrysler leaped away, noisy as a hot-rodder's Ford. Ida Kaufman rolled down her window and let the breeze waft in; she lit a cigarette. After a while she asked, "That was your nephew, wasn't it, that took Linda out Saturday night?"

"Michael? Yes." Epstein flushed, for reasons Ida Kaufman did not know. He felt the red on his neck and coughed to make it appear that some respiratory failure had caused the blood to rush up from his heart.

"He's a very nice boy, extremely polite," she said.

"My brother Sol's," Epstein said, "in Detroit." And he shifted his thoughts to Sol so that the flush might fade: if there had been no words with Sol it would be Michael who would be heir to Epstein Paper Bag. Would he have wanted that? Was it any better than a stranger . . . ?

While Epstein thought, Ida Kaufman smoked, and they drove on without speaking, under the elm trees, the choir of birds, and the new spring sky unfurled like a blue banner.

"He looks like you," she said.

"What? Who?"

"Michael."

"No," Epstein said, "him, he's the image of Sol."

"No, no, don't deny it—" and she exploded with laughter, smoke dragoning out of her mouth; she jerked her head back mightily, "No, no, no, he's got your face!"

Epstein looked at her, wondering: the lips, big and red, over her teeth, grinning. Why? Of course—your little boy looks like the iceman, she'd made that joke. He grinned, mostly at the thought of going to bed with his sister-in-law, whose everything had dropped even lower than his wife's.

Epstein's grin provoked Ida Kaufman into more extravagant mirth. What the hell, he decided, he would try a joke himself.

"Your Linda, who does *she* look like?"

Ida Kaufman's mouth straightened; her lids narrowed, killing the light in her eyes. Had he said the wrong thing? Stepped too far? Defiled the name of a dead man, a man who'd had cancer yet? But no, for suddenly she raised her arms in front of her, and shrugged her shoulders as though to say, "Who knows, Epstein, who knows?"

Epstein roared. It was so long since he had been with a woman who had a sense of humor; his wife took everything he said seriously. Not Ida Kaufman, though—she laughed so hard her breasts swelled over the top of her tan dress. They were not cups but pitchers. The next thing Epstein knew he was telling her another joke, and another, in the middle of which a cop screamed up alongside him and gave him a ticket for a red light which, in his joy, he had not seen. It was the first of three tickets he received that day; he earned a second racing down to Barnegat later that morning, and a third speeding up the Parkway at dusk, trying not to be too late for dinner. The tickets cost him $32 in all, but, as he told Ida, when you're laughing so hard you have tears in your eyes, how can you tell the green lights from the red ones, fast from slow?

At seven o'clock that evening he returned Ida to the bus stop on the corner and squeezed a bill into her hands.

"Here," he said, "Here—buy something"; which brought the day's total to fifty-two.

Then he turned up the street, already prepared with a story for his wife: a man interested in buying Epstein Paper Bag had kept him away all day, a good prospect. As he pulled into his driveway he saw his wife's square shape back of the venetian blinds. She ran one hand across a slat, checking for dust while she awaited her husband's homecoming.

3

Prickly heat?

He clutched his pajama trousers around his knees and looked at himself in the bedroom mirror. Downstairs a key turned in the lock but he was too engaged to hear it. Prickly heat is what Herbie always had—a child's complaint. Was it possible for a grown man to have it? He shuffled closer to the mirror, tripping on his half-hoisted pajamas. Maybe it was a sand rash. Sure, he thought, for during those three warm, sunny weeks, he and Ida Kaufman, when they were through, would rest on the beach in front of the cottage. Sand must have gotten into his trousers and irritated him on the drive up the Parkway. He stepped back now and was squinting at himself in the mirror when Goldie walked into the bedroom. She had just emerged from a hot tub—her bones ached, she had said—and her flesh was boiled red. Her entrance startled Epstein, who had been contemplating his blemish with the intensity of a philosopher. When he turned swiftly from his reflection, his feet caught in his pants leg, he tripped, and the pajamas slipped to the floor. So there they were, naked as Adam and Eve, except that Goldie was red all over, and Epstein had prickly heat, or a sand rash, or—and it came to him as a first principle comes to a metaphysician. Of course! His hands shot down to cover his crotch.

Goldie looked at him, mystified, while Epstein searched for words appropriate to his posture.

At last: "You had a nice bath?"

"Nice, shmice, it was a bath," his wife mumbled.

"You'll catch a cold," Epstein said. "Put something on."

"I'll catch a cold? *You'll* catch a cold!" She looked at the hands laced across his crotch. "Something hurts?"

"It's a little chilly," he said.

"Where?" She motioned towards his protection. "There?"

"All over."

"Then cover all over."

He leaned over to pick up his pajama trousers; the instant he dropped the fig leaf of his hands Goldie let out a short airless gasp. "What is *that*?"

"What?"

"That!"

He could not look into the eyes of her face, so concentrated instead on the purple eyes of her droopy breasts. "A sand rash, I think."

"*Vus far* sand!"

"A rash then," he said.

She stepped up closer and reached out her hand, not to touch but to point. She drew a little circle of the area with her index finger. "A rash, there?"

"Why not there?" Epstein said. "It's like a rash on the hand or the chest. A rash is a rash."

"But how come all of a sudden?" his wife said.

"Look, I'm not a doctor," Epstein said. "It's there today, maybe tomorrow it'll be gone. How do I know! I probably got it from the toilet seat at the shop. The *shvartzes* are pigs—"

Goldie made a clicking sound with her tongue.

"You're calling me a liar?"

She looked up. "Who said liar?" And she gave her own form a swift looking-over, checked limbs, stomach, breast, to see if she had perhaps caught the rash from him. She looked back at her husband, then at her own body again, and suddenly her eyes widened. "You!" she screamed.

"Shah," Epstein said, "you'll wake Michael."

"You pig! Who, who was it!"

"I told you, the *shvartzes*—"

"Liar! Pig!" Wheeling her way back to the bed, she flopped onto it so hard the springs squeaked. "Liar!" And then she was off the bed pulling the sheets from it. "I'll burn them, I'll burn every one!"

Epstein stepped out of the pajamas that roped his ankles and raced to the bed. "What are you doing—it's not catching. Only on the toilet seat. You'll buy a little ammonia—"

"Ammonia!" she yelled, "you should *drink* ammonia!"

"No," Epstein shouted, "no," and he grabbed the sheets from her and threw them back over the bed, tucking them in madly. "Leave it be—" He ran to the back of the bed but as he tucked there Goldie raced around and ripped up what he had tucked in the front; so he raced back to the front while Goldie raced around to the back. "Don't touch me," she screamed, "don't come near me, you filthy pig! Go touch some filthy whore!" Then she yanked the sheets off again in one swoop, held them in a ball before her and spat. Epstein grabbed them back and the tug-of-war began, back and forth, back and forth, until they had torn them to shreds. Then for the first time Goldie cried. With white strips looped over her arms she began to sob. "My sheets, my nice clean sheets—" and she threw herself on the bed.

Two faces appeared in the doorway of the bedroom. Sheila Epstein groaned, "Holy Christ!"; the folk singer peeped in, once, twice, and then bobbed out, his feet scuttling down the stairs. Epstein whipped some white strands about him to cover his privates. He did not say a word as his daughter entered.

"Mamma, what's the matter?"

"Your father," the voice groaned from the bed, "he has—a rash!" And so violently did she begin to sob that the flesh on her white buttocks rippled and jumped.

"That's right," Epstein said, "a rash. That's a crime? Get out of here! Let your mother and father get some sleep."

"Why is she crying?" Sheila demanded. "I want an answer!"

"How do I know! I'm a mind reader? This whole family is crazy, who knows what they think!"

"Don't call my mother crazy!"

"Don't you raise your voice to me! Respect your father!" He pulled the white strips tighter around him. "Now get out of here!"

"No!"

"Then I'll throw you out." He started for the door; his daughter did not move, and he could not bring himself to reach out and push her. Instead he threw back his head and addressed the ceiling. "She's picketing my bedroom! Get out, you lummox!" He took a step towards her and growled, as though to scare away a stray cat or dog. With all her one hundred and sixty pounds she pushed her father back; in his surprise and hurt he dropped

PHILIP ROTH

the sheet. And the daughter looked on the father. Under her lipstick she turned white.

Epstein looked up at her. He pleaded, "I got it from the toilet seat. The *shvartzes—*"

Before he could finish, a new head had popped into the doorway, hair messed and lips swollen and red; it was Michael, home from Linda Kaufman, his regular weekend date. "I heard the noise, is any—" and he saw his aunt naked on the bed. When he turned his eyes away, there was Uncle Lou.

"All of you," Epstein shouted. "Get out!"

But no one obeyed. Sheila blocked the door, politically committed; Michael's legs were rooted, one with shame, the other curiosity.

"Get out!"

Feet now came pounding up the stairs. "Sheila, should I call somebody—" And then the guitar plucker appeared in the doorway, eager, big-nosed. He surveyed the scene and his gaze, at last, landed on Epstein's crotch; the beak opened.

"What's he got? The syph?"

The words hung for a moment, bringing peace. Goldie Epstein stopped crying and raised herself off the bed. The young men in the doorway lowered their eyes. Goldie arched her back, flopped out her breasts, and began to move her lips. "I want . . . " she said. "I want . . . "

"What, Mamma?" Sheila demanded. "What is it?"

"I want . . . a divorce!" She looked amazed when she said it, though not as amazed as her husband; he smacked his palm to his head.

"Divorce! Are you crazy?" Epstein looked around; to Michael he said, "She's crazy!"

"I want one," she said, and then her eyes rolled up into her head and she passed out across the sheetless mattress.

After the smelling salts Epstein was ordered to bed in Herbie's room. He tossed and turned in the narrow bed which he was unused to; in the twin bed beside him he heard Michael breathing. Monday, he thought, Monday he would seek help. A lawyer. No, first a doctor. Surely in a minute a doctor could take a look and tell him what he already knew—that Ida Kaufman was a clean woman. Epstein would swear by it—he had smelled her flesh! The doctor would reassure him: his blemish resulted simply from their rubbing together. It was a temporary thing, produced by two, not transmitted by one. He was innocent! Unless what made him guilty had nothing to do with some dirty bug. But either way the doctor would prescribe for him. And then the lawyer would prescribe. And by then everyone would know, including, he suddenly realized, his brother Sol who would take special pleasure in thinking the worst. Epstein rolled over and looked to Michael's bed.

Pinpoints of light gleamed in the boy's head; he was awake, and wearing the Epstein nose, chin, and brow.

"Michael?"

"Yes."

"You're awake?"

"Yes."

"Me, too," Epstein said, and then apologetically, "all the excitement . . ." He looked back to the ceiling. "Michael?"

"Yes?"

"Nothing . . . " But he was curious as well as concerned. "Michael, you haven't got a rash, have you?"

Michael sat up in bed; firmly he said, "No."

"I just thought," Epstein said quickly. "You know, I have this rash . . . " He dwindled off and looked away from the boy, who, it occurred to him again, might have been heir to the business if that stupid Sol hadn't . . . But what difference did the business make now. The business had never been for him, but for them. And there was no more them.

He put his hands over his eyes. "The change, the change," he said. "I don't even know when it began. Me, Lou Epstein, with a rash. I don't even feel any more like Lou Epstein. All of a sudden, pffft! and things are changed." He looked at Michael again, speaking slowly now, stressing every word, as though the boy were more than a nephew, more, in fact, than a single person. "All my life I tried. I swear it, I should drop dead on the spot, if all my life I didn't try to do right, to give my family what I didn't have . . ."

He stopped; it was not exactly what he wanted to say. He flipped on the bedside light and started again, a new way. "I was seven years old, Michael. I came here I was a boy seven years old, and that day, I can remember it like it was yesterday. Your grandparents and me—your father wasn't born yet, this stuff believe me he doesn't know. With your grandparents I stood on the dock, waiting for Charlie Goldstein to pick us up. He was your grandfather's partner in the old country, the thief. Anyway, we waited, and finally he came to pick us up, to take us where we would live. And when he came he had a big can in his hand. And you know what was in it? Kerosene. We stood there and Charlie Goldstein poured it on all our heads. He rubbed it in, to delouse us. It tasted awful. For a little boy it was awful . . . "

Michael shrugged his shoulder.

"Eh! How can you understand?" Epstein grumbled. "What do you know? Twenty years old . . . "

Michael shrugged again. "Twenty-two," he said softly.

There were more stories Epstein could tell, but he wondered if any of them would bring him closer to what it was he had on his mind but could not find the words for. He got out of bed and walked to the bedroom door. He opened it and stood there listening. On the downstairs sofa he could hear the folk singer snoring. Some night for guests! He shut the door and came back into the room, scratching his thigh. "Believe me, *she's* not losing any sleep . . . She doesn't deserve me. What, she cooks? That's a big deal? She cleans? That deserves a medal? One day I should come home and the house should be a *mess*. I should be able to write my initials in the dust, somewhere, in the basement at least. Michael, after all these years that would be a pleasure!" He grabbed at his gray hair. "How did this happen? My Goldie, that such a woman should become a cleaning machine. Impossible." He walked to the far wall and stared into Herbie's baseball pictures, the long jaw-muscled faces, faded technicolor now, with signatures at the bottom: Charlie Keller, Lou Gehrig, Red Ruffing . . . A long time. How Herbie had loved his Yankees.

"One night," Epstein started again, "it was before the Depression even . . . you know what we did, Goldie and me?" He was staring at Red Ruffing now, through him. "You didn't know my Goldie, what a beautiful beautiful woman she was. And that night we took pictures, photos. I set up the camera—it was in the old house—and we took pictures, in the bedroom." He stopped, remembered. "I wanted a picture of my wife naked, to carry with me. I admit it. The next morning I woke up and there was Goldie tearing up the negatives. She said God forbid I should get in an accident one day and the police would take out my wallet for identification, and then oy-oy-oy!" He smiled. "You know, a woman, she worries . . . But at least we took the pictures, even if we didn't develop them. How many people even do that?" He wondered, and then turned away from Red Ruffing to Michael, who was, faintly, at the corners of his mouth, smiling.

"What, the photos?"

Michael started to giggle.

"Huh?" Epstein smiled. "What, you never had that kind of idea? I admit it. Maybe to someone else it would seem wrong, a sin or something, but who's to say—"

Michael stiffened, at last his father's son. "Somebody's got to say. Some things just aren't right."

Epstein was willing to admit a youthful lapse. "Maybe," he said, "maybe she was even right to tear—"

Michael shook his head vehemently. "No! Some things aren't right. They're just not!"

And Epstein saw the finger pointing not at Uncle Lou the Photographer, but at Uncle Lou the Adulterer. Suddenly he was shouting. "Right, wrong! From you and your father that's all I ever hear. Who are you, what are you, King Solomon!" He gripped the bedposts. "Should I tell you what else happened the night we took pictures? That my Herbie was started that night,

I'm sure of it. Over a year we tried and tried till I was *oysgamitched*, and that was the night. After the pictures, because of the pictures. Who knows!"

"But—"

"But what! But *this*?" He was pointing at his crotch. "You're a boy, you don't understand. When they start taking things away from you, you reach out, you *grab*—maybe like a pig even, but you grab. And right, wrong, who knows! With tears in your eyes, who can even see the difference!" His voice dropped now, but in a minor key the scolding grew more fierce. "Don't call *me* names. I didn't see you with Ida's girl, there's not a name for that? For *you* it's right?"

Michael was kneeling in his bed now. "*You—saw?*"

"I saw!"

"But it's different—"

"Different?" Epstein shouted.

"To be married is different!"

"What's different you don't know about. To have a wife, to be a father, twice a father—and then they start taking things away—" and he fell weak-kneed across Michael's bed. Michael leaned back and looked at his uncle, but he did not know what to do or how to chastise, for he had never seen anybody over fifteen years old cry before.

Usually Sunday morning went like this: at nine-thirty Goldie started the coffee and Epstein walked to the corner for the lox and the Sunday *News*. When the lox was on the table, the bagels in the oven, the rotogravure section of the *News* two inches from Goldie's nose, then Sheila would descend the stairs, yawning, in her toe-length housecoat. They would sit down to eat, Sheila cursing her father for buying the *News* and "putting money in a Fascist's pocket." Outside, the Gentiles would be walking to church. It had always been the same, except, of course, that over the years the *News* had come closer to Goldie's nose and further from Sheila's heart; she had the *Post* delivered.

This Sunday, when he awoke, Epstein smelled coffee bubbling in the kitchen. When he sneaked down the stairs, past the kitchen—he had been ordered to use the basement bathroom until he'd seen a doctor—he could smell lox. And, at last, when he entered the kitchen, shaved and dressed, he heard newspapers rattling. It was as if another Epstein, his ghost, had risen an hour earlier and performed his Sunday duties. Beneath the clock, around the table, sat Sheila, the folk singer, and Goldie. Bagels toasted in the oven, while the folk singer, sitting backwards in a chair, strummed his guitar and sang—

> *I've been down so long*
> *It look like up to me . . .*

Epstein clapped his hands and rubbed them together, preparatory to eating. "Sheila, you went out for this?" He gestured towards the paper and the lox. "Thank you."

The folk singer looked up, and in the same tune, improvised—

I went out for the lox . . .

and grinned, a regular clown.

"Shut up!" Sheila told him.

He echoed her words, plunk! plunk!

"Thank *you*, then, young man," Epstein said.

"His name is Marvin," Sheila said, "for your information."

"Thank you, Martin."

"Mar*vin*," the young man said.

"I don't hear so good."

Goldie Epstein looked up from the paper. "Syphilis softens the brain."

"What!"

"Syphilis softens the brain . . . "

Epstein stood up, raging. "Did you tell her that?" he shouted at his daughter. "Who told her that?"

The folk singer stopped plucking his guitar. Nobody answered; a conspiracy. He grabbed his daughter by the shoulders. "You respect your father, you understand!"

She jerked her shoulder away. "You're not *my* father!"

And the words hurled him back—to the joke Ida Kaufman had made in the car, to her tan dress, the spring sky . . . He leaned across the table to his wife. "Goldie, Goldie, look at me! Look at *me*, Lou!"

She stared back into the newspaper, though she held it far enough from her nose for Epstein to know she could not see the print; with everything else, the optometrist said the muscles in her eyes had loosened. "Goldie," he said, "Goldie, I did the worst thing in the world? Look me in the eyes, Goldie. Tell me, since when do Jewish people get a divorce? Since when?"

She looked up at him, and then at Sheila. "Syphilis makes soft brains. I can't live with a pig!"

"We'll work it out. We'll go to the rabbi—"

"He wouldn't recognize you—"

"But the children, what about the children?"

"What children?"

Herbie was dead and Sheila a stranger; she was right.

"A grown-up child can take care of herself," Goldie said. "If she wants, she can come to Florida with me. I'm thinking I'll move to Miami Beach."

"Goldie!"

"Stop shouting," Sheila said, anxious to enter the brawl. "You'll wake Michael."

Painfully polite, Goldie addressed her daughter. "Michael left early this morning. He took his Linda to the beach for the day, to their place in Belmar."

"Barnegat," Epstein grumbled, retreating from the table.

"What did you say?" Sheila demanded.

"Barnegat." And he decided to leave the house before any further questions were asked.

At the corner luncheonette he bought his own paper and sat alone, drinking coffee and looking out the window beyond which the people walked to church. A pretty young *shiksa* walked by, holding her white round hat in her hand; she bent over to remove her shoe and shake a pebble from it. Epstein watched her bend, and he spilled some coffee on his shirt front. The girl's small behind was round as an apple beneath the close-fitting dress. He looked, and then as though he were praying, he struck himself on the chest with his fist, again and again. "What have I done! Oh, God!"

When he finished his coffee, he took his paper and started up the street. To home? What home? Across the street in her backyard he saw Ida Kaufman, who was wearing shorts and a halter, and was hanging her daughter's underwear on the clothesline. Epstein looked around and saw only the Gentiles walking to church. Ida saw him and smiled. Growing angry, he stepped off the curb and, passionately, began to jaywalk.

At noon in the Epstein house those present heard a siren go off. Sheila looked up from the *Post* and listened; she looked at her watch. "Noon? I'm fifteen minutes slow. This lousy watch, my father's present."

Goldie Epstein was leafing through the ads in the travel section of the *New York Times*, which Marvin had gone out to buy for her. She looked at her watch. "I'm fourteen minutes slow. Also," she said to her daughter, "a watch from him . . ."

The wail grew louder. "God," Sheila said, "it sounds like the end of the world."

And Marvin, who had been polishing his guitar with his red handkerchief, immediately broke into song, a high-pitched, shut-eyed Negro tune about the end of the world.

"Quiet!" Sheila said. She cocked her ear. "But it's Sunday. The sirens are Saturday—"

Goldie shot off the couch. "It's a real air raid? Oy, that's all we need!"

"It's the police," Sheila said, and fiery-eyed she raced to the front door, for she was politically opposed to police. "It's coming up the street—an ambulance!"

She raced out the door, followed by Marvin, whose guitar still hung around his neck. Goldie trailed behind, her feet slapping against her slippers. On the street she suddenly turned back to the house to make sure the door was shut against daytime burglars, bugs, and dust. When she turned again she had not far to run. The ambulance had pulled up across the street in Kaufman's driveway.

Already a crowd had gathered, neighbors in bathrobes, housecoats, carrying the comic sections with them; and too, churchgoers, *shiksas* in white hats. Goldie could not make her way to the front where her daughter and Marvin stood, but even from the rear of the crowd she could see a young doctor leap from the ambulance and race up to the porch, his stethoscope wiggling in his back pocket as he took two steps at a time.

Mrs. Katz arrived. A squat red-faced woman whose stomach seemed to start at her knees, she tugged at Goldie's arm. "Goldie, more trouble here?"

"I don't know, Pearl. All that racket. It sounded like an atomic bomb."

"When it's that, you'll know," Pearl Katz said. She surveyed the crowd, then looked at the house. "Poor woman," she said, remembering that only three months before, on a windy March morning an ambulance had arrived to take Mrs. Kaufman's husband to the nursing home, from which he never returned.

"Troubles, troubles . . ." Mrs. Katz was shaking her head, a pot of sympathy. "Everybody has their little bundle, believe me. I'll bet she had a nervous breakdown. That's not a good thing. Gallstones, you have them out and they're out. But a nervous breakdown, it's very bad . . . You think maybe it's the daughter who's sick?"

"The daughter isn't home," Goldie said. "She's away with my nephew, Michael."

Mrs. Katz saw that no one had emerged from the house yet; she had time to gather a little information. "He's who, Goldie? The son of the brother-in-law that Lou doesn't talk to? That's his father?"

"Yes, Sol in Detroit—"

But she broke off, for the front door had opened, though still no one could be seen. A voice at the front of the crowd was commanding. "A little room here. Please! A little room, damn it!" It was Sheila. "A little room! Marvin, help me!"

"I can't put down my guitar—I can't find a place—"

"Get them back!" Sheila said.

"But my instrument—"

The doctor and his helper were now wiggling and tilting the stretcher through the front door. Behind them stood Mrs. Kaufman, a man's white shirt tucked into her shorts. Her eyes peered out of two red holes; she wore no make-up, Mrs. Katz noted.

"It must be the girl," said Pearl Katz, up on her toes. "Goldie, can you see, who is it—it's the girl?"

"The girl's *away*—"

"Stay back!" Sheila commanded. "Marvin, for crying out loud, help!"

The young doctor and his attendant held the stretcher steady as they walked sideways down the front steps.

Mrs. Katz jumped up and down. "Who *is* it?"

"I can't see," Goldie said. "I can't—" She pushed up on her toes, out of her slippers. "I—oh God! My God!" And she was racing forward, screaming, "Lou! Lou!"

"Mamma, stay back." Sheila found herself fighting off her mother. The stretcher was sliding into the ambulance now.

"Sheila, let me go, it's your father!" She pointed to the ambulance, whose red eye spun slowly on top. For a moment Goldie looked back to the steps. Ida Kaufman stood there yet, her fingers fidgeting at the buttons of the shirt. Then Goldie broke for the ambulance, her daughter beside her, propelling her by her elbows.

"Who are you?" the doctor said. He took a step towards them to stop their forward motion, for it seemed as if they intended to dive right into the ambulance on top of his patient.

"The wife—" Sheila shouted.

The doctor pointed to the porch. "Look, lady—"

"I'm the *wife*," Goldie cried. "Me!"

The doctor looked at her. "Get in."

Goldie wheezed as Sheila and the doctor helped her into the ambulance, and she let out a gigantic gasp when she saw the white face sticking up from the gray blanket; his eyes were closed, his skin grayer than his hair. The doctor pushed Sheila aside, climbed in, and then the ambulance was moving, the siren screaming. Sheila ran after the ambulance a moment, hammering on the door, but then she turned the other way and was headed back through the crowd and up the stairs to Ida Kaufman's house.

Goldie turned to the doctor. "He's dead?"

"No, he had a heart attack."

She smacked her face.

"He'll be all right," the doctor said.

"But a heart attack. Never in his life."

"A man sixty, sixty-five, it happens." The doctor snapped the answers back while he held Epstein's wrist.

"He's only fifty-nine."

"Some only," the doctor said.

The ambulance zoomed through a red light and made a sharp right turn that threw Goldie to the floor. She sat there and spoke. "But how does a healthy man—"

PHILIP ROTH

"Lady, don't ask questions. A grown man can't act like a boy."

She put her hands over her eyes as Epstein opened his.

"He's awake now," the doctor said. "Maybe he wants to hold your hand or something."

Goldie crawled to his side and looked at him. "Lou, you're all right? Does anything hurt?"

He did not answer. "He knows it's me?"

The doctor shrugged his shoulders. "Tell him."

"It's me, Lou."

"It's your wife, Lou," the doctor said. Epstein blinked his eyes. "He knows," the doctor said. "He'll be all right. All he's got to do is live a normal life, normal for sixty."

"You hear the doctor, Lou. All you got to do is live a normal life."

Epstein opened his mouth. His tongue hung over his teeth like a dead snake.

"Don't you talk," his wife said. "Don't you worry about anything. Not even the business. That'll work out. Our Sheila will marry Marvin and that'll be that. You won't have to sell, Lou, it'll be in the family. You can retire, rest, and Marvin can take over. He's a smart boy, Marvin, a *mensch*."

Lou rolled his eyes in his head.

"Don't try to talk. I'll take care. You'll be better soon and we can go someplace. We can go to Saratoga, to the mineral baths, if you want. We'll just go, you and me—" Suddenly she gripped his hand. "Lou, you'll live normal, won't you? *Won't you?*" She was crying. "'Cause what'll happen, Lou, is you'll kill yourself! You'll keep this up and that'll be the end—"

"All right," the young doctor said, "you take it easy now. We don't want two patients on our hands."

The ambulance was pulling down and around into the side entrance of the hospital and the doctor knelt at the back door.

"I don't know why I'm crying." Goldie wiped her eyes. "He'll be all right? You say so, I believe you, you're a doctor." And as the young man swung open the door with the big red cross painted on the back, she asked, softly, "Doctor, you have something that will cure what else he's got—this rash?" She pointed.

The doctor looked at her. Then he lifted for a moment the blanket that covered Epstein's nakedness.

"Doctor, it's bad?"

Goldie's eyes and nose were running.

"An irritation," the doctor said.

She grabbed his wrist. "You can clean it up?"

"So it'll never come back," the doctor said, and hopped out of the ambulance.

133

The Linden Tree

In the early years there had been passion, but now they were just a couple who had grown old together. The last twenty years they had owned a rooming house, where they lived contentedly on the ground floor with their cat, Baby.

Giulio was a great putterer. You could always see him sweeping the front steps or polishing the doorknobs, stopping to gossip with the neighbors. He was a slight, pruny man of sixty-eight, perfectly bald, dressed in heavy trousers, a bright sport shirt with a necktie, and an old man's sweater-jacket, liver-colored and hanging straight to the knees. He had a thick Italian accent and gesticulated wildly when he was excited.

George was quite different. Everything about him was slow and solid, touched by grandeur. Though he was a Negro from the Midwest, he spoke with an accent that sounded British, yet not exactly. He was seventy-four, but looked much younger, with a hard body and a hard face with only a few deep fissures in it. Giulio was a neat dresser, but George was attired. His perfectly creased trousers, his crisp white shirt, smoothly knotted tie, and gray sleeveless sweater seemed out of place in the stuffy little flat.

A home is usually the wife's creation, and so it was in their case. The doilies, the vases with their wax flowers, the prints of saints hanging among gaudy floral calendars—all these were Giulio's. George's contribution was less concrete but more important. He made their life possible, dealing with the rents and taxes, attending to the heavy chores, ousting tenants who drank or brawled. If Giulio were to run the building he would soon come to grief, for he had no real sense of work, and as for the rents, it was all he could do to add two digits together. In addition, he was fussy and fault-finding, so that he often took a dislike to perfectly good tenants, yet countenanced glib bullies.

They were a nicely balanced couple, and for years had been happy. When they were young they had had their troubles—living quarters had been hard to find not only because of George's color, but because of their relationship. In those days Giulio had had fetching ways, too obvious to be ignored. But gradually he passed into a fussy dotage, and now people thought of the pair merely as two lonely old men who lived together. George's color no longer presented problems now that he had proved what was not necessarily demanded of those who asked for proof: that he was a responsible man, an asset to the neighborhood. His building was the best kept on the block, his rents reasonable, his tenants, for the most part, permanent. He would not rent to the fly-by-night element that was slowly invading the district.

The tenants consisted of a pair of raddled, gadabout sisters, a World War I veteran with one leg, and a few clerks and students. Giulio regaled George with facts about these people he gleaned by snooping through their rooms in their absence, and George put him down for this, even threatened him, but it did no good. And in any case, the tenants did not seem to care; there was something so simple about Giulio that his spying was like that of a mouse or a bird. They called him Aunty Nellie (his last name being Antonelli), and the younger ones sometimes invited him into their rooms so that his teeth might be enjoyed. These were ill-fitting, too large for his mouth, and clicked through his speech. When he grew excited, they slipped out of place, at which he would pause in a natural, businesslike way to jam them back in before going on.

Giulio was forever dragging the carpet sweeper up and down the halls, looking for an ear to gossip in. George, on the other hand, talked very little. Only tenants who had lived there a long time got to know him at all, when, once in a great while, he would invite them in for a glass of sherry when they came to pay the rent.

In his flat, the tenants found George to be a different man, less aloof and forbidding. Sitting there with Giulio and Baby, the cat, he had something patient, indulgent, altogether loving in his face. Giulio looked with pride at him, glancing now and then at the guest, as though to say: Isn't he wonderful? Sometimes he would go so far as to confess, "I no good at the paper work, but George, George, he *smart*." Or, "We live together fifty years, never a yell, always happy." And George would give him a look to show him that he was saying too much, and then Giulio would sulk and refuse to rejoin the conversation. But the next day he would be the same as ever, whirling creakily around the steps with his broom, or around his garden with a green visor clamped to his head.

He had a shrine in the garden, with statues of the saints standing in sun-blanched profusion. He was an ardent Catholic, and there was no one with a greater collection of religious objects—rosaries and crosses and vestments, which he kept in his bureau drawer and brought out to enjoy their varied glass, wooden, and satin richness. But religious as he was, he would not divest his beloved garden of one fresh bloom for his saints. It was a skimpy garden, heavily bolstered with potted geraniums, and he was so proud of each green shoot that struggled through the hard ground, and attended its subsequent flowering with such worried care, that it was only when a flower had finally begun to wither on the stem that he would pluck it as an offering to his statues.

George understood this attitude and was properly grateful when once a year on his birthday he received a sacrifice of fresh daisies and marigolds. He was amused by Giulio's niggardliness toward the saints. He himself did not care about them. He, too, was a Catholic, but had become one only so that he and Giulio might be buried together. Two fully paid-for plots, side by side, awaited them under a linden tree in Our Lady of Mercy Cemetery just outside town. Whoever was the first to go, George because he was older, Giulio because he was frailer, the other would join him in due time. Giulio had vague visions of an afterlife. The older man did not.

He had had a good life, everything considered, and he would be content to die and be done with when the time came, and have his bones rest by his friend's forever. Sometimes he thought of the linden tree and gave a satisfied nod.

But lately George had noticed something strange about Giulio. His large red ears seemed to have grown less red.

"Giulio," he said one day, "your ears don't seem to be as red as they used to be."

Giulio touched his ear. When he was young he had been sensitive about their largeness. "Nothing wrong with my ears," he said defensively.

"I'm not criticizing you, Giulio. I think it's just strange." And now he realized that some definite change had been taking place in his friend, but he could not put his finger on it. It was as though he were a little smaller. The jacket seemed to hang lower than it had.

Ah, well, he thought, we're both getting old.

A few days later, as Giulio was raking the leaves in the garden, he complained to George of shortness of breath, and there was the faintest touch of blue in his lips.

"Why don't you go to the doctor for a checkup?" George asked as casually as he could.

Giulio shook his head and continued his raking.

That night, as Giulio was turning on the television set, he suddenly stepped back and dropped into a chair with his hand spread across his chest. "Help!" he shouted into the air. "Help!" and when his friend ran to his side, he gasped, "I gotta pain. Here! Here!" And his hand clutched at his heart so hard that the knuckles were white.

The next day George took him to the doctor, and sat by his side through all the tests. Giulio was terrified, but when it was all over and they came out of the doctor's office he seemed restored.

"See," he said, "I'm okay. The doctor he say no worry."

George's face did not reflect Giulio's good spirits. "I know he says not to worry, but . . . "

"He say no worry," Giulio repeated cheerfully.

But from then on Giulio was visited frequently by the paralyzing pains. He would stop what he was doing and crouch over, his eyes darting frenziedly in their sockets. If George was there he would hurry to his friend's side, but at these moments Giulio seemed totally alone even though his hand grasped George's arm. When it was over he would be stripped of his little ways; he would wander slowly around the room or stand for long moments looking at nothing. Patiently George would wait, and eventually the old Giulio returned. Uneasily, fretfully, he would say, "I no understand. Looka me, I never hurt a fly in all my life, and this pain, he come and scare me. It's not right."

"Well," George would venture soothingly, "if you'd just eat fewer starches and stop worrying, these pains would go away. You've got plenty of years ahead of you . . ."

"Plenty years?" Giulio would break in sharply. "I *know*, I *know* I got plenty years ahead. This pain, he no *important*, he just *scare* me."

In an effort to distract him, George broke a lifelong precedent and invited Myrna and Alice Heppleworth, the two aging sisters who lived on the third floor, down to the flat for the evening. He himself did not like women, but Giulio did, in a way that George could not understand. Giulio loved to gossip with them, and afterward delighted in describing their clothes and manners, which he usually found distressing. He was more interested in the Heppleworth sisters than in anyone else in the building, and always pursed his lips when he saw them going out with their rheumy escorts, and could never forget that he once found a bottle of gin in a dresser drawer ostensibly given over to scarves and stockings.

The Heppleworth sisters came, drank all their wine, and turned the television set up as high as it would go. George grew rigid; Giulio went to bed. The sisters were not asked again.

It seemed to George that Giulio failed daily. His ears were as pale as his face, and this seemed particularly significant to George. He found himself suddenly looking at his friend to check his ears, and each time they looked whiter. He never discussed this with Giulio, because Giulio refused to speak about his fears, as though not daring to give them authority by acknowledging them.

And then one morning Giulio gave up this pretense. As he was getting out of bed he had an attack, and when he recovered this time he let out a piercing wail and began to weep, banging his head from side to side. The rest of the day he spent immobile, wrapped from head to foot in a patchwork quilt.

Toward evening George made him get up and walk in the garden with him. George pointed to the flowers, praising them, and gently turned his friend's face to the shrine. The white plaster faces looked peaceful. Even he,

George, felt it, and he realized that for weeks he had been in need of some comfort, something outside himself.

"Look," he said, and that was all, fearing to sound presumptuous, because the statues belonged to Giulio and the Church—he himself understood nothing of them.

Giulio looked without interest, and then, forgetting them, he took George's arm and his eyes swam with tears. "What can I do?" he asked. "What will happen?"

As they walked slowly back to the house he drew his lips back from his big false teeth and whispered, "I'm gonna die."

"No, no, don't think that way," George soothed, but he felt helpless, and resentful that his friend must go through this terror. And now that Giulio had said the words, his terror would grow, just as the pain of a bad tooth grows when you finally acknowledge the decay and are plunged into a constant probing of it with your tongue.

When they came back inside Giulio went straight to bed. George stood in the kitchen and looked at his face in the little mirror that hung on the wall. He feared Giulio would die this very minute in the bedroom as he was removing his carpet slippers, and he wanted with every muscle to run to him. But it would not do to become as hysterical as Giulio, and he stood still. Presently the sound of the bedsprings released a sigh from his throat. The flat was silent. He looked again at his face in the mirror. It was as though he were one person and the reflection another, and he was uneasy and embarrassed, and yet could not look away. He felt deeply aware of himself standing there, staring, and it seemed he was out of place, lost. He whirled around, catching his breath. He had felt entirely alone for the first time in fifty years.

The next day he decided to call for Father Salmon, the young priest from the neighborhood church Giulio attended. Father Salmon dropped in for friendly chats now and then, and Giulio liked him very much, so much, in fact, that the priest often had to silence him when he got carried away with intimate gossip.

A few days later the priest knocked on the door. He was horse-faced, with thinning hair and rimless glasses, and he was quiet and pleasant.

Giulio was wrapped up in his quilt in the armchair. He did not greet the priest with his usual beam of pleasure; he did not even smile.

"Well, Giulio," the priest said, "how are you feeling? I haven't seen you at church lately."

Giulio said at once, "Father, I'm dying."

"What is the trouble?" the priest asked gently.

"It's my heart," Giulio shot back, his hand scrounging around his shirtfront and fumbling with the buttons until it was clutching his bare chest. He looked as though he were prepared to pull the heart out for inspection. His eyes pleaded with the priest to set it right. The priest sat down next to him.

"What does your doctor say?" he asked.

"Oh, Father," Giulio moaned, "the doctor is a stupid. He never tell me one real thing. In and out and all around, around the bush. He no understand, but *I* understand—this heart, he gonna kill me. You think so, Father? What do you think? You think so?"

"Surely, Giulio," the priest replied, "you must accept the doctor's word. If he says there's no reason to fear . . . "

Giulio looked away, black with melancholy.

The priest sat silently for a moment, then began again. "Giulio, death is as natural as birth. Think of your flowers out there in the garden, how they grow from little seeds and then fade and fall—what could be more natural? God has been with you all your life, and He will not forsake you now . . . "

But Giulio, his eyes shutting tighter and tighter as the priest spoke, got up from his chair and crept into the bedroom, dragging his quilt behind him.

Afterward he said to George, "I no wanna see Father Salmon again."

"Father Salmon is trying to help," George told him.

Giulio shook his head, his fingers rubbing the area of his heart.

What a strange person he is, George thought, looking at him closely. All these years he has been immersed in the church, and now, suddenly, the church means nothing to him. He recalled a conversation he had overheard a few days ago as he was fixing a faulty burner in the second floor kitchen. Two of the students were going down the hall, talking. One had commented on Giulio's bad health. The other had replied, "Don't worry, Aunty Nellie could never do anything so profound as to die."

George had bristled, as he always did whenever anyone made fun of his friend—but it was true that Giulio was not profound. He liked pretty things, and the church gave him its rich symbols; he liked intimate conversation, and the church gave him patient Father Salmon; he liked the idea of an afterlife, and the church gave him that, too. He loved the church, but when you came right down to it, he believed only what he could see with his two eyes, and he could see only his blue lips and wasted face in the mirror. This oddly realistic attitude explained his stinginess toward the saints; they were, after all, only plaster. And yet when Baby had once jumped up on the shrine and relieved himself on St. Francis's foot, Giulio had screamed at the animal until the neighbors hung from the windows.

All these amiable contradictions in Giulio had been known to George for fifty years, and he had always believed that they would sustain his friend through everything. Now the contradictions were gone. All that was left in Giulio was the certainty of death. It made George feel forlorn, on the outside. He sensed that nothing could be set right, that Giulio would live consumed by fear until he died consumed by fear, and the linden tree would not mark two intertwined lives, but forever cast its shadow between two strangers.

They had met for the first time in front of the Minneapolis train station in the first decade of the century. George sat in the driver's seat of a Daimler, in his duster and goggles. His employer had gone inside to meet one Giulio Antonelli, just arrived from Calabria, nephew of the head gardener. When he emerged he had in tow a thin boy of eighteen dressed in a shabby suit and carrying a suitcase that looked like a wicker basket. He wore cherry-colored cigar bands on his fingers, and had a shoot of wilted wild flowers stuck through the buttonhole of his jacket. His eyes were red-rimmed; apparently he had been crying all the way from Calabria. Delicate and terrified, his cigar bands glittering hectically in the sunlight, he crawled into the Daimler and collapsed in a corner.

George had worked as a chauffeur and handyman on his employer's estate for five years, but was originally from an isolated Finnish farming community where God knows what fates had conspired to bring his parents, a bitter, quarreling, aloof, and extremely poor black couple. George became friends with only one thing native to that cold country, the stones that littered the fields. He could not say what attracted him to them, but he felt a great bond with them. When he was ten he built a wall of the stones. It was only a foot high and not very long, and there was nothing in the world for it to guard there in the middle of the empty field, but he knew he had discovered the proper use of the stones, and all his life he had the feeling he was that wall.

In Minneapolis, on the estate, he kept to himself. He liked the Daimler, which he drove with authority, and the appearance of which on the streets caused people to gawk with admiration. He picked up his employer's speech habits, and this, combined with the Finnish accent he had absorbed, gave a peculiar, unplaceable ring to his words, which he relished, because it was his alone.

The Calabrian boy turned out to be a poor gardener, not because he was listless with homesickness, for that soon passed, but because he made favorites of certain flowers and would have nothing to do with the others. The tulips, for instance, he apparently considered stout and silly-looking, and he made disparaging faces at them. He liked the wild flowers that cropped up in odd corners.

George was fascinated by Giulio, although he did not like him. He reminded him of a woman. Women had never respected George's wall, at least a certain type of woman had not—the bold Finnish farm girls, some of the hired women here on the estate. He was well favored, and maybe there was something in his coloring, too, that attracted women, something tawny, reminiscent of the sun, here, where everyone else looked like a peeled banana. In any case, they were always after him. He was not flattered. He felt they were not interested in him as he knew himself, proud and valuable, but in some small part of him that they wanted for their own use, quickly, in a dark corner.

But Giulio, though girlish, had no boldness in him. He would leave the garden and lean against the garage door where George was polishing the Daimler. "*Bella, bella,*" he would murmur, and his face shone with a kind of radiant simplemindedness. There was no calculation in him—sometimes you could see him cocking his head and singing before the wild flowers in the garden. Watching George, the boy spoke foreign words rich in their tones of admiration, and his quick, glittering fingers—he had bought flashy rings with his pay—seemed anxious to catch the sun and make a present of it to the tall, mute figure in the gloom of the garage.

Two months after his arrival Giulio was fired. George, filled with fear for himself, feeling a great chasm opening before him, quit his job, and the two of them, with hardly a word between them, took the train to San Francisco, where Giulio had another uncle. All during the trip George asked himself: "Why am I doing this? Why am I going with him? I don't even like him. He's a silly, ridiculous person; there's something the matter with him."

They got off at the San Francisco depot, and before George was even introduced to the uncle, who stood waiting, he picked up his baggage and, without a word of farewell to Giulio, walked quickly away from him.

First he found odd jobs, and finally he wound up on Rincon Hill with another Daimler. On his half day off each week he would wander around the city, looking at the sights. Whenever he saw a quick, thin figure that reminded him of Giulio his heart would pound, and he would say to himself, "Thank God it's not Giulio, I don't want to see him again." And then he found that what had begun as a casual walk around the city was turning into a passionate weekly search. The day he caught sight of Giulio sadly and ineffectively constructing a pyramid of cabbages in a vegetable market, he had to restrain himself from throwing his arms around him.

Giulio's face had blanched with surprise when he looked up, and then his eyes had filled with a dazzling welcome, and he had extended his hand to his returned friend with a tenderness George never forgot.

They were together from then on. In time they bought a vegetable stand, and as a result of George's frugality and common sense he was able to save in spite of Giulio's extravagances. They worked and invested, and in thirty years they were able to buy, for cash, the old apartment building they now lived in. Life had always been strangely easy for them. They had been incapable of acknowledging affronts, even when they were refused lodgings or openly stared at on the street, and the last twenty years in the security of their own flat had been free from problems, satisfying in all ways.

Now Giulio moaned, "Oh, I gotta pain, I gotta pain."

George would take his hand and say, "I'm here, Giulio, I'm here."

But Giulio would look through him, as though he did not exist.

"Don't we *know* each other?" George finally exploded one day, causing Baby to speed under a table with his ears laid back. "Are we strangers after all these years?"

Giulio closed his eyes, involved with his fear.

George sighed, stroking his friend's hand, thin and waxy as a sliver of soap. "What are you thinking about now, this very minute, Giulio? You must tell me."

"I'm thinking of my dog," Giulio said, after a silence.

"What dog was that?" George asked softly.

"I had him in Nocera."

"And what about him?"

"He died, and my father he dug a hole and put him in." His lips turned down. "I dug him up later, I was lonely for him."

"What a foolish thing to do, my poor Giulio."

"His own mother wouldn'a wanted him. Bones and worms . . . "

"Hush, Giulio."

"Gonna happen to me."

"But your soul . . . "

"What's my soul look like?" Giulio asked quickly.

"Like you, Giulio . . . it's true . . . "

Giulio cast him a look of contempt George would not have thought him capable of.

"The little hole, the bones and worms," Giulio moaned.

"But you've *had* a life!" George suddenly cried with exasperation. "Do you want to live forever?"

"Yes," Giulio said simply.

From then on George felt a fury. In the past all Giulio's little fears had been bearable because he, George, could exorcise them, like a stevedore bearing a small load away. But this final cowardice excluded him. And there was nothing, no one he could turn to. He went halfheartedly to church, but got nothing from it. He began making small overtures to his tenants, but his sociability was stiff with rust. He looked with curiosity at the black people on the street, and thought there were more of them than there used to be. When a young black couple stopped him on a corner one day he listened attentively as they talked of civil rights. He accepted a pamphlet from them and read it thoroughly. But afterward he threw it out. He felt no connection with the problems it presented.

He cursed Giulio as he had cursed him fifty years ago when he had walked away from him at the train depot, and he wished for the oneness with himself that he had known in the empty fields of his youth.

In the daytime he was angrily helpful, like a disapproving orderly, but at night, as they sat in the small living room with Baby flicking his tail back and forth across the blank television screen, he went to Giulio and mutely pleaded with him. Giulio sighed abstractedly; he seemed far away, deep inside himself, listening to every heartbeat, counting every twinge, with a deep frown line between his eyes.

George moved the twin beds together, and Giulio allowed his hand to be held through the night. From then on they slept that way, hand in hand. George slept lightly, waking often. It was almost as if he wished to be awake, to enjoy the only hours of closeness he had with his friend as he held his hand. And also, in the back of his mind was the fear that if he drifted off, Giulio would be released into the arms of death. And so he lay quietly, listening to Giulio's breathing, to the wind in the trees.

Then gradually the bedroom window would turn from black to gray, and the breeze that ruffled the curtain carried in the scent of early morning. Dawn brought him sleep; the rising sun gave him a sense of security. Bad things never happened in the daytime—at least one felt that way. And so his fingers grew lax in Giulio's hand as he trusted his friend to the kindness of the dawning day.

But when he awoke later it would be with a sharp sense of foreboding. Quickly he would turn to look at Giulio, his eyes narrowed against the possible shock. But Giulio would be breathing evenly, his bluish lips parted over his gums, his teeth grinning from a water glass on the bureau. Giulio's clothes were neatly laid out, his liver-colored jacket hung over the back of a chair. How lifeless the jacket looked. George would shut his eyes, knowing that the sight of that empty jacket would be unbearable when Giulio was gone. He shook the thought from his head, wondering if life could be more painful than this. Then Giulio's eyes would open, George's face take on a formal nonchalance. And so another night had passed. Their hands parted.

"How do you feel?" George would ask shortly.

Giulio would sigh.

They took their breakfast. The sun shone through the kitchen window with a taunting golden light. George snapped at Giulio. Giulio was unmoved.

One summer morning George persuaded Giulio to sit outside in the backyard. He hoped that watching him work in the garden, Giulio might be persuaded to putter around again. He settled his friend into a chair and picked up the rake, but as the minutes wore on and he moved around the garden in the hot sun, raking the leaves together, Giulio showed no sign of interest. George stopped and put the rake down. Not knowing if he wished to please Giulio or anger him, he suddenly broke off the largest marigold in the garden and held it out.

Giulio shaded his watering eyes with his hand; then his eyes drifted away from the flower like two soap bubbles in the air. George flung the flower to the ground, staring at Giulio, then strode to the shrine and stood there with his hands in fists, blindly determined to do something that would shake his friend open, break him in two if need be. He grabbed the arm of the Virgin Mary and lifted the statue high, and heard Giulio's voice.

"George."

"That's right," George growled, replacing the statue and breathing threateningly through his nostrils, "I would have smashed it to bits!"

"Smash what?" Giulio asked indifferently, and George saw that under the awning of his thin hand his eyes were closed.

"Were your eyes closed?" George thundered. "Didn't you *see* me?"

"You no care that I can't open my eyes—this sun, he hurt them. You *mean*, George, make me sit out here. Too hot. Make me feel sick. I wanna go inside."

"I was going to smash your Virgin Mary!" George cried.

Giulio shrugged. "I wanna go inside."

And then George's shoulders hunched, his face twisted up, and he broke into a storm of tears. Turning his head aside with shame, he made for the back door; then he turned around and hurried back, glancing up at the windows, where he hoped no one stood watching him cry. He put his arm around Giulio and helped him up from his chair, and the two old men haltingly crossed the garden out of the sun.

"Humiliating," George whispered when they were inside, shaking his head and pressing his eyes with a handkerchief. He slowly folded the handkerchief into a square and replaced it in his pocket. He gave a loud sniff and squared his shoulders, and looked with resignation at his distant friend.

Giulio was settling himself into the armchair, plucking the patchwork quilt around him. "Time for pills," he muttered, reaching next to him, and he poured a glass of water from a decanter and took two capsules, smacking his lips mechanically, like a goldfish. Sitting back, he looked around the room in his usual blank, uninterested way. Then a puzzled expression came into his eyes.

"Why you cry then, George?"

George shook his head silently.

"I do something you no like?"

"You never talk. It's as though we're strangers." And he broke off with a sigh. "I've told you all that before—what's the use?"

"I got big worry, George. No time to talk."

"It would be better than to think and think. What do you think about all day?"

Giulio slowly raised his eyebrows, as though gazing down upon a scene. "Bones and worms."

"Giulio, Giulio."

"Big worry, George."

"You'll drive yourself mad that way."

"I no mad at you. Just him." He lay one thin finger on his heart, lightly, as though afraid of rousing it.

"I don't mean angry . . . "

But Giulio was already tired of talking, and was plucking at the quilt again, ill, annoyed, retreating into sleep.

"Giulio, please, you've talked a little. Talk a little more—stay."

With an effort, his eyes sick and distant, Giulio stayed.

But now that he had his attention, George did not know where to begin, what to say. His mind spun; his tongue formed a few tentative words; then, clubbed by an immense fatigue, he sank into a chair with his head in his hands.

"I'm sick man," Giulio explained tonelessly, closing his eyes. After a silence he opened them and looked over at George, painfully, as though from under a crushing weight. "Tonight I hold your hand in bed again, like always. Hold your hand every night, you know that."

"You hold *my* hand?" George asked softly, lifting his head.

"In daytime," Giulio said slowly, his eyes laboriously fixed on George's attentive face, "in daytime only the bones and worms. But in the night . . . in the night, I see other things, too . . . " He was silent for a moment until a twinge had passed, then spoke again. "See you, George. And I hold your hand. Make you feel better . . . " His eyes still fixed on George's face, he gave an apologetic twitch of the lip as his lids closed, and slowly he nodded off to sleep.

Fallback

An outdoor sign: under the big word FARVIEW
smaller letters spell *Intermediate Care.*

Year-round, now, she focuses at first light
on the sign, a wren of a woman looking out
from her cover. The night girl wakes her
at six for a washcloth, before
the day girls come on.
        In the waking
they've shared for sixty-two years, she watches
Stanton getting his face washed, next to
the window in the same room. Out the window, over
the sign, rain thickens the lake, clouds
lie low on the mountain.
        My body gone,
she thinks, *and his mind.*
        When anyone visits,
his manners rise from the room's one armchair,
in his tweed suit, intact; she lies back
where she's been all day, her backbone so thin
the doctor jokes that X-rays can't find it.
She thinks her daughter may come today.
If she can. Labor Day she couldn't. Today
it's almost Hallowe'en, the Day Room filled
with paper pumpkins. Down at the nurse's station
the girls have carved a real one.
        Out the window
not much color: the oaks dead bronze,
the marshgrass rusty. This morning she plans
how to set their watches tonight:
the old rule: *spring forward,*
        fall back.
        Now the night girl is back,
saying she's doing a double shift, covering
for Elsie.

PHILIP BOOTH

And the loons have been fewer, out
on the lake, and the Red Delicious are far
from what they were. Even at home,
the last year Elmer brought manure,
he said *Somethin's wrong with the bees,*
they're not comin round to spread pollen.
She watches Stanton wanting to talk to
the girl while she cranks up his bed;
watching, his curtain all the way back,
she can see his pale emeritus head risen into
the steel engraving of Harvard College.

His mind,

she thinks, *and my body.*

Bringing trays now,
the night girl looks like a grebe. The woman
sips tea. Watching her husband try cereal,
she thinks back to summers they bird-watched,
Julys on Monhegan, a week once on Skye.

. . . out-of-

style beyond doubt, we were worn but fit.
His old Harris jacket, scratchy only in places.
She tries to smell the peat smell, the jacket he
laid out for picnics. But the night girl, bending
to take her tray, brings her home: the perfume
still lingering from whatever went on
before last night's shift.

And you at twenty,
who look away from us, wearing so cleverly little
(she smiles an idle small smile at her husband)
—how would you know we ever made love
in the sweetfern high on an island.

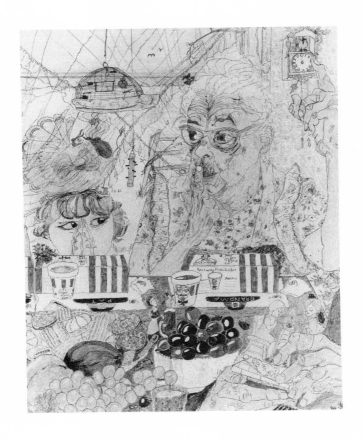

AGING AND THE FAMILY

Introduction

Marge Piercy wrote, "My mother is my mirror and I am hers," in "My Mother's Body," a poem reflecting the confrontive and sometimes assuring knowledge of the biological and emotional ties we have to our parents. Our selective sight often sees family patterns we celebrate—the comforting, connective traits and habits of nature. So matter-of-fact are these connections that they are often unacknowledged or unexpressed. Amy Tan's Jing-Mei Woo recognizes this unspoken connectedness only after her mother's death when she realizes the everydayness of their relationship: "What was that pork stuff she used to make that had the texture of sawdust? What were the names of the uncles who died in Shanghai?" Here and in other stories, we find not moments of drama portraying family life, just moments that reflect the familiarity of families over a lifetime, full of conversations, bus rides, mah jong, dinners.

At other times we shield ourselves from the fact of our aging parents because of the recognition of what we may become. Old photographs, startlingly familiar, remind us that the seamed faces and veined hands were not always so. For some, this may induce fear or an Ivan Ilych–denial of the inevitability of our own aging: "It can't be. It's impossible! But here it is. How is this? How is one to understand it?"

Yet, there may be more here than the self-absorbed fear of aging bodies. As we watch the changes of aging family members, we look but don't want to; we recognize our inability to freeze time, to make them stay where they were in our earliest memories: healthy, brisk, sure of foot, ear, and memory. Our responses may reflect such helplessness, much like the family dinner in Susan Irene Rea's poem, "Stroke," with family members frantically offering disparate objects to an uncle unable to remember the name of what he wants. Sometimes the helplessness is reflected in the well-intentioned act, too often under the assumption that we know what they want: the trip they've never taken, the retirement condominium they've never been able to afford, the reunion with family and friends. Tillie Olsen reminds us how wrong we can be in her story "Tell Me a Riddle." Here the dying Eva cannot escape the oppressiveness of her family's assumptions of how she wants to spend her last months—full of babies, memories, old friends, travel. But all

151

she wants is to go home, and if not that, then peace. While they thought she napped, she would escape to a closet to "hide, hunch behind the dresses deeper," only to be found by a granddaughter ("Is this where you hide too, Grammy?").

Sometimes the fact of aging families leads one to give up ghosts rather than anticipate them. The years of trying to please parents through proper marriages, occupations, and beliefs may cease, replaced by new kinds of relationships marked by the fond antagonism between daughter and father in Grace Paley's "A Conversation With My Father," or the indifference of adult children to their father in Peter Taylor's "Porte-Cochere."

But no matter how family relationships are characterized in literature, there appears to be one constant: relationships between generations remain knotty, often difficult, sometimes ambivalent, and always mysterious.

Tell Me A Riddle

"These Things Shall Be"

1

For forty-seven years they had been married. How deep back the stubborn, gnarled roots of the quarrel reached, no one could say—but only now, when tending to the needs of others no longer shackled them together, the roots swelled up visible, split the earth between them, and the tearing shook even to the children, long since grown.

Why now, why now? wailed Hannah.

As if when we grew up weren't enough, said Paul.

Poor Ma. Poor Dad. It hurts so for both of them, said Vivi. They never had very much; at least in old age they should be happy.

Knock their heads together, insisted Sammy; tell 'em: you're too old for this kind of thing; no reason not to get along now.

Lennie wrote to Clara: They've lived over so much together; what could possibly tear them apart?

Something tangible enough.

Arthritic hands, and such work as he got, occasional. Poverty all his life, and there was little breath left for running. He could not, could not turn away from this desire: to have the troubling of responsibility, the fretting with money, over and done with; to be free, to be *care*free where success was not measured by accumulation, and there was use for the vitality still in him.

There was a way. They could sell the house, and with the money join his lodge's Haven, cooperative for the aged. Happy communal life, and was he not already an official; had he not helped organize it, raise funds, served as a trustee?

But she—would not consider it.

"What do we need all this for?" he would ask loudly, for her hearing aid was turned down and the vacuum was shrilling. "Five rooms" (pushing the sofa so she could get into the corner) "furniture" (smoothing down the rug) "floors and surfaces to make work. Tell me, why do we need it?" And he was glad he could ask in a scream.

153

"Because I'm use't."

"Because you're use't. This is a reason, Mrs. Word Miser? Used to can get unused!"

"Enough unused I have to get used to already. . . . Not enough words?" turning off the vacuum a moment to hear herself answer. "Because soon enough we'll need only a little closet, no windows, no furniture, nothing to make work, but for worms. Because now I want room. . . . Screech and blow like you're doing, you'll need that closet even sooner. . . . Ha, again!" for the vacuum bag wailed, puffed half up, hung stubbornly limp. "This time fix it so it stays; quick before the phone rings and you get too important-busy."

But while he struggled with the motor, it seethed in him. Why fix it? Why have to bother? And if it can't be fixed, have to wring the mind with how to pay the repair? At the Haven they come in with their own machines to clean your room or your cottage; you fish, or play cards, or make jokes in the sun, not with knotty fingers fight to mend vacuums.

Over the dishes, coaxingly: "For once in your life, to be free, to have everything done for you, like a queen."

"I never liked queens."

"No dishes, no garbage, no towel to sop, no worry what to buy, what to eat."

"And what else would I do with my empty hands? Better to eat at my own table when I want, and to cook and eat how I want."

"In the cottages they buy what you ask, and cook it how you like. *You* are the one who always used to say: better mankind born without mouths and stomachs than always to worry for money to buy, to shop, to fix, to cook, to wash, to clean."

"How cleverly you hid that you heard. I said it then because eighteen hours a day I ran. And you never scraped a carrot or knew a dish towel sops. Now—for you and me—who cares? A herring out of a jar is enough. But when *I* want, and nobody to bother." And she turned off her ear button, so she would not have to hear.

But as *he* had no peace, juggling and rejuggling the money to figure: how will I pay for this now?; prying out the storm windows (there they take care of this); jolting in the streetcar on errands (there I would not have to ride to take care of this or that); fending the patronizing relatives just back from Florida (at the Haven it matters what one is, not what one can afford), he gave *her* no peace.

"Look! In their bulletin. A reading circle. Twice a week it meets."

"Haumm," her answer of not listening.

"A reading circle. Chekhov they read that you like, and Peretz. Cultured people at the Haven that you would enjoy."

"Enjoy!" She tasted the word. "Now, when it pleases you, you find a reading circle for me. And forty years ago when the children were morsels and there was a Circle, did you stay home with them once so I could go? Even once? You trained me well. I do not need others to enjoy. Others!" Her voice trembled. "Because *you* want to be there with others. Already it makes me sick to think of you always around others. Clown, grimacer, floormat, yes-man, entertainer, whatever they want of you."

And now it was he who turned on the television loud so he need not hear.

Old scar tissue ruptured and the wounds festered anew. Chekhov indeed. She thought without softness of that young wife, who in the deep night hours while she nursed the current baby, and perhaps held another in her lap, would try to stay awake for the only time there was to read. She would feel again the weather of the outside on his cheek when, coming late from a meeting, he would find her so, and stimulated and ardent, sniffing her skin, coax: "I'll put the baby to bed, and you—put the book away, don't read, don't read."

That had been the most beguiling of all the "don't read, put your book away" her life had been. Chekhov indeed!

"Money?" She shrugged him off. "Could we get poorer than once we were? And in America, who starves?"

But as still he pressed:

"Let me alone about money. Was there ever enough? Seven little ones—for every penny I had to ask—and sometimes, remember, there was nothing. But always *I* had to manage. Now *you* manage. Rub your nose in it good."

But from those years she had had to manage, old humiliations and terrors rose up, lived again, and forced her to relive them. The children's needings; that grocer's face or this merchant's wife she had had to beg credit from when credit was a disgrace; the scenery of the long blocks walked around when she could not pay; school coming, and the desperate going over the old to see what could yet be remade; the soups of meat bones begged "for-the-dog" one winter. . . .

Enough. Now they had no children. Let *him* wrack his head for how they would live. She would not exchange her solitude for anything. *Never again to be forced to move to the rhythms of others.*

For in this solitude she had won to a reconciled peace.

Tranquillity from having the empty house no longer an enemy, for it stayed clean—not as in the days when it was her family, the life in it, that had seemed the enemy: tracking, smudging, littering, dirtying, engaging her in endless defeating battle—and on whom her endless defeat had been spewed.

The few old books, memorized from rereading; the pictures to ponder (the magnifying glass superimposed on her heavy eyeglasses). Or if she wishes, when he is gone, the phonograph, that if she turns up very loud and strains, she can hear: the ordered sounds and the struggling.

Out in the garden, growing things to nurture. Birds to be kept out of the pear tree, and when the pears are heavy and ripe, the old fury of work, for all must be canned, nothing wasted.

And her one social duty (for she will not go to luncheons or meetings) the boxes of old clothes left with her, as with a life-practised eye for finding what is still wearable within the worn (again the magnifying glass superimposed on the heavy glasses) she scans and sorts—this for rag or rummage, that for mending and cleaning, and this for sending away.

Being able at last to live within, and not move to the rhythms of others, as life had forced her to: denying; removing; isolating; taking the children one by one; then deafening, half-blinding—and at last, presenting her solitude.

And in it she had won to a reconciled peace.

Now he was violating it with his constant campaigning: *Sell the house and move to the Haven.* (You sit, you sit—there too you could sit like a stone.) He was making of her a battleground where old grievances tore. (Turn on your ear button—I am talking.) And stubbornly she resisted—so that from wheedling, reasoning, manipulation, it was bitterness he now started with.

And it came to where every happening lashed up a quarrel.

"I will sell the house anyway," he flung at her one night. "I am putting it up for sale. There will be a way to make you sign."

The television blared, as always it did on the evenings he stayed home, and as always it reached her only as noise. She did not know if the tumult was in her or outside. Snap! she turned the sound off. "Shadows," she whispered to him, pointing to the screen, "look, it is only shadows." And in a scream: "Did you say that you will sell the house? Look at me, not at that. I am no shadow. You cannot sell without me."

"Leave on the television. I am watching."

"Like Paulie, like Jenny, a four-year-old. Staring at shadows. *You cannot sell the house.*"

"I will. We are going to the Haven. There you would not hear the television when you do not want it. I could sit in the social room and watch. You could lock yourself up to smell your unpleasantness in a room by yourself—for who would want to come near you?"

"No, no selling." A whisper now.

"The television is shadows. Mrs. Enlightened! Mrs. Cultured! A world comes into your house—and it is shadows. People you would never meet in a thousand lifetimes. Wonders. When you were four years old, yes, like Paulie, like Jenny, did you know of Indian dances, alligators, how they use bamboo in Malaya? No, you scratched in your dirt with the chickens and thought Olshana was the world. Yes, Mrs. Unpleasant, I will sell the house, for there better can we be rid of each other than here."

She did not know if the tumult was outside, or in her. Always a ravening inside, a pull to the bed, to lie down, to succumb.

"Have you thought maybe Ma should let a doctor have a look at her?" asked their son Paul after Sunday dinner, regarding his mother crumpled on the couch, instead of, as was her custom, busying herself in Nancy's kitchen.

"Why not the President, too?"

"Seriously, Dad. This is the third Sunday she's lain down like that after dinner. Is she that way at home?"

"A regular love affair with the bed. Every time I start to talk to her."

Good protective reaction, observed Nancy to herself. The workings of hos-til-ity.

"Nancy could take her. I just don't like how she looks. Let's have Nancy arrange an appointment."

"You think she'll go?" regarding his wife gloomily. "All right, we have to have doctor bills, we have to have doctor bills." Loudly: "Something hurts you?"

She startled, looked to his lips. He repeated: "Mrs. Take It Easy, something hurts?"

"Nothing. . . . Only you."

"A woman of honey. That's why you're lying down?"

"Soon I'll get up to do the dishes, Nancy."

"Leave them, Mother, I like it better this way."

"Mrs. Take It Easy, Paul says you should start ballet. You should go to see a doctor and ask: how soon can you start ballet?"

"A doctor?" she begged. "Ballet?"

"We were talking, Ma," explained Paul, "you don't seem any too well. It would be a good idea for you to see a doctor for a checkup."

"I get up now to do the kitchen. Doctors are bills and foolishness, my son. I need no doctors."

"At the Haven," he could not resist pointing out, "a doctor is *not* bills. He lives beside you. You start to sneeze, he is there before you open up a kleenex. You can be sick there for free, all you want."

"Diarrhea of the mouth, is there a doctor to make you dumb?"

"Ma. Promise me you'll go. Nancy will arrange it."

"It's all of a piece when you think of it," said Nancy, "the way she attacks my kitchen, scrubbing under every cup hook, doing the inside of the oven so I can't enjoy Sunday dinner, knowing that half-blind or not, she's going to find every speck of dirt. . . ."

"Don't, Nancy, I've told you—it's the only way she knows to be useful. What did the *doctor* say?"

"A real fatherly lecture. Sixty-nine is young these days. Go out, enjoy life, find interests. Get a new hearing aid, this one is antiquated. Old age is sickness only if one makes it so. Geriatrics, Inc."

"So there was nothing physical."

"Of course there was. How can you live to yourself like she does without there being? Evidence of a kidney disorder, and her blood count is low. He gave her a diet, and she's to come back for follow-up and lab work. . . . But he was clear enough: Number One prescription—start living like a human being. . . . When I think of your dad, who could really play the invalid with that arthritis of his, as active as a teenager, and twice as much fun. . . . "

"You didn't tell me the doctor says your sickness is in you, how you live." He pushed his advantage. "Life and enjoyments you need better than medicine. And this diet, how can you keep it? To weigh each morsel and scrape away each bit of fat, to make this soup, that pudding. There, at the Haven, they have a dietician, they would do it for you."

She is silent.

"You would feel better there, I know it," he says gently. "There there is life and enjoyments all around."

"What is the matter, Mr. Importantbusy, you have no card game or meeting you can go to?"—turning her face to the pillow.

For a while he cut his meetings and going out, fussed over her diet, tried to wheedle her into leaving the house, brought in visitors:

"I should come to a fashion tea. I should sit and look at pretty babies in clothes I cannot buy. This is pleasure?"

"Always you are better than everyone else. The doctor said you should go out. Mrs. Brem comes to you with goodness and you turn her away."

"Because *you* asked her to, she asked me."

"They won't come back. People you need, the doctor said. Your own cousins I asked; they were willing to come and make peace as if nothing had happened. . . . "

"No more crushers of people, pushers, hypocrites, around me. No more in *my* house. You go to them if you like."

"Kind he is to visit. And you, like ice."

"A babbler. All my life around babblers. Enough!"

"She's even worse, Dad? Then let her stew a while," advised Nancy. "You can't let it destroy you; it's a psychological thing, maybe too far gone for any of us to help."

So he let her stew. More and more she lay silent in bed, and sometimes did not even get up to make the meals. No longer was the tongue-lashing inevitable if he left the coffee cup where it did not belong, or forgot to take out the garbage or mislaid the broom. The birds grew bold that summer and for once pocked the pears, undisturbed.

A bellyful of bitterness and every day the same quarrel in a new way and a different old grievance the quarrel forced her to enter and relive. And the new torment: I am not really sick, the doctor said it, then why do I feel so sick?

One night she asked him: "You have a meeting tonight? Do not go. Stay . . . with me."

He had planned to watch "This Is Your Life," but half sick himself from the heavy heat, and sickening therefore the more after the brooks and woods of the Haven, with satisfaction he grated:

"Hah, Mrs. Live Alone And Like It wants company all of a sudden. It doesn't seem so good the time of solitary when she was a girl exile in Siberia. 'Do not . . . Do not go. Stay with me.' A new song for Mrs. Free As A Bird. Yes, I am going out, and while I am gone chew this aloneness good, and think how you keep us both from where if you want people, you do not need to be alone."

"Go, go. All your life you have gone without me."

After him she sobbed curses he had not heard in years, old-country curses from their childhood: Grow, oh shall you grow like an onion, with your head in the ground. Like the hide of a drum shall you be, beaten in life, beaten in death. Oh shall you be like a chandelier, to hang, and to burn. . . .

She was not in their bed when he came back. She lay on the cot on the sun porch. All week she did not speak or come near him; nor did he try to make peace or care for her.

He slept badly, so used to her next to him. After all the years, old harmonies and dependencies deep in their bodies; she curled to him, or he coiled to her, each warmed, warming, turning as the other turned, the nights a long embrace.

It was not the empty bed or the storm that woke him, but a faint singing. *She* was singing. Shaking off the drops of rain, the lightning riving her lifted face, he saw her so; the cot covers on the floor.

"This is a private concert?" he asked. "Come in, you are wet."

"I can breathe now," she answered; "my lungs are rich." Though indeed the sound was hardly a breath.

"Come in, come in." Loosing the bamboo shades. "Look how wet you are." Half helping, half carrying her, still faint-breathing her song.

A Russian love song of fifty years ago.

He had found a buyer, but before he told her, he called together those children who were close enough to come. Paul, of course, Sammy from New Jersey, Hannah from Connecticut, Vivi from Ohio.

With a kindling of energy for her beloved visitors, she arrayed the house, cooked and baked. She was not prepared for the solemn after-dinner conclave, they too probing in and tearing. Her frightened eyes watched from mouth to mouth as each spoke.

His stories were eloquent and funny of her refusal to go back to the doctor; of the scorned invitations; of her stubborn silence or the bile "like a Niagara"; of her contrariness: "If I clean it's no good how I cleaned; if I don't clean, I'm still a master who thinks he has a slave."

(Vinegar he poured on me all his life; I am well marinated; how can I be honey now?)

Deftly he marched in the rightness for moving to the Haven; their money from social security free for visiting the children, not sucked into daily needs and into the house; the activities in the Haven for him; but mostly the Haven for *her:* her health, her need of care, distraction, amusement, friends who shared her interests.

"This does offer an outlet for Dad," said Paul; "he's always been an active person. And economic peace of mind isn't to be sneezed at, either. I could use a little of that myself."

But when they asked: "And you, Ma, how do you feel about it?" could only whisper:

"For him it is good. It is not for me. I can no longer live between people."

"You lived all your life *for* people," Vivi cried.

"Not with." Suffering doubly for the unhappiness on her children's faces.

"You have to find some compromise," Sammy insisted. "Maybe sell the house and buy a trailer. After forty-seven years there's surely some way you can find to live in peace."

"There is no help, my children. Different things we need."

"Then live alone!" He could control himself no longer. "I have a buyer for the house. Half the money for you, half for me. Either alone or with me to the Haven. You think I can live any longer as we are doing now?"

"Ma doesn't have to make a decision this minute, however you feel, Dad," Paul said quickly, "and you wouldn't want her to. Let's let it lay a few months, and then talk some more."

"I think I can work it out to take Mother home with me for a while," Hannah said. "You both look terrible, but especially you, Mother. I'm going to ask Phil to have a look at you."

"Sure," cracked Sammy. "What's the use of a doctor husband if you can't get free service out of him once in a while for the family? And absence might make the heart . . . you know."

"There was something after all," Paul told Nancy in a colorless voice. "That was Hannah's Phil calling. Her gall bladder. . . . Surgery."

"Her *gall* bladder. If that isn't classic. 'Bitter as gall'—talk of psycho-som——"

He stepped closer, put his hand over her mouth, and said in the same colorless, plodding voice. "We have to get Dad. They operated at once. The cancer was everywhere, surrounding the liver, everywhere. They did what they could . . . at best she has a year. Dad . . . we have to tell him."

2

Honest in his weakness when they told him, and that she was not to know. "I'm not an actor. She'll know right away by how I am. Oh that poor woman. I am old too, it will break me into pieces. Oh that poor woman. She will spit on me: 'So my sickness was how I live.' Oh Paulie, how she will be, that poor woman. Only she should not suffer. . . . I can't stand sickness, Paulie, I can't go with you."

But went. And play-acted.

"A grand opening and you did not even wait for me. . . . A good thing Hannah took you with her."

"Fashion teas I needed. They cut out what tore in me; just in my throat something hurts yet. . . . Look! so many flowers, like a funeral. Vivi called, did Hannah tell you? And Lennie from San Francisco, and Clara; and Sammy is coming." Her gnome's face pressed happily into the flowers.

It is impossible to predict in these cases, but once over the immediate effects of the operation, she should have several months of comparative well-being.

The money, where will come the money?

Travel with her, Dad. Don't take her home to the old associations. The other children will want to see her.

The money, where will I wring the money?

Whatever happens, she is not to know. No, you can't ask her to sign papers to sell the house; nothing to upset her. Borrow instead, then after. . . .

I had wanted to leave you each a few dollars to make life easier, as other fathers do. There will be nothing left now. (Failure! you and your "business is exploitation." Why didn't you make it when it could be made?—Is that what you're thinking, Sammy?)

Sure she's unreasonable, Dad—but you have to stay with her; if there's to be any happiness in what's left of her life, it depends on you.

Prop me up, children, think of me, too. Shuffled, chained with her, bitter woman. No Haven, and the little money going. . . . How happy she looks, poor creature.

The look of excitement. The straining to hear everything (the new hearing aid turned full). Why are you so happy, dying woman?

How the petals are, fold on fold, and the gladioli color. The autumn air.

Stranger grandsons, tall above the little gnome grandmother, the little spry grandfather. Paul in a frenzy of picture-taking before going.

She, wandering the great house. Feeling the books; laughing at the maple shoemaker's bench of a hundred years ago used as a table. The ear turned to music.

"Let us go home. See how good I walk now." "One step from the hospital," he answers, "and she wants to fly. Wait till Doctor Phil says."

"Look—the birds too are flying home. Very good Phil is and will not show it, but he is sick of sickness by the time he comes home."

"Mrs. Telepathy, to read minds," he answers; "read mine what it says: when the trunks of medicines become a suitcase, then we will go."

The grandboys, they do not know what to say to us. . . . Hannah, she runs around here, there, when is there time for herself?

Let us go home. Let us go home.

Musing; gentleness—*but for the incidents of the rabbi in the hospital, and of the candles of benediction.*

Of the rabbi in the hospital:

Now tell me what happened, Mother.

From the sleep I awoke, Hannah's Phil, and he stands there like a devil in a dream and calls me by name. I cannot hear. I think he prays. Go away, please, I tell him, I am not a believer. Still he stands, while my heart knocks with fright.

You scared *him*, Mother. He thought you were delirious.

Who sent him? Why did he come to me?

It is a custom. The men of God come to visit those of their religion they might help. The hospital makes up the list for them— race, religion—and you are on the Jewish list.

Not for rabbis. At once go and make them change. Tell them to write: Race, human; Religion, none.

TILLIE OLSEN

And of the candles of benediction:

Look how you have upset yourself, Mrs. Excited Over Nothing. Pleasant memories you should leave.

Go in, go back to Hannah and the lights. Two weeks I saw candles and said nothing. But she asked me.

So what was so terrible? She forgets you never did, she asks you to light the Friday candles and say the benediction like Phil's mother when she visits. If the candles give her pleasure, why shouldn't she have the pleasure?

Not for pleasure she does it. For emptiness. Because his family does. Because all around her do.

That is not a good reason too? But you did not hear her. For heritage, she told you. For the boys, from the past they should have tradition.

Superstition! From our ancestors, savages, afraid of the dark, of themselves: mumbo words and magic lights to scare away ghosts.

She told you: how it started does not take away the goodness. For centuries, peace in the house it means.

Swindler! does she look back on the dark centuries? Candles bought instead of bread and stuck into a potato for a candlestick? Religion that stifled and said: in Paradise, woman, you will be the footstool of your husband, and in life—poor chosen Jew—ground under, despised, trembling in cellars. And cremated. And cremated.

This is religion's fault? You think you are still an orator of the 1905 revolution? Where are the pills for quieting? Which are they?

Heritage. How have we come from our savage past, how no longer to be savages—this to teach. To look back and learn what humanizes—this to teach. To smash all ghettos that divide us—not to go back, not to go back—this to teach. Learned books in the house, will humankind live or die, and she gives to her boys—superstition.

Hannah that is so good to you. Take your pill, Mrs. Excited For Nothing, swallow.

Heritage! But when did I have time to teach? Of Hannah I asked only hands to help.

Swallow.

Otherwise—musing; gentleness.

Not to travel. To go home.

The children want to see you. We have to show them you are as thorny a flower as ever.

Not to travel.

Vivi wants you should see her new baby. She sent the tickets—airplane tickets—A Mrs. Roosevelt she wants to make of you. To Vivi's we have to go.

A new baby. How many warm, seductive babies. She holds him stiffly, *away* from her, so that he wails. And a long shudder begins, and the sweat beads on her forehead.

"Hush, shush," croons the grandfather, lifting him back. "You should forgive your grandmamma, little prince, she has never held a baby before, only seen them in glass cases. Hush, shush."

"You're tired, Ma," says Vivi. "The travel and the noisy dinner. I'll take you to lie down."

(A long travel from, to, what the feel of a baby evokes.)

In the airplane, cunningly designed to encase from motion (no wind, no feel of flight), she had sat severely and still, her face turned to the sky through which they cleaved and left no scar.

So this was how it looked, the determining, the crucial sky, and this was how man moved through it, remote above the dwindled earth, the concealed human life. Vulnerable life, that could scar.

There was a steerage ship of memory that shook across a great, circular sea: clustered, ill human beings; and through the thick-stained air, tiny fretting waters in a window round like the airplane's—sun round, moon round. (The round thatched roofs of Olshana.) Eye round—like the smaller window that framed distance the solitary year of exile when only her eyes could travel, and no voice spoke. And the polar winds hurled themselves across snows trackless and endless and white—like the clouds which had closed together below and hidden the earth.

Now they put a baby in her lap. Do not ask me, she would have liked to beg. Enough the worn face of Vivi, the remembered grandchildren. I cannot, cannot. . . .

Cannot what? Unnatural grandmother, not able to make herself embrace a baby.

She lay there in the bed of the two little girls, her new hearing aid turned full, listening to the sound of the children going to sleep, the baby's fretful crying and hushing, the clatter of dishes being washed and put away. They thought she slept. Still she rode on.

It was not that she had not loved her babies, her children. The love—the passion of tending—had risen with the need like a torrent; and like a torrent drowned and immolated all else. But when the need was done—oh the power that was lost in the painful damming back and drying up of what still surged, but had nowhere to go. Only the thin pulsing left that could not quiet, suffering over lives one felt, but could no longer hold nor help.

On that torrent she had borne them on their own lives, and the riverbed was desert long years now. Not there would she dwell, a memoried wraith. Surely that was not all, surely there was more. Still the springs, the springs were in her seeking. Somewhere an older power that beat for life. Some-where coherence, transport, meaning. If they would but leave her in the air now stilled of clamor, in the reconciled solitude, to journey on.

And they put a baby in her lap. Immediacy to embrace, and the breath of *that* past: warm flesh like this that had claims and nuzzled away all else and with lovely mouths devoured: hot-living like an animal—intensely and now; the turning maze; the long drunkenness; the drowning into need-ing and being needed. Severely she looked back—and the shudder seized her again, and the sweat. Not that way. Not there, not now could she, not yet. . . .

And all that visit, she could not touch the baby.

"Daddy, is it the . . . sickness she's like that?" asked Vivi. "I was so glad to be having the baby—for her. I told Tim, it'll give her more happiness than anything, being around a baby again. And she hasn't played with him once."

He was not listening. "Aahh little seed of life, little charmer," he crooned, "Hollywood should see you. A heart of ice you would melt. Kick, kick. The future you'll have for a ball. In 2050 still kick. Kick for your gran-daddy then."

Attentive with the older children; sat through their performances (com-mand performance; we command you to be the audience); helped Ann sort autumn leaves to find the best for a school program; listened gravely to Richard tell about his rock collection, while her lips mutely formed the words to remember: *igneous, sedimentary, metamorphic;* looked for miss-ing socks, books, and bus tickets; watched the children whoop after their grandfather who knew how to tickle, chuck, lift, toss, do tricks, tell secrets, make jokes, match riddle for riddle. (Tell me a riddle, Grammy. I know no riddles, child.) Scrubbed sills and woodwork and furniture in every room; folded the laundry; straightened drawers; emptied the heaped baskets wait-ing for ironing (while he or Vivi or Tim nagged: You're supposed to rest here, you've been sick) but to none tended or gave food—and could not touch the baby.

After a week she said: "Let us go home. Today call about the tickets."

"You have important business, Mrs. Inahurry? The President waits to consult with you?" He shouted, for the fear of the future raced in him. "The clothes are still warm from the suitcase, your children cannot show enough how glad they are to see you, and you want home. There is plenty of time for home. We cannot be with the children at home."

"Blind to around you as always: the little ones sleep four in a room be-cause we take their bed. We are two more people in a house with a new baby, and no help."

"Vivi is happy so. The children should have their grandparents a while, she told to me. I should have my mommy and daddy. . . . "

"Babbler and blind. Do you look at her so tired? How she starts to talk and she cries? I am not strong enough yet to help. Let us go home."

(To reconciled solitude.)

For it seemed to her the crowded noisy house was listening to her, listening for her. She could feel it like a great ear pressed under her heart. And everything knocked: quick constant raps: let me in, let me in.

How was it that soft reaching tendrils also became blows that knocked?

C'mon, Grandma, I want to show you. . . .

Tell me a riddle, Grandma. *(I know no riddles.)*

Look, Grammy, he's so dumb he can't even find his hands. (Dody and the baby on a blanket over the fermenting autumn mould.)

I made them—for you. (Ann) (Flat paper dolls with aprons that lifted on scalloped skirts that lifted on flowered pants; hair of yarn and great ringed questioning eyes.)

Watch me, Grandma. (Richard snaking up the tree, hanging exultant, free, with one hand at the top. Below Dody hunching over in pretend-cooking.)

(Climb too, Dody, climb and look.)

Be my nap bed, Grammy. (The "No!" too late.)

Morty's abandoned heaviness, while his fingers ladder up and down her hearing-aid cord to his drowsy chant: eentsiebeentsiespider. *(Children trust.)*

It's to start off your own rock collection, Grandma.

That's a trilobite fossil, 200 million years old (millions of years on a boy's mouth) and that one's obsidian, black glass.

Knocked and knocked.

Mother, I *told* you the teacher said we had to bring it back all filled out this morning. Didn't you even ask Daddy? Then tell *me* which plan and I'll check it: evacuate or stay in the city or wait for you to come and take me away. (Seeing the look of straining to hear.) It's for Disaster, Grandma. *(Children trust.)*

Vivi in the maze of the long, the lovely drunkenness. The old old noises: baby sounds; screaming of a mother flayed to exasperation; children quarreling; children playing; singing; laughter.

And Vivi's tears and memories, spilling so fast, half the words not understood.

She had started remembering out loud deliberately, so her mother would know the past was cherished, still lived in her.

Nursing the baby: My friends marvel, and I tell them, oh it's easy to be such a cow. I remember how beautiful my mother seemed nursing my brother, and the milk just flows. . . . Was that Davy? It must have been Davy. . . .

Lowering a hem: How did you ever . . . when I think how you made everything we wore . . . Tim, just think, seven kids and Mommy sewed everything . . . do I remember you sang while you sewed? That white dress with the red apples on the skirt you fixed over for me, was it Hannah's or Clara's before it was mine?

Washing sweaters: Ma, I'll never forget, one of those days so nice you washed clothes outside; one of the first spring days it must have been. The bubbles just danced while you scrubbed, and we chased after, and you stopped to show us how to blow our own bubbles with green onion stalks . . . you always. . . .

"Strong onion, to still make you cry after so many years," her father said, to turn the tears into laughter.

While Richard bent over his homework: Where is it now, do we still have it, the Book of the Martyrs? It always seemed so, well—exalted, when you'd put it on the round table and we'd all look at it together; there was even a halo from the lamp. The lamp with the beaded fringe you could move up and down; they're in style again, pulley lamps like that, but without the fringe. You know the book I'm talking about, Daddy, the Book of the Martyrs, the first picture was a bust of Spartacus . . . Socrates? I wish there was something like that for the children, Mommy, to give them what you. . . . (And the tears splashed again.)

(What I intended and did not? Stop it, daughter, stop it, leave that time. And he, the hypocrite, sitting there with tears in his eyes—it was nothing to you then, nothing.)

. . . The time you came to school and I almost died of shame because of your accent and because I knew you knew I was ashamed; how could I? . . . Sammy's harmonica and you danced to it once, yes you did, you and Davy squealing in your arms. . . . That time you bundled us up and walked us down to the railway station to stay the night 'cause it was heated and we didn't have any coal, that winter of the strike, you didn't think I remembered that, did you, Mommy? . . . How you'd call us out to see the sunsets. . . .

Day after day, the spilling memories. Worse now, questions, too. Even the grandchildren: grandma, in the olden days, when you were little. . . .

It was the afternoons that saved.

While they thought she napped, she would leave the mosaic on the wall (of children's drawings, maps, calendars, pictures, Ann's cardboard dolls with their great ringed questioning eyes) and hunch in the girls' closet on the low shelf where the shoes stood, and the girls' dresses covered.

For that while she would painfully sheathe against the listening house, the tendrils and noises that knocked, and Vivi's spilling memories. Sometimes it helped to braid and unbraid the sashes that dangled, or to trace the pattern on the hoop slips.

Today she had jacks and children under jet trails to forget. Last night, Ann and Dody silhouetted in the window against a sunset of flaming man-made clouds of jet trail, their jacks ball accenting the peaceful noise of dinner being made. Had she told them, yes she had told them of how they played jacks in her village though there was no ball, no jacks. Six stones, round and flat, toss them out, the seventh on the back of the hand, toss, catch and swoop up as many as possible, toss again. . . .

Of stones (repeating Richard) there are three kinds: earth's fire jetting; rock of layered centuries; crucibled new out of the old (*igneous, sedimentary, metamorphic*). But there was that other—frozen to black glass, never to transform or hold the fossil memory . . . (let not my seed fall on stone). There was an ancient man who fought to heights a great rock that crashed back down eternally—eternal labor, freedom, labor . . . (stone will perish, but the word remain). And you, David, who with a stone slew, screaming: Lord, take my heart of stone and give me flesh

Who was screaming? Why was she back in the common room of the prison, the sun motes dancing in the shafts of light, and the informer being brought in, a prisoner now, like themselves. And Lisa leaping, yes, Lisa, the gentle and tender, biting at the betrayer's jugular. Screaming and screaming.

No, it is the children screaming. Another of Paul and Sammy's terrible fights?

In Vivi's house. Severely: you are in Vivi's house.

Blows, screams, a call: "Grandma!" For her? Oh please not for her. Hide, hunch behind the dresses deeper. But a trembling little body hurls itself beside her—surprised, smothered laughter, arms surround her neck, tears rub dry on her cheek, and words too soft to understand whisper into her ear (Is this where you hide too, Grammy? It's my secret place, we have a secret now).

And the sweat beads, and the long shudder seizes.

It seemed the great ear pressed inside now, and the knocking. "We have to go home," she told him, "I grow ill here."

"It's your own fault, Mrs. Bodybusy, you do not rest, you do too much." He raged, but the fear was in his eyes. "It was a serious operation, they told you to take care. . . . All right, we will go to where you can rest."

But where? Not home to death, not yet. He had thought to Lennie's, to Clara's; beautiful visits with each of the children. She would have to rest first, be stronger. If they could but go to Florida—it glittered before him, the never-realized promise of Florida. California: of course. (The money, the money, dwindling!) Los Angeles first for sun and rest, then to Lennie's in San Francisco.

He told her the next day. "You saw what Nancy wrote: snow and wind back home, a terrible winter. And look at you—all bones and a swollen belly. I called Phil: he said: 'A prescription, Los Angeles sun and rest.'"

She watched the words on his lips. "You have sold the house," she cried, "that is why we do not go home. That is why you talk no more of the Haven, why there is money for travel. After the children you will drag me to the Haven."

"The Haven! Who thinks of the Haven any more? Tell her, Vivi, tell Mrs. Suspicious: a prescription, sun and rest, to make you healthy. . . . And how could I sell the house without *you*?"

At the place of farewells and greetings, of winds of coming and winds of going, they say their good-byes.

They look back at her with the eyes of others before them: Richard with her own blue blaze; Ann with the nordic eyes of Tim; Morty's dreaming brown of a great-grandmother he will never know; Dody with the laughing eyes of him who had been her springtide love (who stands beside her now); Vivi's, all tears.

The baby's eyes are closed in sleep.

Good-bye, my children.

3

It is to the back of the great city he brought her, to the dwelling places of the cast-off old. Bounded by two lines of amusement piers to the north and to the south, and between a long straight paving rimmed with black benches facing the sand—sands so wide the ocean is only a far fluting.

In the brief vacation season, some of the boarded stores fronting the sands open, and families, young people and children, may be seen. A little tasselled tram shuttles between the piers, and the lights of roller coasters prink and tweak over those who come to have sensation made in them.

The rest of the year it is abandoned to the old, all else boarded up and still; seemingly empty, except the occasional days and hours when the sun, like a tide, sucks them out of the low rooming houses, casts them onto the benches and sandy rim of the walk—and sweeps them into decaying enclosures once again.

A few newer apartments glint among the low bleached squares. It is in one of these Lennie's Jeannie has arranged their rooms. "Only a few miles north and south people pay hundreds of dollars a month for just this gorgeous air, Grandaddy, just this ocean closeness."

She had been ill on the plane, lay ill for days in the unfamiliar room. Several times the doctor came by—left medicine she would not take. Several times Jeannie drove in the twenty miles from work, still in her Visiting Nurse uniform, the lightness and brightness of her like a healing.

"Who can believe it is winter?" he asked one morning. "Beautiful it is outside like an ad. Come, Mrs. Invalid, come to taste it. You are well enough to sit in here, you are well enough to sit outside. The doctor said it too."

But the benches were encrusted with people, and the sands at the sidewalk's edge. Besides, she had seen the far ruffle of the sea: "there take me," and though she leaned against him, it was she who led.

Plodding and plodding, sitting often to rest, he grumbling. Patting the sand so warm. Once she scooped up a handful, cradling it close to her better eye; peered, and flung it back. And as they came almost to the brink and she could see the glistening wet, she sat down, pulled off her shoes and stockings, left him and began to run. "You'll catch cold," he screamed, but the sand in his shoes weighed him down—he who had always been the agile one—and already the white spray creamed her feet.

He pulled her back, took a handkerchief to wipe off the wet and the sand. "Oh no," she said, "the sun will dry," seized the square and smoothed it flat, dropped on it a mound of sand, knotted the kerchief corners and tied it to a bag—"to look at with the strong glass" (for the first time in years explaining an action of hers)—and lay down with the little bag against her cheek, looking toward the shore that nurtured life as it first crawled toward consciousness the millions of years ago.

He took her one Sunday in the evil-smelling bus, past flat miles of blister houses, to the home of relatives. Oh what is this? she cried as the light began to smoke and the houses to dim and recede. Smog, he said, everyone knows but you. . . . Outside he kept his arms about her, but she walked with hands pushing the heavy air as if to open it, whispered: who has done this? sat down suddenly to vomit at the curb and for a long while refused to rise.

One's age as seen on the altered face of those known in youth. Is this they he has come to visit? This Max and Rose, smooth and pleasant, introducing them to polite children, disinterested grandchildren, "the whole family, once a month on Sundays. And why not? We have the room, the help, the food."

Talk of cars, of houses, of success: this son that, that daughter this. And *your* children? Hastily skimped over, the intermarriages, the obscure work—"my doctor son-in-law, Phil"—all he has to offer. She silent in a corner. (Car-sick like a baby, he explains.) Years since he has taken her to visit anyone but the children, and old apprehensions prickle: "no incidents," he silently begs, "no incidents." He itched to tell them. "A very sick woman," significantly, indicating her with his eyes, "a very sick woman." Their restricted faces did not react. "Have you thought maybe she'd do better at Palm Springs?" Rose asked. "Or at least a nicer section of the beach, nicer people, a pool." Not to have to say "money" he said instead: "would she have sand to look at through a magnifying glass?" and went on, detail after detail, the old habit betraying of parading the queerness of her for laughter.

After dinner—the others into the living room in men- or women-clusters, or into the den to watch TV—the four of them alone. She sat close to him, and did not speak. Jokes, stories, people they had known, beginning of reminiscence, Russia fifty-sixty years ago. Strange words across the Duncan Phyfe table: *hunger; secret meetings; human rights; spies; betrayals; prison; escape*—interrupted by one of the grandchildren: "Commercial's on; any Coke left? Gee, you're missing a real hair-raiser." And then a granddaughter (Max proudly: "Look at her, an American queen") drove them home on her way back to U.C.L.A. No incident—except that there had been no incidents.

The first few mornings she had taken with her the magnifying glass, but he would sit only on the benches, so she rested at the foot, where slatted bench shadows fell, and unless she turned her hearing aid down, other voices invaded.

Now on the days when the sun shone and she felt well enough, he took her on the tram to where the benches ranged in oblongs, some with tables for checkers or cards. Again the blanket on the sand in the striped shadows, but she no longer brought the magnifying glass. He played cards, and she lay in the sun and looked towards the waters; or they walked—two blocks down to the scaling hotel, two blocks back—past chili-hamburger stands, open-doored bars, Next-to-New and perpetual rummage sale stores.

Once, out of the aimless walkers, slow and shuffling like themselves, someone ran unevenly towards them, embraced, kissed, wept: "dear friends, old friends." A friend of *hers*, not his: Mrs. Mays who had lived next door to them in Denver when the children were small.

Thirty years are compressed into a dozen sentences; and the present, not even in three. All is told: the children scattered; the husband dead; she lives in a room two blocks up from the sing hall—and points to the domed auditorium jutting before the pier. The leg? phlebitis; the heavy breathing? that, one does not ask. She, too, comes to the benches each day to sit. And tomorrow, tomorrow, are they going to the community sing? Of course he would have heard of it, everybody goes—the big doings they wait for all week. They have never been? She will come to them for dinner tomorrow and they will all go together.

So it is that she sits in the wind of the singing, among the thousand various faces of age.

She had turned off her hearing aid at once they came into the auditorium—as she would have wished to turn off sight.

One by one they streamed by and imprinted on her—and though the savage zest of their singing came voicelessly soft and distant, the faces still roared—the faces densened the air—chorded into

children-chants, mother-croons, singing of the chained love serenades, Beethoven storms, mad Lucia's scream drunken joy-songs, keens for the dead, work-singing

while from floor to balcony to dome a bare-footed sore-covered little girl threaded the sound-thronged tumult, danced her ecstasy of grimace to flutes that scratched at a cross-roads village wedding

Yes, faces became sound, and the sound became faces; and faces and sound became weight—pushed, pressed

"Air"—her hands claw his.

"Whenever I enjoy myself. . . . " Then he saw the gray sweat on her face. "Here. Up. Help me, Mrs. Mays," and they support her out to where she can gulp the air in sob after sob.

"A doctor, we should get for her a doctor."

"Tch, it's nothing," says Ellen Mays, "I get it all the time. You've missed the tram; come to my place. Fix your hearing aid, honey . . . close . . . tea. My view. See, she *wants* to come. Steady now, that's how." Adding mysteriously: "Remember your advice, easy to keep your head above water, empty things float. Float."

The singing a fading march for them, tall woman with a swollen leg, weaving little man, and the swollen thinness they help between.

The stench in the hall: mildew? decay? "We sit and rest then climb. My gorgeous view. We help each other and here we are."

The stench along into the slab of room. A washstand for a sink, a box with oilcloth tacked around for a cupboard, a three-burner gas plate. Artificial flowers, colorless with dust. Everywhere pictures foaming: wedding, baby, party, vacation, graduation, family pictures. From the narrow couch under a slit of window, sure enough the view: lurching rooftops and a scallop of ocean heaving, preening, twitching under the moon.

"While the water heats. Excuse me . . . down the hall." Ellen Mays has gone.

"You'll live?" he asks mechanically, sat down to feel his fright; tried to pull her alongside.

She pushed him away. "For air," she said; stood clinging to the dresser. Then, in a terrible voice:

After a lifetime of room. Of many rooms.

Shhh.

You remember how she lived. Eight children. And now one room like a coffin.

She pays rent!

Shrinking the life of her   into one room   like a coffin   Rooms and rooms like this   I lie on the quilt and hear them talk

Please, Mrs. Orator-without-Breath.

Once you went for coffee   I walked   I saw A Balzac   a Chekhov to write it   Rummage Alone On scraps

Better old here than in the old country!

On scraps   Yet they sang like   like   Wondrous!   *Humankind one has to believe*   So strong for what? To rot   not grow?

Your poor lungs beg you. They sob between each word.

Singing.   Unused   the   life in them. She   in this poor room with her pictures   Max   You   The children   Everywhere unused   the life And who has meaning?   Century after century   still all in us   not   to grow?

Coffins, rummage, plants: sick woman. Oh lay down. We will get for you the doctor.

"And when will it end. Oh, *the end.*" *That* nightmare thought, and this time she writhed, crumpled against him, seized his hand (for a moment again the weight, the soft distant roaring of humanity) and on the strangled-for breath, begged: "Man . . . we'll destroy ourselves?"

And looking for answer—in the helpless pity and fear for her (for *her*) that distorted his face—she understood the last months, and knew that she was dying.

4

"Let us go home," she said after several days.

"You are in training for a cross-country run? That is why you do not even walk across the room? Here, like a prescription Phil said, till you are stronger from the operation. You want to break doctor's orders?"

She saw the fiction was necessary to him, was silent; then: "At home I will get better. If the doctor here says?"

"And winter? And the visits to Lennie and to Clara? All right," for he saw the tears in her eyes, "I will write Phil, and talk to the doctor."

Days passed. He reported nothing. Jeannie came and took her out for air, past the boarded concessions, the hooded and tented amusement rides, to the end of the pier. They watched the spent waves feeding the new, the gulls in the clouded sky; even up where they sat, the wind-blown sand stung.

She did not ask to go down the crooked steps to the sea.

Back in her bed, while he was gone to the store, she said: "Jeannie, this doctor, he is not one I can ask questions. Ask him for me, can I go home?"

Jeannie looked at her, said quickly: "Of course, poor Granny. You want your own things around you, don't you? I'll call him tonight. . . . Look, I've something to show you," and from her purse unwrapped a large cookie, intricately shaped like a little girl. "Look at the curls—can you hear me well, Granny?—and the darling eyelashes. I just came from a house where they were baking them."

"The dimples, there in the knees," she marveled, holding it to the better light, turning, studying, "like art. Each singly they cut, or a mold?"

"Singly," said Jeannie, "and if it is a child only the mother can make them. Oh Granny, it's the likeness of a real little girl who died yesterday—Rosita. She was three years old. *Pan del Muerto*, the Bread of the Dead. It was the custom in the part of Mexico they came from."

Still she turned and inspected. "Look, the hollow in the throat, the little cross necklace. . . . I think for the mother it is a good thing to be busy with such bread. You know the family?"

Jeannie nodded. "On my rounds. I nursed. . . . Oh Granny, it is like a party; they play songs she liked to dance to. The coffin is lined with pink velvet and she wears a white dress. There are candles. . . . "

"In the house?" Surprised, "They keep her in the house?"

"Yes," said Jeannie, "and it is against the health law. The father said it would be sad to bury her in this country; in Oaxaca they have a feast night with candles each year; everyone picnics on the graves of those they loved until dawn."

"Yes, Jeannie, the living must comfort themselves." And closed her eyes.

"You want to sleep, Granny?"

"Yes, tired from the pleasure of you. I may keep the Rosita? There stand it, on the dresser, where I can see; something of my own around me."

In the kitchenette, helping her grandfather unpack the groceries, Jeannie said in her light voice:

"I'm resigning my job, Grandaddy."

"Ah, the lucky young man. Which one is he?"

"Too late. You're spoken for." She made a pyramid of cans, unstacked, and built again.

"Something is wrong with the job?"

"With me. I can't be"—she searched for the word—"what they call professional enough. I let myself feel things. And tomorrow I have to report a family. . . . " The cans clicked again. "It's not that, either. I just don't know what I want to do, maybe go back to school, maybe go to art school. I thought if you went to San Francisco I'd come along and talk it over with Momma and Daddy. But I don't see how you can go. She wants to go home. She asked me to ask the doctor."

The doctor told her himself. "Next week you may travel, when you are a little stronger." But next week there was the fever of an infection, and by the time that was over, she could not leave the bed—a rented hospital bed that stood beside the double bed he slept in alone now.

Outwardly the days repeated themselves. Every other afternoon and evening he went out to his newfound cronies, to talk and play cards. Twice a week, Mrs. Mays came. And the rest of the time, Jeannie was there.

By the sickbed stood Jeannie's FM radio. Often into the room the shapes of music came. She would lie curled on her side, her knees drawn up, intense in listening (Jeannie sketched her so, coiled, convoluted like an ear), then thresh her hand out and abruptly snap the radio mute—still to lie in her attitude of listening, concealing tears.

Once Jeannie brought in a young Marine to visit, a friend from high-school days she had found wandering near the empty pier. Because Jeannie asked him to, gravely, without self-consciousness, he sat himself cross-legged on the floor and performed for them a dance of his native Samoa.

Long after they left, a tiny thrumming sound could be heard where, in her bed, she strove to repeat the beckon, flight, surrender of his hands, the fluttering footbeats and his low plaintive calls.

Hannah and Phil sent flowers. To deepen her pleasure, he placed one in her hair. "Like a girl," he said, and brought the hand mirror so she could see. She looked at the pulsing red flower, the yellow skull face; a desolate, excited laugh shuddered from her, and she pushed the mirror away—but let the flower burn.

The week Lennie and Helen came, the fever returned. With it the excited laugh, and incessant words. She, who in her life had spoken but seldom and then only when necessary (never having learned the easy, social uses of words), now in dying, spoke incessantly.

In a half-whisper: "Like Lisa she is, your Jeannie. Have I told you of Lisa who taught me to read? Of the highborn she was, but noble in herself. I was sixteen; they beat me; my father beat me so I would not go to her. It was forbidden, she was a Tolstoyan. At night, past dogs that howled, terrible dogs, my son, in the snows of winter to the road, I to ride in her carriage like a lady, to books. To her, life was holy, knowledge was holy, and she taught me to read. They hung her. Everything that happens one must try to understand why. She killed one who betrayed many. Because of betrayal, betrayed all she lived and believed. In one minute she killed, before my eyes (there is so much blood in a human being, my son), in prison with me. All that happens, one must try to understand.

"The name?" Her lips would work. "The name that was their pole star; the doors of the death houses fixed to open on it; I read of it my year of penal servitude. Thuban!" very excited. "Thuban, in ancient Egypt the pole star. Can you see, look out to see it, Jeannie, if it swings around *our* pole star that seems to *us* not to move.

"Yes, Jeannie, at your age my mother and grandmother had already buried children . . . yes, Jeannie, it is more than oceans between Olshana and you . . . yes, Jeannie, they danced, and for all the bodies they had they might as well be chickens, and indeed, they scratched and flapped their arms and hopped.

"And Andrei Yefimitch, who for twenty years had never known of it and never wanted to know, said as if he wanted to cry: but why my dear friend this malicious laughter?" Telling to herself half-memorized phrases from her few books. "Pain I answer with tears and cries, baseness with indignation, meanness with repulsion . . . for life may be hated or wearied of, but never despised."

Delirious: "Tell me, my neighbor, Mrs. Mays, the pictures never lived, but what of the flowers? Tell them who ask: no rabbis, no ministers, no priests, no speeches, no ceremonies: ah, false—let the living comfort themselves. Tell Sammy's boy, he who flies, tell him to go to Stuttgart and see where Davy has no grave. And what? . . . And what? where millions have no graves—save air."

In delirium or not, wanting the radio on; not seeming to listen, the words still jetting, wanting the music on. Once, silencing it abruptly as of old, she began to cry, unconcealed tears this time. "You have pain, Granny?" Jeannie asked.

"The music," she said, "still it is there and we do not hear; knocks, and our poor human ears too weak. What else, what else we do not hear?"

Once she knocked his hand aside as he gave her a pill, swept the bottles from her bedside table: "no pills, let me feel what I feel," and laughed as on his hands and knees he groped to pick them up.

Nighttimes her hand reached across the bed to hold his.

A constant retching began. Her breath was too faint for sustained speech now, but still the lips moved:

> When no longer necessary   to injure others
> Pick   pick   pick   Blind Chicken
> As a human being   responsibility

"David!" imperious, "Basin!" and she would vomit, rinse her mouth, the wasted throat working to swallow, and begin the chant again.

She will be better off in the hospital now, the doctor said.

He sent the telegrams to the children, was packing her suitcase, when her hoarse voice startled. She had roused, was pulling herself to sitting.

"Where now?" she asked. "Where now do you drag me?"

"You do not even have to have a baby to go this time," he soothed, looking for the brush to pack. "Remember, after Davy you told me—worthy to have a baby for the pleasure of the ten day rest in the hospital?"

"Where now? Not home yet?" Her voice mourned. "Where *is* my home?"

He rose to ease her back. "The doctor, the hospital," he started to explain, but deftly, like a snake, she had slithered out of bed and stood swaying, propped behind the night table.

"Coward," she hissed, "runner."

"You stand," he said senselessly.

"To take me there and run. Afraid of a little vomit."

He reached her as she fell. She struggled against him, half slipped from his arms, pulled herself up again.

"Weakling," she taunted, "to leave me there and run. Betrayer. All your life you have run."

He sobbed, telling Jeannie. "A Marilyn Monroe to run for her virtue. Fifty-nine pounds she weighs, the doctor said, and she beats at me like a Dempsey. Betrayer, she cries, and I running like a dog when she calls; day and night, running to her, her vomit, the bedpan. . . . "

"She needs you, Grandaddy," said Jeannie. "Isn't that what they call love? I'll see if she sleeps, and if she does, poor worn-out darling, we'll have a party, you and I: I brought us rum babas."

They did not move her. By her bed now stood the tall hooked pillar that held the solutions—blood and dextrose—to feed her veins. Jeannie moved down the hall to take over the sickroom, her face so radiant, her grandfather asked her once: "you are in love?" (Shameful the joy, the pure overwhelming joy from being with her grandmother; the peace, the serenity that breathed.) "My darling escape," she answered incoherently, "my darling Granny"—as if that explained.

Now one by one the children came, those that were able. Hannah, Paul, Sammy. Too late to ask: and what did you learn with your living, Mother, and what do we need to know?

Clara, the eldest, clenched:

Pay me back, Mother, pay me back for all you took from me.
Those others you crowded into your heart. The hands I needed to be
for you, the heaviness, the responsibility.

Is this she? Noises the dying make, the crablike hands crawling over the covers. The ethereal singing.

She hears that music, that singing from childhood; forgotten sound—not heard since, since . . . And the hardness breaks like a cry: Where did we lose each other, first mother, singing mother?

Annulled: the quarrels, the gibing, the harshness between; the fall into silence and the withdrawal.

I do not know you, Mother. Mother, I never knew you.

Lennie, suffering not alone for her who was dying, but for that in her which never lived (for that which in him might never live). From him too, unspoken words: *good-bye Mother who taught me to mother myself.*

Not Vivi, who must stay with her children; not Davy, but he is already here, having to die again with *her* this time, for the living take their dead with them when they die.

Light she grew, like a bird, and, like a bird, sound bubbled in her throat while the body fluttered in agony. Night and day, asleep or awake (though indeed there was no difference now) the songs and the phrases leaping.

And he, who had once dreaded a long dying (from fear of himself, from horror of the dwindling money) now desired her quick death profoundly, for *her* sake. He no longer went out, except when Jeannie forced him; no longer laughed, except when in the bright kitchenette, Jeannie coaxed his laughter (and she, who seemed to hear nothing else, would laugh too, conspiratorial wisps of laughter).

Light, like a bird, the fluttering body, the little claw hands, the beaked shadow on her face; and the throat, bubbling, straining.

He tried not to listen, as he tried not to look on the face in which only the forehead remained familiar, but trapped with her the long nights in that little room, the sounds worked themselves into his consciousness, with their punctuation of death swallows, whimpers, gurglings.

Even in reality (swallow) *life's lack of it*
Slaveships   deathtrains   clubs   eeenough
The bell   summon what enables
78,000 in one minute (whisper of a scream) *78,000*
human beings   we'll destroy ourselves?

"Aah, Mrs. Miserable," he said, as if she could hear, "all your life working, and now in bed you lie, servants to tend, you do not even need to call to be tended, and still you work. Such hard work it is to die? Such hard work?"

The body threshed, her hand clung in his. A melody, ghost-thin, hovered on her lips, and like a guilty ghost, the vision of her bent in listening to it, silencing the record instantly he was near. Now, heedless of his presence, she floated the melody on and on.

"Hid it from me," he complained, "how many times you listened to remember it so?" And tried to think when she had first played it, or first begun to silence her few records when he came near—but could reconstruct nothing. There was only this room with its tall hooked pillar and its swarm of sounds.

No man one   except through others
Strong   with the not yet   in the now
Dogma dead   war dead   one country

"It helps, Mrs. Philosopher, words from books? It helps?" And it seemed to him that for seventy years she had hidden a tape recorder, infinitely microscopic, within her, that it had coiled infinite mile on mile, trapping every song, every melody, every word read, heard, and spoken—and that maliciously she was playing back only what said nothing of him, of the children, of their intimate life together.

"Left us indeed, Mrs. Babbler," he reproached, "you who called others babbler and cunningly saved your words. A lifetime you tended and loved, and now not a word of us, for us. Left us indeed? Left me."

And he took out his solitaire deck, shuffled the cards loudly, slapped them down.

Lift high banner of reason (tatter of an orator's voice) *justice   freedom light*
Humankind   life worthy   capacities
Seeks (blur of shudder) *belong   human being*

"Words, words," he accused, "and what human beings did *you* seek around you, Mrs. Live Alone, and what humankind think worthy?"

Though even as he spoke, he remembered she had not always been isolated, had not always wanted to be alone (as he knew there had been a voice before this gossamer one; before the hoarse voice that broke from silence to lash, make incidents, shame him—a girl's voice of eloquence that spoke their holiest dreams). But again he could reconstruct, image, nothing of what had been before, or when, or how, it had changed.

Ace, queen, jack. The pillar shadow fell, so, in two tracks; in the mirror depths glistened a moonlike blob, the empty solution bottle. And it worked in him: *of reason and justice and freedom . . . Dogma dead:* he remembered the full quotation, laughed bitterly. "Hah, good you do not know what you say; good Victor Hugo died and did not see it, his twentieth century."

Deuce, ten, five. Dauntlessly she began a song of their youth of belief:

These things shall be, a loftier race
than e'er the world hath known shall rise

with flame of freedom in their souls
and light of knowledge in their eyes

King, four, jack "In the twentieth century, hah"

They shall be gentle, brave and strong
to spill no drop of blood, but dare
all . . .

on earth and fire and sea and air

"To spill no drop of blood, hah! So, cadaver, and you too, cadaver Hugo, 'in the twentieth century ignorance will be dead, dogma will be dead, war will be dead, and for all humankind one country—of fulfillment?' Hah!"

And every life (long strangling cough) *shall*
be a song

The cards fell from his fingers. Without warning, the bereavement and betrayal he had sheltered—compounded through the years—hidden even from himself—revealed itself,
uncoiled,
released,
sprung

and with it the monstrous shapes of what had actually happened in the century.

A ravening hunger or thirst seized him. He groped into the kitchenette, switched on all three lights, piled a tray—"you have finished your night snack, Mrs. Cadaver, now I will have mine." And he was shocked at the tears that splashed on the tray.

"Salt tears. For free. I forgot to shake on salt?"

Whispered: "Lost, how much I lost."

Escaped to the grandchildren whose childhoods were childish, who had never hungered, who lived unravaged by disease in warm houses of many rooms, had all the school for which they cared, could walk on any street, stood a head taller than their grandparents, towered above—beautiful skins, straight backs, clear straightforward eyes. "Yes, you in Olshana," he said to the town of sixty years ago, "they would be nobility to you."

And was this not the dream then, come true in ways undreamed? he asked.

And are there no other children in the world? he answered, as if in her harsh voice.

And the flame of freedom, the light of knowledge?
And the drop, to spill no drop of blood?
And he thought that at six Jeannie would get up and it would be his turn
to go to her room and sleep, that he could press the buzzer and she would
come now; that in the afternoon Ellen Mays was coming, and this time they
would play cards and he could marvel at how rouge can stand half an inch on
the cheek; that in the evening the doctor would come, and he could beg him
to be merciful, to stop the feeding solutions, to let her die.

To let her die, and with her their youth of belief out of which her bright,
betrayed words foamed; stained words, that on her working lips came
stainless.

Hours yet before Jeannie's turn. He could press the buzzer and wake
her to come now; he could take a pill, and with it sleep; he could pour
more brandy into his milk glass, though what he had poured was not yet
touched.

Instead he went back, checked her pulse, gently tended with his knotty
fingers as Jeannie had taught.

She was whimpering; her hand crawled across the covers for his. Com-
passionately he enfolded it, and with his free hand gathered up the cards
again. Still was there thirst or hunger ravening in him.

That world of their youth—dark, ignorant, terrible with hate and disease—how was it that living in it, in the midst of corruption, filth, treachery,
degradation, they had not mistrusted man nor themselves; had believed so
beautifully, so . . . falsely?

"Aaah, children," he said out loud, "how we believed, how we belonged."
And he yearned to package for each of the children, the grandchildren, for
everyone, *that joyous certainty, that sense of mattering, of moving and being moved, of being one and indivisible with the great of the past, with all
that freed, ennobled.* Package it, stand on corners, in front of stadiums and
on crowded beaches, knock on doors, give it as a fabled gift.

"And why not in cereal boxes, in soap packages?" he mocked himself.
"Aah. You have taken my senses, cadaver."

Words foamed, died unsounded. Her body writhed; she made kissing
motions with her mouth. (Her lips moving as she read, poring over the Book
of the Martyrs, the magnifying glass superimposed over the heavy eyeglasses.) *Still she believed?* "Eva!" he whispered. "Still you believed? You
lived by it? These Things Shall Be?"

"One pound soup meat," she answered distinctly, "one soup bone."

"My ears heard you. Ellen Mays was witness: 'Humankind . . . one has to
believe.'" Imploringly: "Eva!"

"Bread, day-old." She was mumbling. "Please, in a wooden box . . . for
kindling. The thread, hah, the thread breaks. Cheap thread"—and a gur-
gling, enormously loud, began in her throat.

"I ask for stone; she gives me bread—day-old." He pulled his hand away, shouted: "Who wanted questions? Everything you have to wake?" Then dully, "Ah, let me help you turn, poor creature."

Words jumbled, cleared. In a voice of crowded terror:

"Paul, Sammy, don't fight.

"Hannah, have I ten hands?

"How can I give it, Clara, how can I give it if I don't have?"

"You lie," he said sturdily, "there was joy too." Bitterly: "Ah how cheap you speak of us at the last."

As if to rebuke him, as if her voice had no relationship with her flailing body, she sang clearly, beautifully, a school song the children had taught her when they were little; begged:

"Not look   my hair   where they cut. . . . "

(The crown of braids shorn.) And instantly he left the mute old woman poring over the Book of the Martyrs; went past the mother treading at the sewing machine, singing with the children; past the girl in her wrinkled prison dress, hiding her hair with scarred hands, lifting to him her awkward, shamed, imploring eyes of love; and took her in his arms, dear, personal, fleshed, in all the heavy passion he had loved to rouse from her.

"Eva!"

Her little claw hand beat the covers. How much, how much can a man stand? He took up the cards, put them down, circled the beds, walked to the dresser, opened, shut drawers, brushed his hair, moved his hand bit by bit over the mirror to see what of the reflection he could blot out with each move, and felt that at any moment he would die of what was unendurable. Went to press the buzzer to wake Jeannie, looked down, saw on Jeannie's sketch pad the hospital bed, with *her*; the double bed alongside, with him; the tall pillar feeding into her veins, and their hands, his and hers, clasped, feeding each other. And as if he had been instructed he went to his bed, lay down, holding the sketch (as if it could shield against the monstrous shapes of loss, of betrayal, of death) and with his free hand took hers back into his.

So Jeannie found them in the morning.

That last day the agony was perpetual. Time after time it lifted her almost off the bed, so they had to fight to hold her down. He could not endure and left the room; wept as if there never would be tears enough.

Jeannie came to comfort him. In her light voice she said: Grandaddy, Grandaddy don't cry. She is not there, she promised me. On the last day, she said she would go back to when she first heard music, a little girl on the road of the village where she was born. She promised me. It is a wedding and they dance, while the flutes so joyous and vibrant tremble in the air. Leave her there, Grandaddy, it is all right. She promised me. Come back, come back and help her poor body to die.

TILLIE OLSEN

It is a wedding and they dance, while the flutes so joyous and vibrant tremble in the air. Leave her there, Grandaddy, it is all right. She promised me.
Come back, come back and help her poor body to die.

———

For my mother, my father,
and
Two of that generation
Seevya and Genya
Infinite, dauntless, incorruptible

Death deepens the wonder

Porte-Cochere

Clifford and Ben Junior always came for Old Ben's birthday. Clifford came all the way from Dallas. Ben Junior came only from Cincinnati. They usually stayed in Nashville through the following week end, or came the week end before and stayed through the birthday. Old Ben, who was seventy-six and nearly blind—the cataracts had been removed twice since he was seventy—could hear them now on the side porch, their voices louder than the others', Clifford's the loudest and strongest of all. "Clifford's the real man amongst them," he said to himself, hating to say it but needing to say it. There was no knowing what went on in the heads of the other children, but there were certain things Clifford did know and understand. Clifford, being a lawyer, knew something about history—about Tennessee history he knew, for instance, the difference between Chucky Jack Sevier and Judge John Overton and could debate with you the question of whether or not Andy Jackson had played the part of the coward when he and Chucky Jack met in the wilderness that time. Old Ben kept listening for Cliff's voice above the others. All of his grown-up children were down on the octagonal side porch, which was beyond the porte-cochere and which, under its red tile roof, looked like a pagoda stuck out there on the side lawn. Old Ben was in his study.

His study was directly above the porte-cochere, or what his wife, in her day, had called the porte-cochere—he called it the drive-under and the children used to call it the portcullis—but the study was not a part of the second floor; it opened off the landing halfway up the stairs. Under his south window was the red roof of the porch. He sat by the open window, wearing his dark glasses, his watery old eyes focused vaguely on the peak of the roof. He had napped a little since dinner but had not removed his suit coat or even unbuttoned his linen vest. During most of the afternoon, he had been awake and had heard his five children talking down there on the porch—Cliff and Ben Junior had arrived only that morning—talking on and on in such loud voices that his good right ear could catch individual words and sometimes whole sentences.

Midday dinner had been a considerable ordeal for Old Ben. Laura Nell's interminable chatter had been particularly taxing and obnoxious. Afterward, he had hurried to his study for his prescribed nap and had spent a good part of the afternoon dreading the expedition to the country club for supper that had been planned for that evening. Now it was almost time to begin getting ready for that expedition, and simultaneously with the thought of it and with the movement of his hand toward his watch pocket he became aware that Clifford was taking his leave of the group on the side porch. Ah, yes, at dinner time Clifford had said he had a letter to write before supper—to his wife. Yet here it was six and he had dawdled away the afternoon palavering with the others down there on the porch. Old Ben could recognize Cliff's leave-taking and the teasing voices of the others, and then he heard Cliff's footsteps on the cement driveway, below the study—a hurried step. He heard Cliff in the side hall and then his footsteps at the bottom of the stairs. In a moment he would go sailing by Old Ben's door, without a thought for anyone but himself. Old Ben's lower lip trembled. Wasn't there some business matter he could take up with Cliff? Or some personal matter? And now Cliff's footsteps on the stairs—heavy footsteps, like his own. Suddenly, though, the footsteps halted, and Clifford went downstairs again. His father heard him go across the hall and into the living room, where that carpet silenced his footsteps; he was getting writing paper from the desk there. Old Ben hastily pulled the cord that closed the draperies across the south window, leaving only the vague light from the east window in the room. No, sir, he would not advertise his presence when Cliff passed on the landing.

With the draperies drawn, the light in the room had a strange quality—strange because Old Ben seldom drew the draperies before night. For one moment, he felt that his eyes or his glasses were playing him some new trick. Then he dropped his head on the chair back, for the strange quality now seemed strangely familiar, and now no longer strange—only familiar. It was like the light in that cellar where, long ago, he used to go to fetch Mason jars for his great-aunt Nell Partee. Aunt Nell would send for him all the way across town to come fetch her Mason jars, and even when he was ten or twelve, she made him whistle the whole time he was down in the cellar, to make certain he didn't drink her wine. Aunt Nell, dead and gone. Was this something for Clifford's attention? Where Aunt Nell's shackly house had been, the Trust Company now stood—a near-skyscraper. Her cellar, he supposed, had been in the space now occupied by the basement barbershop—not quite so deep or so large as the shop, its area without boundaries now, suspended in the center of the barber shop, where the ceiling fan revolved. Would this be of interest to Cliff, who would soon ascend the stairs with his own train of thoughts and would pass the open door to the study without a word or a glance? And whatever Cliff was thinking about—his law, his golf, or his wife and children—would be of no real interest to Old Ben. But did not Clifford know that merely the sound of his voice gave his father hope, that his attention gave him comfort? What would old age be without children? Desolation, desolation. But what would old age be with children who chose to ignore the small demands that he would make upon them, that he had ever made upon them? A nameless torment! And with his thoughts Old Ben Brantley's white head rocked on his shoulders and his smoked glasses went so crooked on his nose that he had to frown them back into position.

But now Clifford was hurrying up the stairs again. He was on the landing outside the open study door. It was almost despite himself that the old man cleared his throat and said hoarsely, "The news will be on in five minutes, if you want to listen to it." Then as though he might have sounded too cordial (he would not be reduced to toadying to his own boy), "But if you don't want to, don't say you do." Had Cliff seen his glasses slip down his nose? Cliff, no less than the others, would be capable of laughing at him in his infirmity.

"I wouldn't be likely to, would I, Papa?" Cliff had stopped at the doorway and was stifling a yawn as he spoke, half-covering his face with the envelope and the folded sheet of paper. Old Ben nodded his head to indicate that he had heard what Cliff had said, but also, to himself, he was nodding that yes, this was the way he had raised his children to talk to him.

"Just the hourly newscast," Old Ben said indifferently. "But it don't matter."

"Naw, can't make it, Papa. I got to go and write Sue Alice. The stupid woman staying with her while I'm away bores her pretty much." As he spoke, he looked directly into the dark lenses of his father's glasses, and for a brief second he rested his left hand on the door jamb. His manner was self-possessed and casual, but Old Ben felt that he didn't need good sight to detect his son's ill-concealed haste to be off and away. Cliff had, in fact, turned back to the stairs when his father stopped him with a question, spoken without expression and almost under his breath.

"Why did you come at all? Why did you even bother to come if you weren't going to bring Sue Alice and the grandchildren? Did you think I wanted to see you without them?"

Clifford stopped with one foot on the first step of the second flight. "By God, Papa!" He turned on the ball of the other foot and reappeared in the doorway. "Ever travel with two small kids?" The motion of his body as he turned back from the steps had been swift and sure, calculated to put him exactly facing his father. "And in hot weather like we're having in Texas?"

Despite the undeniable thickness in Clifford's hips and the thin spot on the back of his head, his general appearance was still youthful; about this particular turning on the stairs there had been something decidedly athletic. Imperceptibly, behind the dark glasses, Old Ben lifted his eyebrows in admiration. Clifford was the only boy he had who had ever made any team at the university or done any hunting worth speaking of. For a moment, his eyes rested gently on Cliff's white summer shoes, set wide apart in the doorway. Then, jerking his head up, as though he had just heard Cliff's last words, he began: "Two small *kids?* (Why don't you use the word *brats?* It's more elegant.) I have traveled considerably with five—from here to the mountain and back every summer for fifteen years, from my thirty-first to my forty-sixth year."

"I remember," Cliff said stoically. Then, after a moment: "But now I'm going up to my room and write Sue Alice."

"Then go on up! Who's holding you?" He reached for his smoking stand and switched on the radio. It was a big cabinet radio with a dark mahogany finish, a piece from the late twenties, like all the other furniture in the room, and the mechanism was slow to warm up.

Clifford took several steps toward his father. "Papa, we're due to leave for the club in thirty minutes—less than that now—and I intend to scratch off a note to my wife." He held up the writing paper, as though to prove his intention.

"No concern of mine! No concern of mine! To begin with, I, personally, am not going to the club or anywhere else for supper."

Clifford came even closer. "You may go to the club or not, as you like, Papa. But unless I misunderstand, there is not a servant on the place, and we are all going."

"That is, you are going after you scratch off a note to your wife."

"Papa, Ben Junior and I have each come well over five hundred miles—"

"Not to see me, Clifford."

"Don't be so damned childish, Papa." Cliff was turning away again. Old Ben held his watch in his hand, and he glanced down at it quickly.

"I'm getting childish, am I, Clifford?"

This time, Clifford's turning back was not accomplished in one graceful motion but by a sudden jerking and twisting of his shoulder and leg muscles. Behind the spectacles, Old Ben's eyes narrowed and twitched. His fingers were folded over the face of the watch. Clifford spoke very deliberately. "I didn't say *getting* childish, Papa. When ever in your life have you been anything but that? There's not a senile bone in your brain. It's your children that have got old, and you've stayed young—and not in any good sense, Papa, only in a bad one! You play sly games with us still or you quarrel with us. What the hell do you want of us, Papa? I've thought about it a lot. Why haven't you ever asked for what it is you want? Or are *we* all blind and it's really obvious? You've never given but one piece of advice to us, and that's to be direct and talk up to you like men—as equals. And we've done that, all right, and listened to your wrangling, but somehow it has never satisfied you! What is it?"

"Go on up to your letter-writing; go write your spouse," said Old Ben.

The room had been getting darker while they talked. Old Ben slipped his watch back into his vest pocket nervously, then slipped it out again, constantly running his fingers over the gold case, as though it were a piece of money.

"Thanks for your permission, sir." Clifford took a step backward. During his long speech he had advanced all the way across the room until he was directly in front of his father.

"My permission?" Old Ben said. "Let us not forget one fact, Clifford. No child of mine has ever had to ask my permission to do anything whatsoever he took a mind to do. You have all been free as the air, to come and go in this house. . . . You still are!"

Clifford smiled. "Free to come and go, with you perched here on the landing registering every footstep on the stairs and every car that passed underneath. I used to turn off the ignition and coast through the drive-under, and then think how foolish it was, since there was no back stairway. No back stairway in a house this size!" He paused a moment, running his eyes over the furniture and the other familiar objects in the shadowy room. "And how like the old times this was, Papa—your listening in here in the dark when I came up! By God, Papa, I wouldn't have thought when I was growing up that I'd ever come back and fuss with you once I was grown. But here I am, and, Papa—"

Old Ben pushed himself up from the chair. He put his watch in the vest pocket and buttoned his suit coat with an air of satisfaction. "I'm going along to the club for supper," he said, "since there's to be no-un here to serve me." As he spoke, he heard the clock chiming the half-hour downstairs. And Ben Junior was shouting to Old Ben and Clifford from the foot of the stairs, "Get a move on up there."

Clifford went out on the landing and called down the steps. "Wait till I change my shirt. I believe Papa's all ready."

"No letter written?" Ben Junior asked.

Clifford was hurrying up the second flight with the blank paper. "Nope, no letter this day of Our Lord."

Old Ben heard Ben Junior say, "What did I tell you?" and heard the others laughing. He stood an instant by his chair without putting on a light. Then he reached out his hand for one of the walking canes in the umbrella stand by the radio. His hand lighting on the carved head of a certain oak stick, he felt the head with trembling fingers and quickly released it, and quickly, in three strides, without the help of any cane, he crossed the room to the south window. For several moments, he stood motionless at the window, his huge, soft hands held tensely at his sides, his long body erect, his almost freakishly large head at a slight angle, while he seemed to peer between the open draperies and through the pane of the upper sash, out into the twilight of the wide, shady park that stretched from his great yellow brick house to the Pike. Old Ben's eyes, behind the smoked lenses, were closed, and he was visualizing the ceiling fan in the barber shop. Presently, opening his eyes, he reflected, almost with a smile, that his aunt's cellar was not the only Nashville cellar that had disappeared. Many a cellar! His father's cellar, round like a dungeon; it had been a cistern in the very earliest days, before Old Ben's time, and when he was a boy, he would go down on a ladder with a lantern, and his father's voice, directing him, would seem to go around and around the brick walls and then come back with a hollow sound, as though the cistern were still half-full of water. One time, ah—Old Ben drew back from the window with a grimace—one time he had been so sure there was water below! In fright at the very thought of the water, he had clasped a rung of the ladder tightly with one hand and swung the lantern out, expecting certainly to see the light reflected in the depths below. But the lantern had struck the framework that supported the circular shelves and gone whirling and flaming to the brick floor, which Ben had never before seen. Crashing on the floor, it sent up yellow flames that momentarily lit the old cistern to its very top, and when Ben looked upward, he saw the furious face of his father with the flames casting jagged shadows on the long, black beard and high, white forehead. "Come out of there before you burn out my cellar and my whole damn house to the ground!" He had climbed upward toward his father, wishing the flames might engulf him before he came within reach of those arms. But as his father jerked him up onto the back porch, he saw that the flames had already died out. The whole cellar was pitch-black dark again, and the boy Ben stood with his face against the whitewashed brick wall while his father went to the carriage house to find the old plow line. Presently, he heard his father step up on the porch again. He braced himself for the first blow, but instead there was only the deafening command from his father: "Attention!" Ben whirled about and stood erect, with his chin in the air, his eyes on the ceiling. "Where have you hidden my plow lines?" "I don't know, sir." And then the old man, with his coattails somehow clinging close to his buttocks and thighs, so that his whole powerful form was outlined—his black figure against the white brick and the door—stepped over to the doorway, reached around to the cane stand in the hall, and drew out the oak stick that had his own bearded face carved upon the head. "About face!" he commanded. The boy drew back his toe and made a quick, military turn. The old man dealt him three sharp blows across the upper part of his back. . . . Tears had run down young Ben Brantley's cheeks, even streaking down his neck under his open collar and soaking the neckline binding of his woolen underwear, but he had uttered not a sound. When his father went into the house, Ben remained for a long while standing with his face to the wall. At last, he quietly left the porch and walked through the yard beneath the big shade trees, stopping casually to watch a gray squirrel and then to listen to Aunt Sally Ann's soft nigger voice whispering to him out the kitchen window. He did not answer or turn around but walked on to the latticed summerhouse, between the house and the kitchen garden. There he had lain down on a bench, looked back at the house through the latticework, and said to himself that when he got to be a grown man, he would go away to another country, where there would be no maple trees and no oak trees, no elms, not even sycamores or poplars; where there would be no squirrels and no niggers, no houses that resembled this one; and, most of all, where there would be no children and no fathers.

In the hall, now, Old Ben could hear, very faintly, Ben Junior's voice and Laura Nell's and Katie's and Lawrence's. He stepped to the door and looked down the dark flight of steps at his four younger children. They stood in a circle directly beneath the overhead light, which one of them had just switched on. Their faces were all turned upward in the direction of the open doorway where he was standing, yet he knew in reason that they could not see him there. They were talking about him! Through his dark lenses, their figures were indistinct, their faces mere blurs, and it was hard for him to distinguish their lowered voices one from another. But they were talking about him! And from upstairs he could hear Clifford's footsteps. Clifford, with his letter to Sue Alice unwritten, was thinking about him! Never once in his life had he punished or restrained them in any way! He had given them a freedom unknown to children in the land of his childhood, yet from the time they could utter a word they had despised him and denied his right to any affection or gratitude. Suddenly, stepping out onto the landing, he screamed down the stairs to them, "I've a right to some gratitude!"

They were silent and motionless for a moment. Then he could hear them speaking in lowered voices again, and moving slowly toward the stairs. At the same moment he heard Clifford's footsteps in the upstairs hall. Presently, a light went on up there, and he could dimly see Clifford at the head of the stairs. The four children were advancing up the first flight, and Clifford was coming down from upstairs. Old Ben opened his mouth to call to them, "I'm not afraid of you!" But his voice had left him, and in his momentary fright, in his fear that his wrathful, merciless children might do him harm, he suddenly pitied them. He pitied them for all they had suffered at his hands. And while he stood there, afraid, he realized, or perhaps recalled, how he had tortured and plagued them in all the ways that his resentment of their very good fortune had taught him to do. He even remembered the day when it had occurred to him to build his study above the drive-under and off the stairs, so that he could keep tab on them. He had declared that he wanted his house to be as different from his father's house as a house could be, and so it was! And now he stood in the half-darkness, afraid that he was a man about to be taken by his children and at the same time pitying them, until one of them, ascending the steps switched on the light above the landing.

In the sudden brightness, Old Ben felt that his senses had returned to him. Quickly, he stepped back into the study, closed the door, and locked it. As the lock clicked, he heard Clifford say, "Papa!" Then he heard them all talking at once, and while they talked, he stumbled through the dark study to the umbrella stand. He pulled out the stick with his father's face carved on the head, and in the darkness, while he heard his children's voices, he stumbled about the room beating the upholstered chairs with the stick and calling the names of his children under his breath.

Everything That Rises Must Converge

Her doctor had told Julian's mother that she must lose twenty pounds on account of her blood pressure, so on Wednesday nights Julian had to take her downtown on the bus for a reducing class at the Y. The reducing class was designed for working girls over fifty, who weighed from 165 to 200 pounds. His mother was one of the slimmer ones, but she said ladies did not tell their age or weight. She would not ride the buses by herself at night since they had been integrated, and because the reducing class was one of her few pleasures, necessary for her health, and *free*, she said Julian could at least put himself out to take her, considering all she did for him. Julian did not like to consider all she did for him, but every Wednesday night he braced himself and took her.

She was almost ready to go, standing before the hall mirror, putting on her hat, while he, his hands behind him, appeared pinned to the door frame, waiting like Saint Sebastian for the arrows to begin piercing him. The hat was new and had cost her seven dollars and a half. She kept saying, "Maybe I shouldn't have paid that for it. No, I shouldn't have. I'll take it off and return it tomorrow. I shouldn't have bought it."

Julian raised his eyes to heaven. "Yes, you should have bought it," he said. "Put it on and let's go." It was a hideous hat. A purple velvet flap came down on one side of it and stood up on the other; the rest of it was green and looked like a cushion with the stuffing out. He decided it was less comical than jaunty and pathetic. Everything that gave her pleasure was small and depressed him.

She lifted the hat one more time and set it down slowly on top of her head. Two wings of gray hair protruded on either side of her florid face, but her eyes, sky-blue, were as innocent and untouched by experience as they must have been when she was ten. Were it not that she was a widow who had struggled fiercely to feed and clothe and put him through school and who was supporting him still, "until he got on his feet," she might have been a little girl that he had to take to town.

"It's all right, it's all right," he said. "Let's go." He opened the door himself and started down the walk to get her going. The sky was a dying violet and the houses stood out darkly against it, bulbous liver-colored monstrosities of a uniform ugliness though no two were alike. Since this had been a fashionable neighborhood forty years ago, his mother persisted in thinking they did well to have an apartment in it. Each house had a narrow collar of dirt around it in which sat, usually, a grubby child. Julian walked with his hands in his pockets, his head down and thrust forward and his eyes glazed with the determination to make himself completely numb during the time he would be sacrificed to her pleasure.

The door closed and he turned to find the dumpy figure, surmounted by the atrocious hat, coming toward him. "Well," she said, "you only live once and paying a little more for it, I at least won't meet myself coming and going."

"Some day I'll start making money," Julian said gloomily—he knew he never would—"and you can have one of those jokes whenever you take the fit." But first they would move. He visualized a place where the nearest neighbors would be three miles away on either side.

"I think you're doing fine," she said, drawing on her gloves. "You've only been out of school a year. Rome wasn't built in a day."

She was one of the few members of the Y reducing class who arrived in hat and gloves and who had a son who had been to college. "It takes time," she said, "and the world is in such a mess. This hat looked better on me than any of the others, though when she brought it out I said, 'Take that thing back. I wouldn't have it on my head,' and she said, 'Now wait till you see it on,' and when she put it on me, I said, 'We-ull,' and she said, 'If you ask me, that hat does something for you and you do something for the hat, and besides,' she said, 'with that hat, you won't meet yourself coming and going.' "

Julian thought he could have stood his lot better if she had been selfish, if she had been an old hag who drank and screamed at him. He walked along, saturated in depression, as if in the midst of his martyrdom he had lost his faith. Catching sight of his long, hopeless, irritated face, she stopped suddenly with a grief-stricken look, and pulled back on his arm. "Wait on me," she said. "I'm going back to the house and take this thing off and to-morrow I'm going to return it. I was out of my head. I can pay the gas bill with that seven-fifty."

He caught her arm in a vicious grip. "You are not going to take it back," he said. "I like it."

"Well," she said, "I don't think I ought . . . "

"Shut up and enjoy it," he muttered, more depressed than ever.

"With the world in the mess it's in," she said, "it's a wonder we can enjoy anything. I tell you, the bottom rail is on the top."

Julian sighed.

"Of course," she said, "if you know who you are, you can go anywhere." She said this every time he took her to the reducing class. "Most of them in it are not our kind of people," she said, "but I can be gracious to anybody. I know who I am."

"They don't give a damn for your graciousness," Julian said savagely. "Knowing who you are is good for one generation only. You haven't the foggiest idea where you stand now or who you are."

She stopped and allowed her eyes to flash at him. "I most certainly do know who I am," she said, "and if you don't know who you are, I'm ashamed of you."

"Oh hell," Julian said.

"Your great-grandfather was a former governor of this state," she said. "Your grandfather was a prosperous landowner. Your grandmother was a Godhigh."

"Will you look around you," he said tensely, "and see where you are now?" and he swept his arm jerkily out to indicate the neighborhood, which the growing darkness at least made less dingy.

"You remain what you are," she said. "Your great-grandfather had a plantation and two hundred slaves."

"There are no more slaves," he said irritably.

"They were better off when they were," she said. He groaned to see that she was off on that topic. She rolled onto it every few days like a train on an open track. He knew every stop, every junction, every swamp along the way, and knew the exact point at which her conclusion would roll majestically into the station: "It's ridiculous. It's simply not realistic. They should rise, yes, but on their own side of the fence."

"Let's skip it," Julian said.

"The ones I feel sorry for," she said, "are the ones that are half white. They're tragic."

"Will you skip it?"

"Suppose we were half white. We would certainly have mixed feelings."

"I have mixed feelings now," he groaned.

"Well let's talk about something pleasant," she said. "I remember going to Grandpa's when I was a little girl. Then the house had double stairways that went up to what was really the second floor—all the cooking was done on the first. I used to like to stay down in the kitchen on account of the way the walls smelled. I would sit with my nose pressed against the plaster and take deep breaths. Actually the place belonged to the Godhighs but your grandfather Chestny paid the mortgage and saved it for them. They were in reduced circumstances," she said, "but reduced or not, they never forgot who they were."

"Doubtless that decayed mansion reminded them," Julian muttered. He never spoke of it without contempt or thought of it without longing. He had seen it once when he was a child before it had been sold. The double stairways had rotted and been torn down. Negroes were living in it. But it remained in his mind as his mother had known it. It appeared in his dreams regularly. He would stand on the wide porch, listening to the rustle of oak leaves, then wander through the high-ceilinged hall into the parlor that opened onto it and gaze at the worn rugs and faded draperies. It occurred to him that it was he, not she, who could have appreciated it. He preferred its threadbare elegance to anything he could name and it was because of it that all the neighborhoods they had lived in had been a torment to him—whereas she had hardly known the difference. She called her insensitivity "being adjustable."

"And I remember the old darky who was my nurse, Caroline. There was no better person in the world. I've always had a great respect for my colored friends," she said. "I'd do anything in the world for them and they'd . . . "

"Will you for God's sake get off that subject?" Julian said. When he got on a bus by himself, he made it a point to sit down beside a Negro, in reparation as it were for his mother's sins.

"You're mighty touchy tonight," she said. "Do you feel all right?"

"Yes I feel all right," he said. "Now lay off."

She pursed her lips. "Well, you certainly are in a vile humor," she observed. "I just won't speak to you at all."

They had reached the bus stop. There was no bus in sight and Julian, his hands still jammed in his pockets and his head thrust forward, scowled down the empty street. The frustration of having to wait on the bus as well as ride on it began to creep up his neck like a hot hand. The presence of his mother was borne in upon him as she gave a pained sigh. He looked at her bleakly. She was holding herself very erect under the preposterous hat, wearing it like a banner of her imaginary dignity. There was in him an evil urge to break her spirit. He suddenly unloosened his tie and pulled it off and put it in his pocket.

She stiffened. "Why must you look like *that* when you take me to town?" she said. "Why must you deliberately embarrass me?"

"If you'll never learn where you are," he said, "you can at least learn where I am."

"You look like a—thug," she said.

"Then I must be one," he murmured.

"I'll just go home," she said. "I will not bother you. If you can't do a little thing like that for me . . . "

Rolling his eyes upward, he put his tie back on. "Restored to my class," he muttered. He thrust his face toward her and hissed, "True culture is in the mind, the *mind*," he said, and tapped his head, "the mind."

"It's in the heart," she said, "and in how you do things and how you do things is because of who you *are*."

"Nobody in the damn bus cares who you are."

"I care who I am," she said icily.

The lighted bus appeared on the top of the next hill and as it approached, they moved out into the street to meet it. He put his hand under her elbow and hoisted her up on the creaking step. She entered with a little smile, as if she were going into a drawing room where everyone had been waiting for her. While he put in the tokens, she sat down on one of the broad front seats for three which faced the aisle. A thin woman with protruding teeth and long yellow hair was sitting on the end of it. His mother moved up beside her and left room for Julian beside herself. He sat down and looked at the floor across the aisle where a pair of thin feet in red and white canvas sandals were planted.

His mother immediately began a general conversation meant to attract anyone who felt like talking. "Can it get any hotter?" she said and removed from her purse a folding fan, black with a Japanese scene on it, which she began to flutter before her.

"I reckon it might could," the woman with the protruding teeth said, "but I know for a fact my apartment couldn't get no hotter."

"It must get the afternoon sun," his mother said. She sat forward and looked up and down the bus. It was half filled. Everybody was white. "I see we have the bus to ourselves," she said. Julian cringed.

"For a change," said the woman across the aisle, the owner of the red and white canvas sandals. "I come on one the other day and they were thick as fleas—up front and all through."

"The world is in a mess everywhere," his mother said. "I don't know how we've let it get in this fix."

"What gets my goat is all those boys from good families stealing automobile tires," the woman with the protruding teeth said. "I told my boy, I said you may not be rich but you been raised right and if I ever catch you in any such mess, they can send you on to the reformatory. Be exactly where you belong."

"Training tells," his mother said. "Is your boy in high school?"

"Ninth grade," the woman said.

"My son just finished college last year. He wants to write but he's selling typewriters until he gets started," his mother said.

The woman leaned forward and peered at Julian. He threw her such a malevolent look that she subsided against the seat. On the floor across the aisle there was an abandoned newspaper. He got up and got it and opened it out in front of him. His mother discreetly continued the conversation in a lower tone but the woman across the aisle said in a loud voice, "Well that's nice. Selling typewriters is close to writing. He can go right from one to the other."

"I tell him," his mother said, "that Rome wasn't built in a day."

Behind the newspaper Julian was withdrawing into the inner compartment of his mind where he spent most of his time. This was a kind of mental bubble in which he established himself when he could not bear to be a part of what was going on around him. From it he could see out and judge but in it he was safe from any kind of penetration from without. It was the only place where he felt free of the general idiocy of his fellows. His mother had never entered it but from it he could see her with absolute clarity.

The old lady was clever enough and he thought that if she had started from any of the right premises, more might have been expected of her. She lived according to the laws of her own fantasy world, outside of which he had never seen her set foot. The law of it was to sacrifice herself for him after she had first created the necessity to do so by making a mess of things. If he had permitted her sacrifices, it was only because her lack of foresight had made them necessary. All of her life had been a struggle to act like a Chestny without the Chestny goods, and to give him everything she thought a Chestny ought to have; but since, said she, it was fun to struggle, why complain? And when you had won, as she had won, what fun to look back on the hard times! He could not forgive her that she had enjoyed the struggle and that she thought *she* had won.

What she meant when she said she had won was that she had brought him up successfully and had sent him to college and that he had turned out so well—good looking (her teeth had gone unfilled so that his could be straightened), intelligent (he realized he was too intelligent to be a success), and with a future ahead of him (there was of course no future ahead of him). She excused his gloominess on the grounds that he was still growing up and his radical ideas on his lack of practical experience. She said he didn't yet know a thing about "life," that he hadn't even entered the real world—when already he was as disenchanted with it as a man of fifty.

The further irony of all this was that in spite of her, he had turned out so well. In spite of going to only a third-rate college, he had, on his own initiative, come out with a first-rate education; in spite of growing up dominated by a small mind, he had ended up with a large one; in spite of all her foolish views, he was free of prejudice and unafraid to face facts. Most miraculous of all, instead of being blinded by love for her as she was for him, he had cut himself emotionally free of her and could see her with complete objectivity. He was not dominated by his mother.

The bus stopped with a sudden jerk and shook him from his meditation. A woman from the back lurched forward with little steps and barely escaped falling in his newspaper as she righted herself. She got off and a large Negro got on. Julian kept his paper lowered to watch. It gave him a certain satisfaction to see injustice in daily operation. It confirmed his view that with a few exceptions there was no one worth knowing within a radius of three hundred miles. The Negro was well dressed and carried a briefcase. He looked around and then sat down on the other end of the seat where the woman with the red and white canvas sandals was sitting. He immediately unfolded a newspaper and obscured himself behind it. Julian's mother's elbow at once prodded insistently into his ribs. "Now you see why I won't ride on these buses by myself," she whispered.

The woman with the red and white canvas sandals had risen at the same time the Negro sat down and had gone further back in the bus and taken the seat of the woman who had got off. His mother leaned forward and cast her an approving look.

Julian rose, crossed the aisle, and sat down in the place of the woman with the canvas sandals. From this position, he looked serenely across at his mother. Her face had turned an angry red. He stared at her, making his eyes the eyes of a stranger. He felt his tension suddenly lift as if he had openly declared war on her.

He would have liked to get in conversation with the Negro and to talk with him about art or politics or any subject that would be above the comprehension of those around them, but the man remained entrenched behind his paper. He was either ignoring the change of seating or had never noticed it. There was no way for Julian to convey his sympathy.

His mother kept her eyes fixed reproachfully on his face. The woman with the protruding teeth was looking at him avidly as if he were a type of monster new to her.

"Do you have a light?" he asked the Negro.

Without looking away from his paper, the man reached in his pocket and handed him a packet of matches.

"Thanks," Julian said. For a moment he held the matches foolishly. A NO SMOKING sign looked down upon him from over the door. This alone would not have deterred him; he had no cigarettes. He had quit smoking some months before because he could not afford it. "Sorry," he muttered and handed back the matches. The Negro lowered the paper and gave him an annoyed look. He took the matches and raised the paper again.

His mother continued to gaze at him but she did not take advantage of his momentary discomfort. Her eyes retained their battered look. Her face seemed to be unnaturally red, as if her blood pressure had risen. Julian allowed no glimmer of sympathy to show on his face. Having got the advantage, he wanted desperately to keep it and carry it through. He would have liked to teach her a lesson that would last her a while, but there seemed no way to continue the point. The Negro refused to come out from behind his paper.

Julian folded his arms and looked stolidly before him, facing her but as if he did not see her, as if he had ceased to recognize her existence. He visualized a scene in which, the bus having reached their stop, he would remain in his seat and when she said, "Aren't you going to get off?" he would look at her as at a stranger who had rashly addressed him. The corner they got off on was usually deserted, but it was well lighted and it would not hurt her to walk by herself the four blocks to the Y. He decided to wait until the time came and then decide whether or not he would let her get off by herself. He would have to be at the Y at ten to bring her back, but he could leave her wondering if he was going to show up. There was no reason for her to think she could always depend on him.

He retired again into the high-ceilinged room sparsely settled with large pieces of antique furniture. His soul expanded momentarily but then he became aware of his mother across from him and the vision shriveled. He studied her coldly. Her feet in little pumps dangled like a child's and did not quite reach the floor. She was training on him an exaggerated look of reproach. He felt completely detached from her. At that moment he could with pleasure have slapped her as he would have slapped a particularly obnoxious child in his charge.

He began to imagine various unlikely ways by which he could teach her a lesson. He might make friends with some distinguished Negro professor or lawyer and bring him home to spend the evening. He would be entirely justified but her blood pressure would rise to 300. He could not push her to the extent of making her have a stroke, and moreover, he had never been successful at making any Negro friends. He had tried to strike up an acquaintance on the bus with some of the better types, with ones that looked like professors or ministers or lawyers. One morning he had sat down next to a distinguished-looking dark brown man who had answered his questions with a sonorous solemnity but who had turned out to be an undertaker. Another day he had sat down beside a cigar-smoking Negro with a diamond ring on his finger, but after a few stilted pleasantries, the Negro had rung the buzzer and risen, slipping two lottery tickets into Julian's hand as he climbed over him to leave.

He imagined his mother lying desperately ill and his being able to secure only a Negro doctor for her. He toyed with that idea for a few minutes and then dropped it for a momentary vision of himself participating as a sympathizer in a sit-in demonstration. This was possible but he did not linger with it. Instead, he approached the ultimate horror. He brought home a beautiful suspiciously Negroid woman. Prepare yourself, he said. There is nothing you can do about it. This is the woman I've chosen. She's intelligent, dignified, even good, and she's suffered and she hasn't thought it *fun*. Now persecute us, go ahead and persecute us. Drive her out of here, but remember, you're driving me too. His eyes were narrowed and through the indignation he had generated, he saw his mother across the aisle, purple-faced, shrunken to the dwarf-like proportions of her moral nature, sitting like a mummy beneath the ridiculous banner of her hat.

He was tilted out of his fantasy again as the bus stopped. The door opened with a sucking hiss and out of the dark a large, gaily dressed, sullen-looking colored woman got on with a little boy. The child, who might have been four, had on a short plaid suit and a Tyrolean hat with a blue feather in it. Julian hoped that he would sit down beside him and that the woman would push in beside his mother. He could think of no better arrangement.

As she waited for her tokens, the woman was surveying the seating possibilities—he hoped with the idea of sitting where she was least wanted. There was something familiar-looking about her but Julian could not place what it was. She was a giant of a woman. Her face was set not only to meet opposition but to seek it out. The downward tilt of her large lower lip was like a warning sign: DON'T TAMPER WITH ME. Her bulging figure was encased in a green crepe dress and her feet overflowed in red shoes. She had on a hideous hat. A purple velvet flap came down on one side of it and stood up on the other; the rest of it was green and looked like a cushion with the stuffing out. She carried a mammoth red pocketbook that bulged throughout as if it were stuffed with rocks.

To Julian's disappointment, the little boy climbed up on the empty seat beside his mother. His mother lumped all children, black and white, into the common category, "cute," and she thought little Negroes were on the whole cuter than little white children. She smiled at the little boy as he climbed on the seat.

Meanwhile the woman was bearing down upon the empty seat beside Julian. To his annoyance, she squeezed herself into it. He saw his mother's face change as the woman settled herself next to him and he realized with satisfaction that this was more objectionable to her than it was to him. Her face seemed almost gray and there was a look of dull recognition in her eyes, as if suddenly she had sickened at some awful confrontation. Julian saw that it was because she and the woman had, in a sense, swapped sons. Though his mother would not realize the symbolic significance of this, she would feel it. His amusement showed plainly on his face.

The woman next to him muttered something unintelligible to herself. He was conscious of a kind of bristling next to him, a muted growling like that of an angry cat. He could not see anything but the red pocketbook upright on the bulging green thighs. He visualized the woman as she had stood waiting for her tokens—the ponderous figure, rising from the red shoes upward over the solid hips, the mammoth bosom, the haughty face, to the green and purple hat.

His eyes widened.

The vision of the two hats, identical, broke upon him with the radiance of a brilliant sunrise. His face was suddenly lit with joy. He could not believe that Fate had thrust upon his mother such a lesson. He gave a loud chuckle so that she would look at him and see that he saw. She turned her eyes on him slowly. The blue in them seemed to have turned a bruised purple. For a moment he had an uncomfortable sense of her innocence, but it lasted only a second before principle rescued him. Justice entitled him to laugh. His grin hardened until it said to her as plainly as if he were saying aloud: Your punishment exactly fits your pettiness. This should teach you a permanent lesson.

Her eyes shifted to the woman. She seemed unable to bear looking at him and to find the woman preferable. He became conscious again of the bristling presence at his side. The woman was rumbling like a volcano about to become active. His mother's mouth began to twitch slightly at one corner. With a sinking heart, he saw incipient signs of recovery on her face and realized that this was going to strike her suddenly as funny and was going to be no lesson at all. She kept her eyes on the woman and an amused smile came over her face as if the woman were a monkey that had stolen her hat. The little Negro was looking up at her with large fascinated eyes. He had been trying to attract her attention for some time.

"Carver!" the woman said suddenly. "Come heah!"

When he saw that the spotlight was on him at last, Carver drew his feet up and turned himself toward Julian's mother and giggled.

"Carver!" the woman said. "You heah me? Come heah!"

Carver slid down from the seat but remained squatting with his back against the base of it, his head turned slyly around toward Julian's mother, who was smiling at him. The woman reached a hand across the aisle and snatched him to her. He righted himself and hung backwards on her knees, grinning at Julian's mother. "Isn't he cute?" Julian's mother said to the woman with the protruding teeth.

"I reckon he is," the woman said without conviction.

The Negress yanked him upright but he eased out of her grip and shot across the aisle and scrambled, giggling wildly, onto the seat beside his love.

"I think he likes me," Julian's mother said, and smiled at the woman. It was the smile she used when she was being particularly gracious to an inferior. Julian saw everything lost. The lesson had rolled off her like rain on a roof.

The woman stood up and yanked the little boy off the seat as if she were snatching him from contagion. Julian could feel the rage in her at having no weapon like his mother's smile. She gave the child a sharp slap across his leg. He howled once and then thrust his head into her stomach and kicked his feet against her shins. "Be-have," she said vehemently.

The bus stopped and the Negro who had been reading the newspaper got off. The woman moved over and set the little boy down with a thump between herself and Julian. She held him firmly by the knee. In a moment he put his hands in front of his face and peeped at Julian's mother through his fingers.

"I see yoooooooo!" she said and put her hand in front of her face and peeped at him.

The woman slapped his hand down. "Quit yo' foolishness," she said, "before I knock the living Jesus out of you!"

Julian was thankful that the next stop was theirs. He reached up and pulled the cord. The woman reached up and pulled it at the same time. Oh my God, he thought. He had the terrible intuition that when they got off the bus together, his mother would open her purse and give the little boy a nickel. The gesture would be as natural to her as breathing. The bus stopped and the woman got up and lunged to the front, dragging the child, who wished to stay on, after her. Julian and his mother got up and followed. As they neared the door, Julian tried to relieve her of her pocketbook.

"No," she murmured, "I want to give the little boy a nickel."

"No!" Julian hissed. "No!"

She smiled down at the child and opened her bag. The bus door opened and the woman picked him up by the arm and descended with him, hanging at her hip. Once in the street she set him down and shook him.

Julian's mother had to close her purse while she got down the bus step but as soon as her feet were on the ground, she opened it again and began to rummage inside. "I can't find but a penny," she whispered, "but it looks like a new one."

"Don't do it!" Julian said fiercely between his teeth. There was a streetlight on the corner and she hurried to get under it so that she could better see into her pocketbook. The woman was heading off rapidly down the street with the child still hanging backward on her hand.

"Oh little boy!" Julian's mother called and took a few quick steps and caught up with them just beyond the lamppost. "Here's a bright new penny for you," and she held out the coin, which shone bronze in the dim light.

The huge woman turned and for a moment stood, her shoulders lifted and her face frozen with frustrated rage, and stared at Julian's mother. Then all at once she seemed to explode like a piece of machinery that had been given one ounce of pressure too much. Julian saw the black fist swing out with the red pocketbook. He shut his eyes and cringed as he heard the woman shout, "He don't take nobody's pennies!" When he opened his eyes, the woman was disappearing down the street with the little boy staring wide-eyed over her shoulder. Julian's mother was sitting on the sidewalk.

"I told you not to do that," Julian said angrily. "I told you not to do that!"

He stood over her for a minute, gritting his teeth. Her legs were stretched out in front of her and her hat was on her lap. He squatted down and looked her in the face. It was totally expressionless. "You got exactly what you deserved," he said. "Now get up."

He picked up her pocketbook and put what had fallen out back in it. He picked the hat up off her lap. The penny caught his eye on the sidewalk and he picked that up and let it drop before her eyes into the purse. Then he stood up and leaned over and held his hands out to pull her up. She remained immobile. He sighed. Rising above them on either side were black apartment buildings, marked with irregular rectangles of light. At the end of the block a man came out of a door and walked off in the opposite direction. "All right," he said, "suppose somebody happens by and wants to know why you're sitting on the sidewalk?"

She took the hand and, breathing hard, pulled heavily up on it and then stood for a moment, swaying slightly as if the spots of light in the darkness were circling around her. Her eyes, shadowed and confused, finally settled on his face. He did not try to conceal his irritation. "I hope this teaches you a lesson," he said. She leaned forward and her eyes raked his face. She seemed trying to determine his identity. Then, as if she found nothing familiar about him, she started off with a headlong movement in the wrong direction.

"Aren't you going on to the Y?" he asked.

"Home," she muttered.

"Well, are we walking?"

For answer she kept going. Julian followed along, his hands behind him. He saw no reason to let the lesson she had had go without backing it up with an explanation of its meaning. She might as well be made to understand what had happened to her. "Don't think that was just an uppity Negro woman," he said. "That was the whole colored race which will no longer take your condescending pennies. That was your black double. She can wear the same hat as you, and to be sure," he added gratuitously (because he thought it was funny), "it looked better on her than it did on you. What all this means," he said, "is that the old world is gone. The old manners are obsolete and your graciousness is not worth a damn." He thought bitterly of the house that had been lost for him. "You aren't who you think you are," he said.

She continued to plow ahead, paying no attention to him. Her hair had come undone on one side. She dropped her pocketbook and took no notice. He stooped and picked it up and handed it to her but she did not take it.

"You needn't act as if the world had come to an end," he said, "because it hasn't. From now on you've got to live in a new world and face a few realities for a change. Buck up," he said, "it won't kill you."

She was breathing fast.

"Let's wait on the bus," he said.

"Home," she said thickly.

"I hate to see you behave like this," he said. "Just like a child. I should be able to expect more of you." He decided to stop where he was and make her stop and wait for a bus. "I'm not going any farther," he said, stopping. "We're going on the bus."

She continued to go on as if she had not heard him. He took a few steps and caught her arm and stopped her. He looked into her face and caught his breath. He was looking into a face he had never seen before. "Tell Grandpa to come get me," she said.

He stared, stricken.

"Tell Caroline to come get me," she said.

Stunned, he let her go and she lurched forward again, walking as if one leg were shorter than the other. A tide of darkness seemed to be sweeping her from him. "Mother!" he cried. "Darling, sweetheart, wait!" Crumpling, she fell to the pavement. He dashed forward and fell at her side, crying, "Mamma, Mamma!" He turned her over. Her face was fiercely distorted. One eye, large and staring, moved slightly to the left as if it had become unmoored. The other remained fixed on him, raked his face again, found nothing and closed.

"Wait here, wait here!" he cried and jumped up and began to run for help toward a cluster of lights he saw in the distance ahead of him. "Help, help!" he shouted, but his voice was thin, scarcely a thread of sound. The lights drifted farther away the faster he ran and his feet moved numbly as if they carried him nowhere. The tide of darkness seemed to sweep him back to her, postponing from moment to moment his entry into the world of guilt and sorrow.

The Jewbird

The window was open so the skinny bird flew in. Flappity-flap with its frazzled black wings. That's how it goes. It's open, you're in. Closed, you're out and that's your fate. The bird wearily flapped through the open kitchen window of Harry Cohen's top-floor apartment of First Avenue near the lower East River. On a rod on the wall hung an escaped canary cage, its door wide open, but this black-type longbeaked bird—its ruffled head and small dull eyes, crossed a little, making it look like a dissipated crow—landed if not smack on Cohen's thick lamb chop, at least on the table, close by. The frozen foods salesman was sitting at supper with his wife and young son on a hot August evening a year ago. Cohen, a heavy man with hairy chest and beefy shorts; Edie, in skinny yellow shorts and red halter; and their ten-year-old Morris (after her father)—Maurie, they called him, a nice kid though not overly bright—were all in the city after two weeks out, because Cohen's mother was dying. They had been enjoying Kingston, New York, but drove back when Mama got sick in her flat in the Bronx.

"Right on the table," said Cohen, putting down his beer glass and swatting at the bird. "Son of a bitch."

"Harry, take care with your language," Edie said, looking at Maurie, who watched every move.

The bird cawed hoarsely and with a flap of its bedraggled wings—feathers tufted this way and that—rose heavily to the top of the open kitchen door, where it perched staring down.

"Gevalt, a pogrom!"

"It's a talking bird," said Edie in astonishment.

"In Jewish," said Maurie.

"Wise guy," muttered Cohen. He gnawed on his chop, then put down the bone. "So if you can talk, say what's your business. What do you want here?"

"If you can't spare a lamb chop," said the bird, "I'll settle for a piece of herring with a crust of bread. You can't live on your nerve forever."

"This ain't a restaurant," Cohen replied. "All I'm asking is what brings you to this address?"

"The window was open," the bird sighed; adding after a moment, "I'm running. I'm flying but I'm also running."

"From whom?" asked Edie with interest.

"Anti-Semeets."

"Anti-Semites?" they all said.

"That's from who."

"What kind of anti-Semites bother a bird?" Edie asked.

"Any kind," said the bird, "also including eagles, vultures, and hawks. And once in a while some crows will take your eyes out."

"But aren't you a crow?"

"Me? I'm a Jewbird."

Cohen laughed heartily. "What do you mean by that?"

The bird began dovening. He prayed without Book or tallith, but with passion. Edie bowed her head though not Cohen. And Maurie rocked back and forth with the prayer, looking up with one wide-open eye.

When the prayer was done Cohen remarked, "No hat, no phylacteries?"

"I'm an old radical."

"You're sure you're not some kind of a ghost or dybbuk?"

"Not a dybbuk," answered the bird, "though one of my relatives had such an experience once. It's all over now, thanks God. They freed her from a former lover, a crazy jealous man. She's now the mother of two wonderful children."

"Birds?" Cohen asked slyly.

"Why not?"

"What kind of birds?"

"Like me. Jewbirds."

Cohen tipped back in his chair and guffawed. "That's a big laugh. I've heard of a Jewfish but not a Jewbird."

"We're once removed." The bird rested on one skinny leg, then on the other. "Please, could you spare maybe a piece of herring with a small crust of bread?"

Edie got up from the table.

"What are you doing?" Cohen asked her.

"I'll clear the dishes."

Cohen turned to the bird. "So what's your name, if you don't mind saying?"

"Call me Schwartz."

"He might be an old Jew changed into a bird by somebody," said Edie, removing a plate.

"Are you?" asked Harry, lighting a cigar.

"Who knows?" answered Schwartz. "Does God tell us everything?"

Maurie got up on his chair. "What kind of herring?" he asked the bird in excitement.

"Get down, Maurie, or you'll fall," ordered Cohen.

"If you haven't got matjes, I'll take schmaltz," said Schwartz.

"All we have is marinated, with slices of onion—in a jar," said Edie.

"If you'll open for me the jar I'll eat marinated. Do you have also, if you don't mind, a piece of rye bread—the spitz?"

Edie thought she had.

"Feed him out on the balcony," Cohen said. He spoke to the bird. "After that take off."

Schwartz closed both bird eyes. "I'm tired and it's a long way."

"Which direction are you headed, north or south?"

Schwartz, barely lifting his wings, shrugged.

"You don't know where you're going?"

"Where there's charity I'll go."

"Let him stay, papa," said Maurie. "He's only a bird."

"So stay the night," Cohen said, "but no longer."

In the morning Cohen ordered the bird out of the house but Maurie cried, so Schwartz stayed for a while. Maurie was still on vacation from school and his friends were away. He was lonely and Edie enjoyed the fun he had, playing with the bird.

"He's no trouble at all," she told Cohen, "and besides his appetite is very small."

"What'll you do when he makes dirty?"

"He flies across the street in a tree when he makes dirty, and if nobody passes below, who notices?"

"So all right," said Cohen, "but I'm dead set against it. I warn you he ain't gonna stay here long."

"What have you got against the poor bird?"

"Poor bird, my ass. He's a foxy bastard. He thinks he's a Jew."

"What difference does it make what he thinks?"

"A Jewbird, what a chuzpah. One false move and he's out on his drumsticks."

At Cohen's insistence Schwartz lived out on the balcony in a new wooden birdhouse Edie had bought him.

"With many thanks," said Schwartz, "though I would rather have a human roof over my head. You know how it is at my age. I like the warm, the windows, the smell of cooking. I would also be glad to see once in a while the *Jewish Morning Journal* and have now and then a schnapps because it helps my breathing, thanks God. But whatever you give me, you won't hear complaints."

However, when Cohen brought home a bird feeder full of dried corn, Schwartz said, "Impossible."

Cohen was annoyed. "What's the matter, crosseyes, is your life getting too good for you? Are you forgetting what it means to be migratory? I'll bet a helluva lot of crows you happen to be acquainted with, Jews or otherwise, would give their eyeteeth to eat this corn."

Schwartz did not answer. What can you say to a grubber yung?

"Not for my digestion," he later explained to Edie. "Cramps. Herring is better even if it makes you thirsty. At least rainwater don't cost anything." He laughed sadly in breathy caws.

And herring, thanks to Edie, who knew where to shop, was what Schwartz got, with an occasional piece of potato pancake, and even a bit of soupmeat when Cohen wasn't looking.

When school began in September, before Cohen would once again suggest giving the bird the boot, Edie prevailed on him to wait a little while until Maurie adjusted.

"To deprive him right now might hurt his school work, and you know what trouble we had last year."

"So okay, but sooner or later the bird goes. That I promise you."

Schwartz, though nobody had asked him, took on full responsibility for Maurie's performance in school. In return for favors granted, when he was let in for an hour or two at night, he spent most of his time overseeing the boy's lessons. He sat on top of the dresser near Maurie's desk as he laboriously wrote out his homework. Maurie was a restless type and Schwartz gently kept him to his studies. He also listened to him practice his screechy violin, taking a few minutes off now and then to rest his ears in the bathroom. And they afterwards played dominoes. The boy was an indifferent checker player and it was impossible to teach him chess. When he was sick, Schwartz read him comic books though he personally disliked them. But Maurie's work improved in school and even his violin teacher admitted his playing was better. Edie gave Schwartz credit for these improvements though the bird pooh-poohed them.

Yet he was proud there was nothing lower than C minuses on Maurie's report card, and on Edie's insistence celebrated with a little schnapps.

"If he keeps up like this," Cohen said, "I'll get him in an Ivy League college for sure."

"Oh I hope so," sighed Edie.

But Schwartz shook his head. "He's a good boy—you don't have to worry. He won't be a shicker or a wifebeater, God forbid, but a scholar he'll never be, if you know what I mean, although maybe a good mechanic. It's no disgrace in these times."

"If I were you," Cohen said, angered, "I'd keep my big snoot out of other people's private business."

"Harry, please," said Edie.

"My goddamn patience is wearing out. That crosseyes butts into everything."

Though he wasn't exactly a welcome guest in the house, Schwartz gained a few ounces although he did not improve in appearance. He looked bedraggled as ever, his feathers unkempt, as though he had just flown out of a snowstorm. He spent, he admitted, little time taking care of himself. Too much to think about. "Also outside plumbing," he told Edie. Still there was more glow to his eyes so that though Cohen went on calling him crosseyes he said it less emphatically.

Liking his situation, Schwartz tried tactfully to stay out of Cohen's way, but one night when Edie was at the movies and Maurie was taking a hot shower, the frozen foods salesman began a quarrel with the bird.

"For Christ sake, why don't you wash yourself sometimes? Why must you always stink like a dead fish?"

"Mr. Cohen, if you'll pardon me, if somebody eats garlic he will smell from garlic. I eat herring three times a day. Feed me flowers and I will smell like flowers."

"Who's obligated to feed you anything at all? You're lucky to get herring."

"Excuse me, I'm not complaining," said the bird. "You're complaining."

"What's more," said Cohen, "even from out on the balcony I can hear you snoring away like a pig. It keeps me awake at night."

"Snoring," said Schwartz, "isn't a crime, thanks God."

"All in all you are a goddamn pest and free loader. Next thing you'll want to sleep in bed next to my wife."

"Mr. Cohen," said Schwartz, "on this rest assured. A bird is a bird."

"So you say, but how do I know you're a bird and not some kind of a goddamn devil?"

"If I was a devil you would know already. And I don't mean because your son's good marks."

"Shut up, you bastard bird," shouted Cohen.

"Grubber yung," cawed Schwartz, rising to the tips of his talons, his long wings outstretched.

Cohen was about to lunge for the bird's scrawny neck but Maurie came out of the bathroom, and for the rest of the evening until Schwartz's bedtime on the balcony, there was pretended peace.

But the quarrel had deeply disturbed Schwartz and he slept badly. His snoring woke him, and awake, he was fearful of what would become of him. Wanting to stay out of Cohen's way, he kept to the birdhouse as much as possible. Cramped by it, he paced back and forth on the balcony ledge, or sat on the birdhouse roof, staring into space. In the evenings, while overseeing Maurie's lessons, he often fell asleep. Awakening, he nervously hopped around exploring the four corners of the room. He spent much time in Maurie's closet, and carefully examined his bureau drawers when they were left open. And once when he found a large paper bag on the floor, Schwartz poked his way into it to investigate what possibilities were. The boy was amused to see the bird in the paper bag.

"He wants to build a nest," he said to his mother.

Edie, sensing Schwartz's unhappiness, spoke to him quietly.

"Maybe if you did some of the things my husband wants you, you would get along better with him."

"Give me a for instance," Schwartz said.

"Like take a bath, for instance."

"I'm too old for baths," said the bird. "My feathers fall out without baths."

"He says you have a bad smell."

"Everybody smells. Some people smell because of their thoughts or because who they are. My bad smell comes from the food I eat. What does his come from?"

"I better not ask him or it might make him mad," said Edie.

In late November Schwartz froze on the balcony in the fog and cold, and especially on rainy days he woke with stiff joints and could barely move his wings. Already he felt twinges of rheumatism. He would have liked to spend more time in the warm house, particularly when Maurie was in school and Cohen at work. But though Edie was goodhearted and might have sneaked him in in the morning, just to thaw out, he was afraid to ask her. In the meantime Cohen, who had been reading articles about the migration of birds, came out on the balcony one night after work when Edie was in the kitchen preparing pot roast, and peeking into the birdhouse, warned Schwartz to be on his way soon if he knew what was good for him. "Time to hit the flyways."

"Mr. Cohen, why do you hate me so much?" asked the bird. "What did I do to you?"

"Because you're an A-number-one trouble maker, that's why. What's more, whoever heard of a Jewbird? Now scat or it's open war."

But Schwartz stubbornly refused to depart so Cohen embarked on a campaign of harassing him, meanwhile hiding it from Edie and Maurie. Maurie hated violence and Cohen didn't want to leave a bad impression. He thought maybe if he played dirty tricks on the bird he would fly off without being physically kicked out. The vacation was over, let him make his easy living off the fat of somebody else's land. Cohen worried about the effect of the bird's departure on Maurie's schooling but decided to take the chance, first, because the boy now seemed to have the knack of studying—give the black bird-bastard credit—and second, because Schwartz was driving him bats by being there always, even in his dreams.

The frozen foods salesman began his campaign against the bird by mixing watery cat food with the herring slices in Schwartz's dish. He also blew up and popped numerous paper bags outside the birdhouse as the bird slept, and when he had got Schwartz good and nervous, though not enough to leave, he brought a full-grown cat into the house, supposedly a gift for little Maurie, who had always wanted a pussy. The cat never stopped springing up at Schwartz whenever he saw him, one day managing to claw out several of his tailfeathers. And even at lesson time, when the cat was usually excluded from Maurie's room, though somehow or other he quickly found his way in at the end of the lesson, Schwartz was desperately fearful of his life and flew from pinnacle to pinnacle—light fixture to clothestree to door-top—in order to elude the beast's wet jaws.

Once when the bird complained to Edie how hazardous his existence was, she said, "Be patient, Mr. Schwartz. When the cat gets to know you better he won't try to catch you any more."

"When he stops trying we will both be in Paradise," Schwartz answered. "Do me a favor and get rid of him. He makes my whole life worry. I'm losing feathers like a tree loses leaves."

"I'm awfully sorry but Maurie likes the pussy and sleeps with it."

What could Schwartz do? He worried but came to no decision, being afraid to leave. So he ate the herring garnished with cat food, tried hard not to hear the paper bags bursting like fire crackers outside the birdhouse at night, and lived terror-stricken closer to the ceiling than the floor, as the cat, his tail flicking, endlessly watched him.

Weeks went by. Then on the day after Cohen's mother had died in her flat in the Bronx, when Maurie came home with a zero on an arithmetic test, Cohen, enraged, waited until Edie had taken the boy to his violin lesson, then openly attacked the bird. He chased him with a broom on the balcony and Schwartz frantically flew back and forth, finally escaping into his birdhouse. Cohen triumphantly reached in, and grabbing both skinny legs, dragged the bird out, cawing loudly, his wings wildly beating. He whirled the bird around and around his head. But Schwartz, as he moved in circles, managed to swoop down and catch Cohen's nose in his beak, and hung on for dear life. Cohen cried out in great pain, punched the bird with his fist, and tugging at its legs with all his might, pulled his nose free. Again he swung the yawking Schwartz around until the bird grew dizzy, then with a furious heave, flung him into the night. Schwartz sank like stone into the street. Cohen then tossed the birdhouse and feeder after him, listening at the ledge until they crashed on the sidewalk below. For a full hour, broom in hand, his heart palpitating and nose throbbing with pain, Cohen waited for Schwartz to return but the broken hearted bird didn't.

That's the end of that dirty bastard, the salesman thought and went in. Edie and Maurie had come home.

"Look," said Cohen, pointing to his bloody nose swollen three times its normal size, "what that sonofabitchy bird did. It's a permanent scar."

"Where is he now?" Edie asked, frightened.

"I threw him out and he flew away. Good riddance."

Nobody said no, though Edie touched a handkerchief to her eyes and Maurie rapidly tried the nine times table and found he knew approximately half.

In the spring when the winter's snow had melted, the boy, moved by a memory, wandered in the neighborhood, looking for Schwartz. He found a dead black bird in a small lot near the river, his two wings broken, neck twisted, and both bird-eyes plucked clean.

"Who did it to you, Mr. Schwartz?" Maurie wept.

"Anti-Semeets," Edie said later.

Maggie of the Green Bottles

Maggie had not intended to get sucked in on this thing, sleeping straight through the christening, steering clear of the punch bowl, and refusing to dress for company. But when she glanced over my grandfather's shoulder and saw "Aspire, Enspire, Perspire" scrawled across the first page in that hard-core Protestant hand, and a grease stain from the fried chicken too, something snapped in her head. She snatched up the book and retired rapidly to her room, locked my mother out, and explained through the door that my mother was a fool to encourage a lot of misspelled nonsense from Mr. Tyler's kin, and an even bigger fool for having married the monster in the first place.

I imagine that Maggie sat at her great oak desk, rolled the lace cuffs gently back, and dipped her quill into the lavender ink pot with all the ceremony due the Emancipation Proclamation, which was, after all, exactly what she was drafting. Writing to me, she explained, was serious business, for she felt called upon to liberate me from all historical and genealogical connections except the most divine. In short, the family was a disgrace, degrading Maggie's and my capacity for wings, as they say. I can only say that Maggie was truly inspired. And she probably ruined my life from the get-go.

There is a photo of the two of us on the second page. There's Maggie in Minnie Mouse shoes and a long polka-dot affair with her stockings rolled up at the shins, looking like muffins. There's me with nothing much at all on, in her arms, and looking almost like a normal, mortal, everyday-type baby— raw, wrinkled, ugly. Except that it must be clearly understood straightaway that I sprang into the world full wise and invulnerable and gorgeous like a goddess. Behind us is the player piano with the spooky keys. And behind that, the window outlining Maggie's crosshatched face and looking out over the yard, overgrown even then, where later I lay lost in the high grass, never hoping to be found till Maggie picked me up into her hair and told me all about the earth's moons.

Once just a raggedy thing holding telegrams from well-wishers, the book was pleasant reading on those rainy days when I didn't risk rusting my skates, or maybe just wasn't up to trailing up and down the city streets with the kids, preferring to study Maggie's drawings and try to grab hold of the fearsome machinery which turned the planets and coursed the stars and told me in no uncertain terms that as an Aries babe I was obligated to carry on the work of other Aries greats from Alexander right on down to anyone you care to mention. I could go on to relate all the wise-alecky responses I gave to Maggie's document as an older child rummaging in the trunks among the canceled checks and old sheet music, looking for some suspicioned love letters or some small proof that my mother had once had romance in her life, and finding instead the raggedy little book I thought was just a raggedy little book. But it is much too easy to smile at one's ignorant youth just to flatter one's present wisdom, but I digress.

Because, on my birthday, Saturn was sitting on its ass and Mars was taken unawares, getting bumped by Jupiter's flunkies, I would not be into my own till well past twenty. But according to the cards, and my palm line bore it out, the hangman would spare me till well into my hundredth year. So all in all, the tea leaves having had their say and the coffee-ground patterns being what they were, I was destined for greatness. She assured me. And I was certain of my success, as I was certain that my parents were not my parents, that I was descended, anointed and ready to gobble up the world from urgent, noble Olympiads.

I am told by those who knew her, whose memories consist of something more substantial than a frantic gray lady who poured coffee into her saucer, that Margaret Cooper Williams wanted something she could not have. And it was the sorrow of her life that all her children and theirs and theirs were uncooperative—worse, squeamish. Too busy taking in laundry, buckling at the knees, putting their faith in Jesus, mute and sullen in their sorrow, too squeamish to band together and take the world by storm, make history, or even to appreciate the calling of Maggie the Ram, or the Aries that came after. Other things they told me too, things I put aside to learn later though I always knew, perhaps, but never quite wanted to, the way you hold your breath and steady yourself to the knowledge secretly, but never let yourself understand. They called her crazy.

It is to Maggie's guts that I bow forehead to the floor and kiss her hand, because she'd tackle the lot of them right there in the yard, blood kin or by marriage, and neighbors or no. And anybody who'd stand up to my father, gross Neanderthal that he was, simply had to be some kind of weird combination of David, Aries, and lunatic. It began with the cooking usually, especially the pots of things Maggie concocted. Witchcraft, he called it. Home cooking, she'd counter. Then he'd come over to the stove, lift a lid with an incredible face, and comment about cesspools and fertilizers. But she'd remind him of his favorite dish, chitlins, addressing the bread box, though. He'd turn up the radio and make some remark about good church music and her crazy voodoo records. Then she'd tell the curtains that some men, who put magic down with nothing to replace it and nothing much to recommend them in the first place but their magic wand, lived a runabout life, practicing black magic on other men's wives. Then he'd say something about freeloading relatives and dancing to the piper's tune. And she'd whisper to the kettles that there wasn't no sense in begging from a beggar. Depending on how large an audience they drew, this could go on for hours until my father would cock his head to the side, listening, and then try to make his getaway.

"Ain't nobody calling you, Mr. Tyler, cause don't nobody want you." And I'd feel kind of bad about my father like I do about the wolf man and the phantom of the opera. Monsters, you know, more than anybody else, need your pity cause they need beauty and love so bad.

One day, right about the time Maggie would say something painful that made him bring up freeloaders and piper's tunes, he began to sputter so bad it made me want to cry. But Maggie put the big wooden spoon down and whistled for Mister T—at least that's what Maggie and my grandmother, before she died, insisted on calling him. The dog, always hungry, came bounding through the screen door, stopped on a dime by the sink, and slinked over to Maggie's legs the way beat-up dogs can do, their tails all confused as to just what to do, their eyes unblinkingly watchful. Maggie offered him something from the pot. And when Mister T had finished, he licked Maggie's hand. She began to cackle. And then, before I could even put my milk down, up went Maggie's palm, and *bam*, Mister T went skidding across the linoleum and banged all the seltzer bottles down.

"Damn-fool mutt," said Maggie to her wooden spoon, "too dumb to even know you're supposed to bite the hand that feeds you."

My father threw his hand back and yelled for my mother to drop whatever she was doing, which was standing in the doorway shaking her head, and pack up the old lady's things posthaste. Maggie went right on laughing and talking to the spoon. And Mister T slinked over to the table so Baby Jason could pet him. And then it was name-calling time. And again I must genuflect and kiss her ring, because my father was no slouch when it came to names. He could malign your mother and work your father's lineage over in one short breath, describing in absolute detail all the incredible alliances made between your ancestors and all sorts of weird creatures. But Maggie had him beat there too, old lady in lace talking to spoons or no.

My mother came in weary and worn and gave me a nod. I slid my peanut-butter sandwich off the icebox, grabbed Baby Jason by his harness, and dragged him into our room, where I was supposed to read to him real loud. But I listened, I always listened to my mother's footfalls on the porch to the gravel path and down the hard mud road to the woodshed. Then I could give my attention to the kitchen, for "Goldilocks," keep in mind, never was enough to keep the brain alive. Then, right in the middle of some fierce curse or other, my father did this unbelievable thing. He stomped right into Maggie's room—that sanctuary of heaven charts and incense pots and dream books and magic stuffs. Only Jason, hiding from an August storm, had ever been allowed in there, and that was on his knees crawling. But in he stomped all big and bad like some terrible giant, this man whom Grandma Williams used to say was just the sort of size man put on this earth for the "'spress purpose of clubbing us all to death." And he came out with these green bottles, one in each hand, snorting and laughing at the same time. And I figured, peeping into the kitchen, that these bottles were enchanted, for they had a strange effect on Maggie, she shut right up. They had a strange effect on me too, gleaming there up in the air, nearly touching the ceiling, glinting off the shots of sunshine, grasped in the giant's fist. I was awed.

Whenever I saw them piled in the garbage out back I was tempted to touch them and make a wish, knowing all the while that the charm was all used up and that that was why they were in the garbage in the first place. But there was no doubt that they were special. And whenever Baby Jason managed to drag one out from under the bed, there was much whispering and shuffling on my mother's part. And when Sweet Basil, the grocer's boy, delivered these green bottles to Maggie, it was all hush-hush and backdoor and in the corner dealings, slipping it in and out of innumerable paper bags, holding it up to the light, then off she'd run to her room and be gone for hours, days sometimes, and when she did appear, looking mysterious and in a trance, her face all full of shadows. And she'd sit at the sideboard with that famous cup from the World's Fair, pouring coffee into the saucer and blowing on it very carefully, nodding and humming and swirling the grinds. She called me over once to look at the grinds.

"What does this look like, Peaches?"

"Looks like a star with a piece out of it."

"Hmm," she mumbled, and swirled again. "And now?"

Me peering into the cup and lost for words. "Looks like a face that lost its eyes."

"Hmm," again, as she thrust the cup right under my nose, and me wishing it was a box of falling glass I could look at where I knew what was what instead of looking into the bottom of a fat yellow cup at what looked like nothing but coffee grinds.

"Looks like a mouth losing its breath, Great Granny."

"Let's not get too outrageous, Peaches. This is serious business."

"Yes ma'am." Peering again and trying to be worthy of Alexander and the Ram and all my other forebears. "What it really seems to be"—stalling for time and praying for inspiration—"is an upside-down bird, dead on its back with his heart chopped out and the hole bleeding."

She flicked my hand away when I tried to point the picture out which by now I was beginning to believe. "Go play somewhere, girl," she said. She was mad. "And quit calling me Granny."

"What happened here today?" my mother kept asking all evening, thumping out the fragrant dough and wringing the dishtowel, which was supposed to help the dough rise, wringing it to pieces. I couldn't remember anything particular, following her gaze to Maggie's door. "Was Sweet Basil here this afternoon?" Couldn't remember that either, but tried to show I was her daughter by staring hard at the closed door too. "Was Great Granny up and around at all today?" My memory failed me there too. "You ain't got much memory to speak of at all, do you?" said my father. I hung onto my mother's apron and helped her wring the dishtowel to pieces.

They told me she was very sick, so I had to drag Baby Jason out to the high grass and play with him. It was a hot day and the smell of the kerosene soaking the weeds that were stubborn about dying made my eyes tear. I was face down in the grass just listening, waiting for the afternoon siren which last year I thought was Judgement Day because it blew so long to say that the war was over and that we didn't have to eat Spam any more and that there was a circus coming and a parade and Uncle Bubba too, but with only one leg to show for it all. Maggie came into the yard with her basket of vegetables. She sat down at the edge of the gravel path and began stringing the peppers, red and green, red and green. And, like always, she was humming one of those weird songs of hers which always made her seem holier and blacker than she could've been. I tied Baby Jason to a tree so he wouldn't crawl into her lap, which always annoyed her. Maggie didn't like baby boys, or any kind of boys I'm thinking, but especially baby boys born in Cancer and Pisces or anything but in Aries.

"Look here, Peaches," she called, working the twine through the peppers and dropping her voice real low. "I want you to do this thing for your Great Granny."

"What must I do?" I waited a long time till I almost thought she'd fallen asleep, her head rolling around on her chest and her hands fumbling with the slippery peppers, ripping them.

"I want you to go to my room and pull out the big pink box from under the bed." She looked around and woke up a bit. "This is a secret you-and-me thing now, Peaches." I nodded and waited some more. "Open the box and you'll see a green bottle. Wrap this apron around it and tuck it under your arm like so. Then grab up the mushrooms I left on the side board like that's what you came for in the first place. But get yourself back here right quick." I repeated the instructions, flopped a necklace of peppers around me, and dashed into the hot and dusty house. When I got back she dumped the mushrooms into her lap, tucked the bottle under her skirt, and smiled at the poor little peppers her nervous hands had strung. They hung wet and ruined off the twine like broken-necked little animals.

I was down in the bottoms playing with the state-farm kids when Uncle Bubba came sliding down the sand pile on his one good leg. Jason was already in the station wagon hanging onto my old doll. We stayed at Aunt Min's till my father came to get us in the pickup. Everybody was in the kitchen dividing up Maggie's things. The linen chest went to Aunt Thelma. And the souvenirs from Maggie's honeymoons went to the freckle-faced cousins from town. The clothes were packed for the church. And Reverend Elson was directing the pianist's carrying from the kitchen window. The scattered sopranos, who never ever seemed to get together on their high notes or on their visits like this, were making my mother drink tea and kept nodding at me, saying she was sitting in the mourner's seat, which was just like all the other chairs in the set; same as the amen corner was no better or any less dusty than the rest of the church and not even a corner. Then Reverend Elson turned to say that no matter how crazy she'd been, no matter how hateful she'd acted toward the church in general and him in particular, no matter how spiteful she'd behaved towards her neighbors and even her blood kin, and even though everyone was better off without her, seeing how she died as proof of her heathen character, and right there in the front yard too, with a bottle under her skirts, the sopranos joined in scattered as ever, despite all that, the Reverend Elson continued, God rest her soul, if He saw fit, that is.

The china darning egg went into Jason's overalls. And the desk went into my room. Bubba said he wanted the books for his children. And they all gave him such a look. My mother just sat in the kitchen chair called the mourner's seat and said nothing at all except that they were selling the house and moving to the city.

"Well, Peaches," my father said. "You were her special, what you want?"

"I'll take the bottles," I said.

"Let us pray," said the Reverend.

That night I sat at the desk and read the baby book for the first time. It sounded like Maggie for the world, holding me in her lap and spreading the charts on the kitchen table. I looked my new bottle collection over. There were purple bottles with glass stoppers and labels. There were squat blue bottles with squeeze tops but nothing in them. There were flat red bottles that could hold only one flower at a time. I had meant the green bottles. I was going to tell them and then I didn't. I was too small for so much enchantment anyway. I went to bed feeling much too small. And it seemed a shame that the hope of the Aries line should have to sleep with a light on still, and blame it on Jason and cry with balled fists in the eyes just like an ordinary, mortal, everyday-type baby.

The Joy Luck Club

My father has asked me to be the fourth corner at the Joy Luck Club. I am to replace my mother, whose seat at the mah jong table has been empty since she died two months ago. My father thinks she was killed by her own thoughts.

"She had a new idea inside her head," said my father. "But before it could come out of her mouth, the thought grew too big and burst. It must have been a very bad idea."

The doctor said she died of a cerebral aneurysm. And her friends at the Joy Luck Club said she died just like a rabbit: quickly and with unfinished business left behind. My mother was supposed to host the next meeting of the Joy Luck Club.

The week before she died, she called me, full of pride, full of life: "Auntie Lin cooked red bean soup for Joy Luck. I'm going to cook black sesame-seed soup."

"Don't show off," I said.

"It's not showoff." She said the two soups were almost the same, *chabudwo*. Or maybe she said *butong*, not the same thing at all. It was one of those Chinese expressions that means the better half of mixed intentions. I can never remember things I didn't understand in the first place.

My mother started the San Francisco version of the Joy Luck Club in 1949, two years before I was born. This was the year my mother and father left China with one stiff leather trunk filled only with fancy silk dresses. There was no time to pack anything else, my mother had explained to my father after they boarded the boat. Still his hands swam frantically between the slippery silks, looking for his cotton shirts and wool pants.

When they arrived in San Francisco, my father made her hide those shiny clothes. She wore the same brown-checked Chinese dress until the Refugee Welcome Society gave her two hand-me-down dresses, all too large in sizes for American women. The society was composed of a group of white-haired American missionary ladies from the First Chinese Baptist Church. And because of their gifts, my parents could not refuse their invitation to join the church. Nor could they ignore the old ladies' practical advice to improve

219

their English through Bible study class on Wednesday nights and, later, through choir practice on Saturday mornings. This was how my parents met the Hsus, the Jongs, and the St. Clairs. My mother could sense that the women of these families also had unspeakable tragedies they had left behind in China and hopes they couldn't begin to express in their fragile English. Or at least, my mother recognized the numbness in these women's faces. And she saw how quickly their eyes moved when she told them her idea for the Joy Luck Club.

Joy Luck was an idea my mother remembered from the days of her first marriage in Kweilin, before the Japanese came. That's why I think of Joy Luck as her Kweilin story. It was the story she would always tell me when she was bored, when there was nothing to do, when every bowl had been washed and the Formica table had been wiped down twice, when my father sat reading the newspaper and smoking one Pall Mall cigarette after another, a warning not to disturb him. This is when my mother would take out a box of old ski sweaters sent to us by unseen relatives from Vancouver. She would snip the bottom of a sweater and pull out a kinky thread of yarn, anchoring it to a piece of cardboard. And as she began to roll with one sweeping rhythm, she would start her story. Over the years, she told me the same story, except for the ending, which grew darker, casting long shadows into her life, and eventually into mine.

"I dreamed about Kweilin before I ever saw it," my mother began, speaking Chinese. "I dreamed of jagged peaks lining a curving river, with magic moss greening the banks. At the tops of these peaks were white mists. And if you could float down this river and eat the moss for food, you would be strong enough to climb the peak. If you slipped, you would only fall into a bed of soft moss and laugh. And once you reached the top, you would be able to see everything and feel such happiness it would be enough to never have worries in your life ever again.

"In China, everybody dreamed about Kweilin. And when I arrived, I realized how shabby my dreams were, how poor my thoughts. When I saw the hills, I laughed and shuddered at the same time. The peaks looked like giant fried fish heads trying to jump out of a vat of oil. Behind each hill, I could see shadows of another fish, and then another and another. And then the clouds would move just a little and the hills would suddenly become monstrous elephants marching slowly toward me! Can you see this? And at the root of the hill were secret caves. Inside grew hanging rock gardens in the shapes and colors of cabbage, winter melons, turnips, and onions. These were things so strange and beautiful you can't ever imagine them.

"But I didn't come to Kweilin to see how beautiful it was. The man who was my husband brought me and our two babies to Kweilin because he thought we would be safe. He was an officer with the Kuomintang, and after he put us down in a small room in a two-story house, he went off to the northwest, to Chungking.

"We knew the Japanese were winning, even when the newspapers said they were not. Every day, every hour, thousands of people poured into the city, crowding the sidewalks, looking for places to live. They came from the East, West, North, and South. They were rich and poor, Shanghainese, Cantonese, northerners, and not just Chinese, but foreigners and missionaries of every religion. And there was, of course, the Kuomintang and their army officers who thought they were top level to everyone else.

"We were a city of leftovers mixed together. If it hadn't been for the Japanese, there would have been plenty of reason for fighting to break out among these different people. Can you see it? Shanghai people with north-water peasants, bankers with barbers, rickshaw pullers with Burma refugees. Everybody looked down on someone else. It didn't matter that everybody shared the same sidewalk to spit on and suffered the same fast-moving diarrhea. We all had the same stink, but everybody complained someone else smelled the worst. Me? Oh, I hated the American air force officers who said habba-habba sounds to make my face turn red. But the worst were the northern peasants who emptied their noses into their hands and pushed people around and gave everybody their dirty diseases.

"So you can see how quickly Kweilin lost its beauty for me. I no longer climbed the peaks to say, How lovely are these hills! I only wondered which hills the Japanese had reached. I sat in the dark corners of my house with a baby under each arm, waiting with nervous feet. When the sirens cried out to warn us of bombers, my neighbors and I jumped to our feet and scurried to the deep caves to hide like wild animals. But you can't stay in the dark for so long. Something inside of you starts to fade and you become like a starving person, crazy-hungry for light. Outside I could hear the bombing. Boom! Boom! And then the sound of raining rocks. And inside I was no longer hungry for the cabbage or the turnips of the hanging rock garden. I could only see the dripping bowels of an ancient hill that might collapse on top of me. Can you imagine how it is, to want to be neither inside nor outside, to want to be nowhere and disappear?

"So when the bombing sounds grew farther away, we would come back out like newborn kittens scratching our way back to the city. And always, I would be amazed to find the hills against the burning sky had not been torn apart.

"I thought up Joy Luck on a summer night that was so hot even the moths fainted to the ground, their wings were so heavy with the damp heat. Every place was so crowded there was no room for fresh air. Unbearable smells from the sewers rose up to my second-story window and the stink had nowhere else to go but into my nose. At all hours of the night and day, I heard scream-ing sounds. I didn't know if it was a peasant slitting the throat of a runaway pig or an officer beating a half-dead peasant for lying in his way on the side-walk. I didn't go to the window to find out. What use would it have been? And that's when I thought I needed something to do to help me move.

"My idea was to have a gathering of four women, one for each corner of my mah jong table. I knew which women I wanted to ask. They were all young like me, with wishful faces. One was an army officer's wife, like my-self. Another was a girl with very fine manners from a rich family in Shang-hai. She had escaped with only a little money. And there was a girl from Nanking who had the blackest hair I have ever seen. She came from a low-class family, but she was pretty and pleasant and had married well, to an old man who died and left her with a better life.

"Each week one of us would host a party to raise money and to raise our spirits. The hostess had to serve special *dyansyin* foods to bring good fortune of all kinds—dumplings shaped like silver money ingots, long rice noodles for long life, boiled peanuts for conceiving sons, and of course, many good-luck oranges for a plentiful, sweet life.

"What fine food we treated ourselves to with our meager allowances! We didn't notice that the dumplings were stuffed mostly with stringy squash and that the oranges were spotted with wormy holes. We ate sparingly, not as if we didn't have enough, but to protest how we could not eat another bite, we had already bloated ourselves from earlier in the day. We knew we had lux-uries few people could afford. We were the lucky ones.

"After filling our stomachs, we would then fill a bowl with money and put it where everyone could see. Then we would sit down at the mah jong table. My table was from my family and was of a very fragrant red wood, not what you call rosewood, but *hong mu*, which is so fine there's no English word for it. The table had a very thick pad, so that when the mah jong *pai* were spilled onto the table the only sound was of ivory tiles washing against one another.

"Once we started to play, nobody could speak, except to say 'Pung!' or 'Chr!' when taking a tile. We had to play with seriousness and think of noth-ing else but adding to our happiness through winning. But after sixteen rounds, we would again feast, this time to celebrate our good fortune. And then we would talk into the night until the morning, saying stories about good times in the past and good times yet to come.

"Oh, what good stories! Stories spilling out all over the place! We almost laughed to death. A rooster that ran into the house screeching on top of din-ner bowls, the same bowls that held him quietly in pieces the next day! And one about a girl who wrote love letters for two friends who loved the same man. And a silly foreign lady who fainted on a toilet when firecrackers went off next to her.

"People thought we were wrong to serve banquets every week while many people in the city were starving, eating rats and, later, the garbage that the poorest rats used to feed on. Others thought we were possessed by demons—to celebrate when even within our own families we had lost generations, had lost homes and fortunes, and were separated, husband from wife, brother from sister, daughter from mother. Hnnnh! How could we laugh, people asked.

"It's not that we had no heart or eyes for pain. We were all afraid. We all had our miseries. But to despair was to wish back for something already lost. Or to prolong what was already unbearable. How much can you wish for a favorite warm coat that hangs in the closet of a house that burned down with your mother and father inside of it? How long can you see in your mind arms and legs hanging from telephone wires and starving dogs running down the streets with half-chewed hands dangling from their jaws? What was worse, we asked among ourselves, to sit and wait for our own deaths with proper somber faces? Or to choose our own happiness?

"So we decided to hold parties and pretend each week had become the new year. Each week we could forget past wrongs done to us. We weren't allowed to think a bad thought. We feasted, we laughed, we played games, lost and won, we told the best stories. And each week, we could hope to be lucky. That hope was our only joy. And that's how we came to call our little parties Joy Luck."

My mother used to end the story on a happy note, bragging about her skill at the game. "I won many times and was so lucky the others teased that I had learned the trick of a clever thief," she said. "I won tens of thousands of *yuan*. But I wasn't rich. No. By then paper money had become worthless. Even toilet paper was worth more. And that made us laugh harder, to think a thousand-*yuan* note wasn't even good enough to rub on our bottoms."

I never thought my mother's Kweilin story was anything but a Chinese fairy tale. The endings always changed. Sometimes she said she used that worthless thousand-*yuan* note to buy a half-cup of rice. She turned that rice into a pot of porridge. She traded that gruel for two feet from a pig. Those two feet became six eggs, those eggs six chickens. The story always grew and grew.

And then one evening, after I had begged her to buy me a transistor radio, after she refused and I had sulked in silence for an hour, she said, "Why do you think you are missing something you never had?" And then she told me a completely different ending to the story.

"An army officer came to my house early one morning," she said, "and told me to go quickly to my husband in Chungking. And I knew he was telling me to run away from Kweilin. I knew what happened to officers and their families when the Japanese arrived. How could I go? There were no trains leaving Kweilin. My friend from Nanking, she was so good to me. She bribed a man to steal a wheelbarrow used to haul coal. She promised to warn our other friends.

"I packed my things and my two babies into this wheelbarrow and began pushing to Chungking four days before the Japanese marched into Kweilin. On the road I heard news of the slaughter from people running past me. It was terrible. Up to the last day, the Kuomintang insisted that Kweilin was safe, protected by the Chinese army. But later that day, the streets of Kweilin were strewn with newspapers reporting great Kuomintang victories, and on top of these papers, like fresh fish from a butcher, lay rows of people—men, women, and children who had never lost hope, but had lost their lives instead. When I heard this news, I walked faster and faster, asking myself at each step, Were they foolish? Were they brave?

"I pushed toward Chungking, until my wheel broke. I abandoned my beautiful mah jong table of *hong mu*. By then I didn't have enough feeling left in my body to cry. I tied scarves into slings and put a baby on each side of my shoulder. I carried a bag in each hand, one with clothes, the other with food. I carried these things until deep grooves grew in my hands. And I finally dropped one bag after the other when my hands began to bleed and became too slippery to hold onto anything.

"Along the way, I saw others had done the same, gradually given up hope. It was like a pathway inlaid with treasures that grew in value along the way. Bolts of fine fabric and books. Paintings of ancestors and carpenter tools. Until one could see cages of ducklings now quiet with thirst and, later still, silver urns lying in the road, where people had been too tired to carry them for any kind of future hope. By the time I arrived in Chungking I had lost everything except for three fancy silk dresses which I wore one on top of the other."

"What do you mean by 'everything'?" I gasped at the end. I was stunned to realize the story had been true all along. "What happened to the babies?"

She didn't even pause to think. She simply said in a way that made it clear there was no more to the story: "Your father is not my first husband. You are not those babies."

When I arrive at the Hsus' house, where the Joy Luck Club is meeting tonight, the first person I see is my father. "There she is! Never on time!" he announces. And it's true. Everybody's already here, seven family friends in their sixties and seventies. They look up and laugh at me, always tardy, a child still at thirty-six.

I'm shaking, trying to hold something inside. The last time I saw them, at the funeral, I had broken down and cried big gulping sobs. They must wonder now how someone like me can take my mother's place. A friend once told me that my mother and I were alike, that we had the same wispy hand gestures, the same girlish laugh and sideways look. When I shyly told my mother this, she seemed insulted and said, "You don't even know little percent of me! How can you be me?" And she's right. How can I be my mother at Joy Luck?

"Auntie, Uncle," I say repeatedly, nodding to each person there. I have always called these old family friends Auntie and Uncle. And then I walk over and stand next to my father.

He's looking at the Jongs' pictures from their recent China trip. "Look at that," he says politely, pointing to a photo of the Jongs' tour group standing on wide slab steps. There is nothing in this picture that shows it was taken in China rather than San Francisco, or any other city for that matter. But my father doesn't seem to be looking at the picture anyway. It's as though everything were the same to him, nothing stands out. He has always been politely indifferent. But what's the Chinese word that means indifferent because you can't *see* any differences? That's how troubled I think he is by my mother's death.

"Will you look at that," he says, pointing to another nondescript picture.

The Hsus' house feels heavy with greasy odors. Too many Chinese meals cooked in a too small kitchen, too many once fragrant smells compressed onto a thin layer of invisible grease. I remember how my mother used to go into other people's houses and restaurants and wrinkle her nose, then whisper very loudly: "I can see and feel the stickiness with my nose."

I have not been to the Hsus' house in many years, but the living room is exactly the same as I remember it. When Auntie An-mei and Uncle George moved to the Sunset district from Chinatown twenty-five years ago, they bought new furniture. It's all there, still looking mostly new under yellowed plastic. The same turquoise couch shaped in a semicircle of nubby tweed. The colonial end tables made out of heavy maple. A lamp of fake cracked porcelain. Only the scroll-length calendar, free from the Bank of Canton, changes every year.

I remember this stuff, because when we were children, Auntie An-mei didn't let us touch any of her new furniture except through the clear plastic coverings. On Joy Luck nights, my parents brought me to the Hsus'. Since I was the guest, I had to take care of all the younger children, so many children it seemed as if there were always one baby who was crying from having bumped its head on a table leg.

"You are responsible," said my mother, which meant I was in trouble if anything was spilled, burned, lost, broken, or dirty. I was responsible, no matter who did it. She and Auntie An-mei were dressed up in funny Chinese dresses with stiff stand-up collars and blooming branches of embroidered silk sewn over their breasts. These clothes were too fancy for real Chinese people, I thought, and too strange for American parties. In those days, before my mother told me her Kweilin story, I imagined Joy Luck was a shameful Chinese custom, like the secret gathering of the Ku Klux Klan or the tom-tom dances of TV Indians preparing for war.

But tonight, there's no mystery. The Joy Luck aunties are all wearing slacks, bright print blouses, and different versions of sturdy walking shoes. We are all seated around the dining room table under a lamp that looks like a Spanish candelabra. Uncle George puts on his bifocals and starts the meeting by reading the minutes:

"Our capital account is $24,825, or about $6,206 a couple, $3,103 per person. We sold Subaru for a loss at six and three-quarters. We bought a hundred shares of Smith International at seven. Our thanks to Lindo and Tin Jong for the goodies. The red bean soup was especially delicious. The March meeting had to be canceled until further notice. We were sorry to have to bid a fond farewell to our dear friend Suyuan and extended our sympathy to the Canning Woo family. Respectfully submitted, George Hsu, president and secretary."

That's it. I keep thinking the others will start talking about my mother, the wonderful friendship they shared, and why I am here in her spirit, to be the fourth corner and carry on the idea my mother came up with on a hot day in Kweilin.

But everybody just nods to approve the minutes. Even my father's head bobs up and down routinely. And it seems to me my mother's life has been shelved for new business.

Auntie An-mei heaves herself up from the table and moves slowly to the kitchen to prepare the food. And Auntie Lin, my mother's best friend, moves to the turquoise sofa, crosses her arms, and watches the men still seated at the table. Auntie Ying, who seems to shrink even more every time I see her, reaches into her knitting bag and pulls out the start of a tiny blue sweater.

The Joy Luck uncles begin to talk about stocks they are interested in buying. Uncle Jack, who is Auntie Ying's younger brother, is very keen on a company that mines gold in Canada.

"It's a great hedge on inflation," he says with authority. He speaks the best English, almost accentless. I think my mother's English was the worst, but she always thought her Chinese was the best. She spoke Mandarin slightly blurred with a Shanghai dialect.

"Weren't we going to play mah jong tonight?" I whisper loudly to Auntie Ying, who's slightly deaf.

"Later," she says, "after midnight."

"Ladies, are you at this meeting or not?" says Uncle George.

After everybody votes unanimously for the Canada gold stock, I go into the kitchen to ask Auntie An-mei why the Joy Luck Club started investing in stocks.

"We used to play mah jong, winner take all. But the same people were always winning, the same people always losing," she says. She is stuffing wonton, one chopstick jab of gingery meat dabbed onto a thin skin and then a single fluid turn with her hand that seals the skin into the shape of a tiny nurse's cap. "You can't have luck when someone else has skill. So long time ago, we decided to invest in the stock market. There's no skill in that. Even your mother agreed."

Auntie An-mei takes count of the tray in front of her. She's already made five rows of eight wonton each. "Forty wonton, eight people, ten each, five row more," she says aloud to herself, and then continues stuffing. "We got smart. Now we can all win and lose equally. We can have stock market luck. And we can play mah jong for fun, just for a few dollars, winner take all. Losers take home leftovers! So everyone can have some joy. Smart-hanh?"

I watch Auntie An-mei make more wonton. She has quick, expert fingers. She doesn't have to think about what she is doing. That's what my mother used to complain about, that Auntie An-mei never thought about what she was doing.

"She's not stupid," said my mother on one occasion, "but she has no spine. Last week, I had a good idea for her. I said to her, Let's go to the consulate and ask for papers for your brother. And she almost wanted to drop her things and go right then. But later she talked to someone. Who knows who? And that person told her she can get her brother in bad trouble in China. That person said FBI will put her on a list and give her trouble in the U.S. the rest of her life. That person said, You ask for a house loan and they say no loan, because your brother is a communist. I said, You already have a house! But still she was scared."

"Auntie An-mei runs this way and that," said my mother, "and she doesn't know why."

As I watch Auntie An-mei, I see a short bent woman in her seventies, with a heavy bosom and thin, shapeless legs. She has the flattened soft fingertips of an old woman. I wonder what Auntie An-mei did to inspire a life-long stream of criticism from my mother. Then again, it seemed my mother was always displeased with all her friends, with me, and even with my father. Something was always missing. Something always needed improving. Something was not in balance. This one or that had too much of one element, not enough of another.

The elements were from my mother's own version of organic chemistry. Each person is made of five elements, she told me.

Too much fire and you had a bad temper. That was like my father, whom my mother always criticized for his cigarette habit and who always shouted back that she should keep her thoughts to herself. I think he now feels guilty that he didn't let my mother speak her mind.

Too little wood and you bent too quickly to listen to other people's ideas, unable to stand on your own. This was like my Auntie An-mei.

Too much water and you flowed in too many directions, like myself, for having started half a degree in biology, then half a degree in art, and then finishing neither when I went off to work for a small ad agency as a secretary, later becoming a copywriter.

I used to dismiss her criticisms as just more of her Chinese superstitions, beliefs that conveniently fit the circumstances. In my twenties, while taking Introduction to Psychology, I tried to tell her why she shouldn't criticize so much, why it didn't lead to a healthy learning environment.

"There's a school of thought," I said, "that parents shouldn't criticize children. They should encourage instead. You know, people rise to other people's expectations. And when you criticize, it just means you're expecting failure."

"That's the trouble," my mother said. "You never rise. Lazy to get up. Lazy to rise to expectations."

"Time to eat," Auntie An-mei happily announces, bringing out a steaming pot of the wonton she was just wrapping. There are piles of food on the table, served buffet style, just like at the Kweilin feasts. My father is digging into the chow mein, which still sits in an oversize aluminum pan surrounded by little plastic packets of soy sauce. Auntie An-mei must have bought this on Clement Street. The wonton soup smells wonderful with delicate sprigs of cilantro floating on top. I'm drawn first to a large platter of *chaswei*, sweet barbecued pork cut into coin-sized slices, and then to a whole assortment of what I've always called finger goodies—thin-skinned pastries filled with chopped pork, beef, shrimp, and unknown stuffings that my mother used to describe as "nutritious things."

Eating is not a gracious event here. It's as though everybody had been starving. They push large forkfuls into their mouths, jab at more pieces of pork, one right after the other. They are not like the ladies of Kweilin, who I always imagined savored their food with a certain detached delicacy.

And then, almost as quickly as they started, the men get up and leave the table. As if on cue, the women peck at last morsels and then carry plates and bowls to the kitchen and dump them in the sink. The women take turns washing their hands, scrubbing them vigorously. Who started this ritual? I too put my plate in the sink and wash my hands. The women are talking about the Jongs' China trip, then they move toward a room in the back of the apartment. We pass another room, what used to be the bedroom shared by the four Hsu sons. The bunk beds with their scuffed, splintery ladders are still there. The Joy Luck uncles are already seated at the card table. Uncle

George is dealing out cards, fast, as though he learned this technique in a casino. My father is passing out Pall Mall cigarettes, with one already dangling from his lips.

And then we get to the room in the back, which was once shared by the three Hsu girls. We were all childhood friends. And now they've all grown and married and I'm here to play in their room again. Except for the smell of camphor, it feels the same—as if Rose, Ruth, and Janice might soon walk in with their hair rolled up in big orange-juice cans and plop down on their identical narrow beds. The white chenille bedspreads are so worn they are almost translucent. Rose and I used to pluck the nubs out while talking about our boy problems. Everything is the same, except now a mahogany-colored mah jong table sits in the center. And next to it is a floor lamp, a long black pole with three oval spotlights attached like the broad leaves of a rubber plant.

Nobody says to me, "Sit here, this is where your mother used to sit." But I can tell even before everyone sits down. The chair closest to the door has an emptiness to it. But the feeling doesn't really have to do with the chair. It's her place on the table. Without having anyone tell me, I know her corner on the table was the East.

The East is where things begin, my mother once told me, the direction from which the sun rises, where the wind comes from.

Auntie An-mei, who is sitting on my left, spills the tiles onto the green felt tabletop and then says to me, "Now we wash tiles." We swirl them with our hands in a circular motion. They make a cool swishing sound as they bump into one another.

"Do you win like your mother?" asks Auntie Lin across from me. She is not smiling.

"I only played a little in college with some Jewish friends."

"Annh! Jewish mah jong," she says in disgusted tones. "Not the same thing." This is what my mother used to say, although she could never explain exactly why.

"Maybe I shouldn't play tonight. I'll just watch," I offer.

Auntie Lin looks exasperated, as though I were a simple child: "How can we play with just three people? Like a table with three legs, no balance. When Auntie Ying's husband died, she asked her brother to join. Your father asked you. So it's decided."

"What's the difference between Jewish and Chinese mah jong?" I once asked my mother. I couldn't tell by her answer if the games were different of just her attitude toward Chinese and Jewish people.

"Entirely different kind of playing," she said in her English explanation voice. "Jewish mah jong, they watch only for their own tile, play only with their eyes."

Then she switched to Chinese: "Chinese mah jong, you must play using your head, very tricky. You must watch what everybody else throws away and keep that in your head as well. And if nobody plays well, then the game becomes like Jewish mah jong. Why play? There's no strategy. You're just watching people make mistakes."

These kinds of explanations made me feel my mother and I spoke two different languages, which we did. I talked to her in English, she answered back in Chinese.

"So what's the difference between Chinese and Jewish mah jong?" I ask Auntie Lin.

"Aii-ya," she exclaims in a mock scolding voice. "Your mother did not teach you anything?"

Auntie Ying pats my hand. "You a smart girl. You watch us, do the same. Help us stack the tiles and make four walls."

I follow Auntie Ying, but mostly I watch Auntie Lin. She is the fastest, which means I can almost keep up with the others by watching what she does first. Auntie Ying throws the dice and I'm told that Auntie Lin has become the East wind. I've become the North wind, the last hand to play. Auntie Ying is the South and Auntie An-mei is the West. And then we start taking tiles, throwing the dice, counting back on the wall to the right number of spots where our chosen tiles lie. I rearrange my tiles, sequences of bamboo and balls, doubles of colored number tiles, odd tiles that do not fit anywhere.

"Your mother was the best, like a pro," says Auntie An-mei while slowly sorting her tiles, considering each piece carefully.

Now we begin to play, looking at our hands, casting tiles, picking up others at an easy, comfortable pace. The Joy Luck aunties begin to make small talk, not really listening to each other. They speak in their special language, half in broken English, half in their own Chinese dialect. Auntie Ying mentions she bought yarn at half price, somewhere out in the avenues. Auntie An-mei brags about a sweater she made for her daughter Ruth's new baby. "She thought it was store-bought," she says proudly.

Auntie Lin explains how mad she got at a store clerk who refused to let her return a skirt with a broken zipper. "I was *chiszle*," she says, still fuming, "mad to death."

"But Lindo, you are still with us. You didn't die," teases Auntie Ying, and then as she laughs Auntie Lin says '*Pung!*' and '*Mah jong!*' and then spreads her tiles out, laughing back at Auntie Ying while counting up her points. We start washing tiles again and it grows quiet. I'm getting bored and sleepy.

"Oh, I have a story," says Auntie Ying loudly, startling everybody. Auntie Ying has always been the weird auntie, someone lost in her own world. My mother used to say, "Auntie Ying is not hard of hearing. She is hard of listening."

"Police arrested Mrs. Emerson's son last weekend," Auntie Ying says in a way that sounds as if she were proud to be the first with this big news. "Mrs. Chan told me at church. Too many TV set found in his car."

Auntie Lin quickly says, "Aii-ya, Mrs. Emerson good lady," meaning Mrs. Emerson didn't deserve such a terrible son. But now I see this is also said for the benefit of Auntie An-mei, whose own youngest son was arrested two years ago for selling stolen car stereos. Auntie An-mei is rubbing her tile carefully before discarding it. She looks pained.

"Everybody has TVs in China now," says Auntie Lin, changing the subject. "Our family there all has TV sets—not just black-and-white, but color and remote! They have everything. So when we asked them what we should buy them, they said nothing, it was enough that we would come to visit them. But we bought them different things anyway, VCR and Sony Walkman for the kids. They said, No, don't give it to us, but I think they liked it."

Poor Auntie An-mei rubs her tiles ever harder. I remember my mother telling me about the Hsus' trip to China three years ago. Auntie An-mei had saved two thousand dollars, all to spend on her brother's family. She had shown my mother the insides of her heavy suitcases. One was crammed with See's Nuts & Chews, M & M's, candy-coated cashews, instant hot chocolate with miniature marshmallows. My mother told me the other bag contained the most ridiculous clothes, all new: bright California-style beachwear, baseball caps, cotton pants with elastic waists, bomber jackets, Stanford sweatshirts, crew socks.

My mother had told her, "Who wants those useless things? They just want money." But Auntie An-mei said her brother was so poor and they were so rich by comparison. So she ignored my mother's advice and took the heavy bags and their two thousand dollars to China. And when their China tour finally arrived in Hangzhou, the whole family from Ningbo was there to meet them. It wasn't just Auntie An-mei's little brother, but also his wife's stepbrothers and stepsisters, and a distant cousin, and that cousin's husband and that husband's uncle. They had all brought their mothers-in-law and children, and even their village friends who were not lucky enough to have overseas Chinese relatives to show off.

As my mother told it, "Auntie An-mei had cried before she left for China, thinking she would make her brother very rich and happy by communist standards. But when she got home, she cried to me that everyone had a palm out and she was the only one who left with an empty hand."

My mother confirmed her suspicions. Nobody wanted the sweatshirts, those useless clothes. The M & M's were thrown in the air, gone. And when the suitcases were emptied, the relatives asked what else the Hsus had brought.

Auntie An-mei and Uncle George were shaken down, not just for two thousand dollars' worth of TVs and refrigerators but also for a night's lodging for twenty-six people in the Overlooking the Lake Hotel, for three banquet tables at a restaurant that catered to rich foreigners, for three special gifts for each relative, and finally, for a loan of five thousand *yuan* in foreign exchange to a cousin's so-called uncle who wanted to buy a motorcycle but who later disappeared for good along with the money. When the train pulled out of Hangzhou the next day, the Hsus found themselves depleted of some nine thousand dollars' worth of goodwill. Months later, after an inspiring Christmastime service at the First Chinese Baptist Church, Auntie An-mei tried to recoup her loss by saying it truly was more blessed to give than to receive, and my mother agreed, her longtime friend had blessings for at least several lifetimes.

Listening now to Auntie Lin bragging about the virtues of her family in China, I realize that Auntie Lin is oblivious to Auntie An-mei's pain. Is Auntie Lin being mean, or is it that my mother never told anybody but me the shameful story of Auntie An-mei's greedy family?

"So, Jing-mei, you go to school now?" says Auntie Lin.

"Her name is June. They all go by their American names," says Auntie Ying.

"That's okay," I say, and I really mean it. In fact, it's even becoming fashionable for American-born Chinese to use their Chinese names.

"I'm not in school anymore, though," I say. "That was more than ten years ago."

Auntie Lin's eyebrows arch. "Maybe I'm thinking of someone else daughter," she says, but I know right away she's lying. I know my mother probably told her I was going back to school to finish my degree, because somewhere back, maybe just six months ago, we were again having this argument about my being a failure, a "college drop-off," about my going back to finish.

Once again I had told my mother what she wanted to hear: "You're right. I'll look into it."

I had always assumed we had an unspoken understanding about these things: that she didn't really mean I was a failure, and I really meant I would try to respect her opinions more. But listening to Auntie Lin tonight reminds me once again: My mother and I never really understood one another. We translated each other's meanings and I seemed to hear less than what was said, while my mother heard more. No doubt she told Auntie Lin I was going back to school to get a doctorate.

Auntie Lin and my mother were both best friends and arch enemies who spent a lifetime comparing their children. I was one month older than Waverly Jong, Auntie Lin's prized daughter. From the time we were babies, our mothers compared the creases in our belly buttons, how shapely our earlobes were, how fast we healed when we scraped our knees, how thick and dark our hair, how many shoes we wore out in one year, and later, how smart Waverly was at playing chess, how many trophies she had won last month, how many newspapers had printed her name, how many cities she had visited.

I know my mother resented listening to Auntie Lin talk about Waverly when she had nothing to come back with. At first my mother tried to cultivate some hidden genius in me. She did housework for an old retired piano teacher down the hall who gave me lessons and free use of a piano to practice on in exchange. When I failed to become a concert pianist, or even an accompanist for the church youth choir, she finally explained that I was late-blooming, like Einstein, who everyone thought was retarded until he discovered a bomb.

Now it is Auntie Ying who wins this hand of mah jong, so we count points and begin again.

"Did you know Lena move to Woodside?" asks Auntie Ying with obvious pride, looking down at the tiles, talking to no one in particular. She quickly erases her smile and tries for some modesty. "Of course, it's not best house in neighborhood, not million-dollar house, not yet. But it's good investment. Better than paying rent. Better than somebody putting you under their thumb to rub you out."

So now I know Auntie Ying's daughter, Lena, told her about my being evicted from my apartment on lower Russian Hill. Even though Lena and I are still friends, we have grown naturally cautious about telling each other too much. Still, what little we say to one another often comes back in another guise. It's the same old game, everybody talking in circles.

"It's getting late," I say after we finish the round. I start to stand up, but Auntie Lin pushes me back down into the chair.

"Stay, stay. We talk awhile, get to know you again," she says. "Been a long time."

I know this is a polite gesture on the Joy Luck aunties' part—a protest when actually they are just as eager to see me go as I am to leave. "No, I really must go now, thank you, thank you," I say, glad I remembered how the pretense goes.

"But you must stay! We have something important to tell you, from your mother," Auntie Ying blurts out in her too-loud voice. The others look uncomfortable, as if this were not how they intended to break some sort of bad news to me.

I sit down. Auntie An-mei leaves the room quickly and returns with a bowl of peanuts, then quietly shuts the door. Everybody is quiet, as if nobody knew where to begin.

It is Auntie Ying who finally speaks. "I think your mother die with an important thought on her mind," she says in halting English. And then she begins to speak in Chinese, calmly, softly.

"Your mother was a very strong woman, a good mother. She loved you very much, more than her own life. And that's why you can understand why a mother like this could never forget her other daughters. She knew they were alive, and before she died she wanted to find her daughters in China."

The babies in Kweilin, I think. I was not those babies. The babies in a sling on her shoulder. Her other daughters. And now I feel as if I were in Kweilin amidst the bombing and I can see these babies lying on the side of the road, their red thumbs popped out of their mouths, screaming to be reclaimed. Somebody took them away. They're safe. And now my mother's left me forever, gone back to China to get these babies. I can barely hear Auntie Ying's voice.

"She had searched for years, written letters back and forth," says Auntie Ying. "And last year she got an address. She was going to tell your father soon. Aii-ya, what a shame. A lifetime of waiting."

Auntie An-mei interrupts with an excited voice: "So your aunties and I, we wrote to this address," she says. "We say that a certain party, your mother, want to meet another certain party. And this party write back to us. They are your sisters, Jing-mei."

My sisters, I repeat to myself, saying these two words together for the first time.

Auntie An-mei is holding a sheet of paper as thin as wrapping tissue. In perfectly straight vertical rows I see Chinese characters written in blue fountain-pen ink. A word is smudged. A tear? I take the letter with shaking hands, marveling at how smart my sisters must be to be able to read and write Chinese.

The aunties are all smiling at me, as though I had been a dying person who has now miraculously recovered. Auntie Ying is handing me another envelope. Inside is a check made out to June Woo for $1,200. I can't believe it.

"My sisters are sending *me* money?" I ask.

"No, no," says Auntie Lin with her mock exasperated voice. "Every year we save our mah jong winnings for big banquet at fancy restaurant. Most times your mother win, so most is her money. We add just a little, so you can go Hong Kong, take a train to Shanghai, see your sisters. Besides, we all getting too rich, too fat." She pats her stomach for proof.

"See my sisters," I say numbly. I am awed by this prospect, trying to imagine what I would see. And I am embarrassed by the end-of-the-year-banquet lie my aunties have told to mask their generosity. I am crying now, sobbing and laughing at the same time, seeing but not understanding this loyalty to my mother.

"You must see your sisters and tell them about your mother's death," says Auntie Ying. "But most important, you must tell them about her life. The mother they did not know, they must now know."

"See my sisters, tell them about my mother," I say, nodding. "What will I say? What can I tell them about my mother? I don't know anything. She was my mother."

The aunties are looking at me as if I had become crazy right before their eyes.

"Not know your own mother?" cries Auntie An-mei with disbelief. "How can you say? Your mother is in your bones!"

"Tell them stories of your family here. How she became success," offers Auntie Lin.

"Tell them stories she told you, lessons she taught, what you know about her mind that has become your mind," says Auntie Ying. "You mother very smart lady."

I hear more choruses of "Tell them, tell them" as each Auntie frantically tries to think what should be passed on.

"Her kindness."

"Her smartness."

"Her dutiful nature to family."

"Her hopes, things that matter to her."

"The excellent dishes she cooked."

"Imagine, a daughter not knowing her own mother!"

And then it occurs to me. They are frightened. In me, they see their own daughters, just as ignorant, just as unmindful of all the truths and hopes they have brought to America. They see daughters who grow impatient when their mothers talk in Chinese, who think they are stupid when they explain things in fractured English. They see that joy and luck do not mean the same to their daughters, that to these closed American-born minds "joy luck" is not a word, it does not exist. They see daughters who will bear grandchildren born without any connecting hope passed from generation to generation.

"I will tell them everything," I say simply, and the aunties look at me with doubtful faces.

"I will remember everything about her and tell them," I say more firmly. And gradually, one by one, they smile and pat my hand. They still look troubled, as if something were out of balance. But they also look hopeful that what I say will become true. What more can they ask? What more can I promise?

They go back to eating their soft boiled peanuts, saying stories among themselves. They are young girls again, dreaming of good times in the past and good times yet to come. A brother from Ningbo who makes his sister cry with joy when he returns nine thousand dollars plus interest. A youngest son whose stereo and TV repair business is so good he sends leftovers to China. A daughter whose babies are able to swim like fish in a fancy pool in Woodside. Such good stories. The best. They are the lucky ones.

And I am sitting at my mother's place at the mah jong table, on the East, where things begin.

Grandfather in the Old Men's Home

Gentle at last, and as clean as ever,
He did not even need drink any more,
And his good sons unbent and brought him
Tobacco to chew, both times when they came
To be satisfied he was well cared for.
And he smiled all the time to remember
Grandmother, his wife, wearing the true faith
Like an iron nightgown, yet brought to birth
Seven times and raising the family
Through her needle's eye while he got away
Down the green river, finding directions
For boats. And himself coming home sometimes
Well-heeled but blind drunk, to hide all the bread
And shoot holes in the bucket while he made
His daughters pump. Still smiled as kindly in
His sleep beside the other clean old men
To see Grandmother, every night the same,
Huge in her age, with her thumbed-down mouth, come
Hating the river, filling with her stare
His gliding dream, while he turned to water,
While the children they both had begotten,
With old faces now, but themselves shrunken
To child-size again, stood ranged at her side,
Beating their little Bibles till he died.

My Father-in-Law's Contract

I find him in the kitchen, slipping
our senile dog yet another treat.
I ask, "How many's that, today?"
"Aaah," he says, "eight or nine.
Who's keeping track?" He is, I know.

I've brought him the *Globe*. He turns to
the stocks, writes in a black notebook
now almost full of calculations. He shows me
what's happened since the breakup of Ma Bell:
his shares have doubled, split. His diaspora
near an end, this is what he thinks he has
to pass on: meticulous writ, proving he kept his
wits, died with his stocks on the rise.

I try to look interested. But I can't
even balance my checkbook. He suspects as much,
shuts his book with a sigh that says everything
these days appears darker under the aspect of eternity.

He reaches for my shoulder to steady himself.
"Weaker," he says, "and not weaker every week,
but every day." His blood is cutting
its losses, beating a strategic retreat
from his extremities. His legs, saplings
stranded in a dry time. And his brain,
"I can't remember my neighbor's names.
But somebody from sixty, seventy years ago,
I can't forget. . . . Take my Hebrew teacher.
His name was . . . Max . . . Max Lazarus.
I used to pay him quarters, maybe
it was dimes, not to squeal about my skipping shul."

I hope he missed the lessons on the Book of Job.
He's eighty now and doesn't need a Torah archetype
to amplify his fear how far a man whose golfing handicap
was three can slip—to thirty-six, and more.
He's veering off the fairway like a slice.
His smoker's cough is raw. What's more,
he's got me for a son-in-law, a goy
who doesn't know from borscht about finance. And yet
he loves me. So he tells me
about his contract with God and another guy
who's eighty at the Club: "We've agreed to settle
for two more years—with an option to renew."

I laugh. I've heard and heard the story,
the last time, yesterday. He sighs,
"You know, I think my contract used to run
for five. . . . But aaah, so what!"
he swings his arm backhand across his body
in the timeless arc of a sower, or someone clearing
the air, or swiping at a dybbuk.
"Contracts schmontracts. What a lotta bullshit,"
he says and laughs the same anarchic laugh
my wife, his daughter, laughs,
the laugh of a kid on roller-skates
who's skipping shul.
                    The sound's a magnet
to his granddaughter, one year old today.

She crawls up to Grandpah, her eyes Chinese
with smiles. He dandles her, then notices
the dog, past reverie, who's docked his head
between the garbage can and wall.
He looks at all of us and says his favorite
benediction, "You should only live and be well."
And as he does, he squeezes my shoulder,
hard as he can. It's nothing more
or less than a caress.

Stroke

After the family dinner, language
is trivial and easy—
until you lose it entirely, Uncle,
asking for something you want
which suddenly has no name.
"Goddam," you moan, "gimme a. . . .
All I want's a . . . Jesus Christ,
ain't you got one?"
The family hands you sweaters,
pills, icepicks, glasses of brandy,
knives. Nothing will do.
Afraid of empty hands,
they rush at you with objects,
determined to interpret what you've said,
afraid to name this dying
and to watch you
leave them, word by word.

Grandmother and Grandson

As I hear it, now when there is company
Always the spindly granddam, stuck standing
In her corner like a lady clock long
Silent, out of some hole in the talk
Is apt to clack cup, clatter teeth, and with
Saucer gesturing to no one special,
Shake out her paper voice concerning
That pimply boy her last grandson: "Now who,
Who does he remind you of?"

                      (Who stuffs there
With cake his puffed face complected half
Of yellow crumbs, his tongue loving over
His damp hands to lick the sticky
From bitten fingers; chinless; all boneless but
His neck and knees; and who now rolls his knowing
Eyes to their attention.)

                    In vain, in vain,
One after the other, their lusterless
Suggestions of faint likenesses; she
Nods at none, her gaze absent and more
Absent, as though watching for someone through
A frosted window, until they are aware
She has forgotten her own question.

When he is alone, though, with only her
And her hazy eyes in the whole house
To mind him, his way is to take himself
Just out of her small sight and there stay
Till she starts calling; let her call till she
Sounds in pain; and as though in pain, at last,
His answers, each farther, leading her
Down passages, up stairs, with her worry
Hard to swallow as a scarf-end, her pace

A spun child's in a blindfold, to the piled
Dust-coop, trunk- and junk-room at the top
Of all the stairs, where he hides till she sways
Clutching her breath in the very room, then
Behind her slips out, locking the door. His
Laughter down stair after stair she hears
Being forgotten. In the unwashed light,
Lost, she turns among the sheeted mounds
Fingering hems and murmuring, "Where, where
Does it remind me of?" Till someone comes.

A Conversation with My Father

My father is eighty-six years old and in bed. His heart, that bloody motor, is equally old and will not do certain jobs any more. It still floods his head with brainy light. But it won't let his legs carry the weight of his body around the house. Despite my metaphors, this muscle failure is not due to his old heart, he says, but to a potassium shortage. Sitting on one pillow, leaning on three, he offers last-minute advice and makes a request.

"I would like you to write a simple story just once more," he says, "the kind de Maupassant wrote, or Chekhov, the kind you used to write. Just recognizable people and then write down what happened to them next."

I say, "Yes, why not? That's possible." I want to please him, though I don't remember writing that way. I *would* like to try to tell such a story, if he means the kind that begins: "There was a woman . . . " followed by plot, the absolute line between two points which I've always despised. Not for literary reasons, but because it takes all hope away. Everyone, real or invented, deserves the open destiny of life.

Finally I thought of a story that had been happening for a couple of years right across the street. I wrote it down, then read it aloud. "Pa," I said, "how about this? Do you mean something like this?"

> Once in my time there was a woman and she had a son. They lived nicely, in a small apartment in Manhattan. This boy at about fifteen became a junkie, which is not unusual in our neighborhood. In order to maintain her close friendship with him, she became a junkie too. She said it was part of the youth culture, with which she felt very much at home. After a while, for a number of reasons, the boy gave it all up and left the city and his mother in disgust. Hopeless and alone, she grieved. We all visit her.

"O.K., Pa, that's it," I said, "an unadorned and miserable tale."

"But that's not what I mean," my father said. "You misunderstood me on purpose. You know there's a lot more to it. You know that. You left everything out. Turgenev wouldn't do that. Chekhov wouldn't do that. There are in fact Russian writers you never heard of, you don't have an inkling of, as good as anyone, who can write a plain ordinary story, who would not leave

GRACE PALEY

out what you have left out. I object not to facts but to people sitting in trees talking senselessly, voices from who knows where . . . "

"Forget that one, Pa, what have I left out now? In this one?"

"Her looks, for instance."

"Oh. Quite handsome, I think. Yes."

"Her hair?"

"Dark, with heavy braids, as though she were a girl or a foreigner."

"What were her parents like, her stock? That she became such a person. It's interesting, you know."

"From out of town. Professional people. The first to be divorced in their county. How's that? Enough?" I asked.

"With you, it's all a joke," he said. "What about the boy's father? Why didn't you mention him? Who was he? Or was the boy born out of wedlock?"

"Yes," I said. "He was born out of wedlock."

"For Godsakes, doesn't anyone in your stories get married? Doesn't anyone have the time to run down to City Hall before they jump into bed?"

"No," I said. "In real life, yes. But in my stories, no."

"Why do you answer me like that?"

"Oh, Pa, this is a simple story about a smart woman who came to N.Y.C. full of interest love trust excitement very up to date, and about her son, what a hard time she had in this world. Married or not, it's of small consequence."

"It is of great consequence," he said.

"O.K.," I said.

"O.K. O.K. yourself," he said, "but listen. I believe you that she's good-looking, but I don't think she was so smart."

"That's true," I said. "Actually that's the trouble with stories. People start out fantastic. You think they're extraordinary, but it turns out as the work goes along, they're just average with a good education. Sometimes the other way around, the person's a kind of dumb innocent, but he outwits you and you can't even think of an ending good enough."

"What do you do then?" he asked. He had been a doctor for a couple of decades and then an artist for a couple of decades and he's still interested in details, craft, technique.

"Well, you just have to let the story lie around till some agreement can be reached between you and the stubborn hero."

"Aren't you talking silly, now?" he asked. "Start again," he said. "It so happens I'm not going out this evening. Tell the story again. See what you can do this time."

"O.K.," I said. "But it's not a five-minute job." Second attempt:

Once, across the street from us, there was a fine handsome woman, our neighbor. She had a son whom she loved because she'd known him since birth (in helpless chubby infancy, and in the wrestling, hugging ages, seven

243

to ten, as well as earlier and later). This boy, when he fell into the fist of adolescence, became a junkie. He was not a hopeless one. He was in fact hopeful, an ideologue and successful converter. With his busy brilliance, he wrote persuasive articles for his high-school newspaper. Seeking a wider audience, using important connections, he drummed into Lower Manhattan newsstand distribution a periodical called *Oh! Golden Horse!*

In order to keep him from feeling guilty (because guilt is the stony heart of nine tenths of all clinically diagnosed cancers in America today, she said), and because she had always believed in giving bad habits room at home where one could keep an eye on them, she too became a junkie. Her kitchen was famous for a while—a center for intellectual addicts who knew what they were doing. A few felt artistic like Coleridge and others were scientific and revolutionary like Leary. Although she was often high herself, certain good mothering reflexes remained, and she saw to it that there was lots of orange juice around and honey and milk and vitamin pills. However, she never cooked anything but chili, and that no more than once a week. She explained, when we talked to her, seriously, with neighborly concern, that it was her part in the youth culture and she would rather be with the young, it was an honor, than with her own generation.

One week, while nodding through an Antonioni film, this boy was severely jabbed by the elbow of a stern and proselytizing girl, sitting beside him. She offered immediate apricots and nuts for his sugar level, spoke to him sharply, and took him home.

She had heard of him and his work and she herself published, edited, and wrote a competitive journal called *Man Does Live By Bread Alone.* In the organic heat of her continuous presence he could not help but become interested once more in his muscles, his arteries, and nerve connections. In fact he began to love them, treasure them, praise them with funny little songs in *Man Does Live . . .*

> *the fingers of my flesh transcend*
> *my transcendental soul*
> *the tightness in my shoulders end*
> *my teeth have made me whole*

To the mouth of his head (that glory of will and determination) he brought hard apples, nuts, wheat germ, and soybean oil. He said to his old friends, From now on, I guess I'll keep my wits about me. I'm going on the natch. He said he was about to begin a spiritual deep-breathing journey. How about you too, Mom? he asked kindly.

His conversion was so radiant, splendid, that neighborhood kids his age began to say that he had never been a real addict at all, only a journalist along for the smell of the story. The mother tried several times to give up what had become without her son and his friends a lonely habit. This effort only brought it to supportable levels. The boy and his girl took their electronic mimeograph and moved to the bushy edge of another borough. They were very strict. They said they would not see her again until she had been off drugs for sixty days.

At home alone in the evening, weeping, the mother read and reread the seven issues of *Oh! Golden Horse!* They seemed to her as truthful as ever. We often crossed the street to visit and console. But if we mentioned any of our children who were at college or in the hospital or dropouts at home, she would cry out, My baby! My baby! and burst into terrible, face-scarring, time-consuming tears. The End.

First my father was silent, then he said, "Number One: You have a nice sense of humor. Number Two: I see you can't tell a plain story. So don't waste time." Then he said sadly, "Number Three: I suppose that means she was alone, she was left like that, his mother. Alone. Probably sick?"

I said, "Yes."

"Poor woman. Poor girl, to be born in a time of fools, to live among fools. The end. The end. You were right to put that down. The end."

I didn't want to argue, but I had to say, "Well, it is not necessarily the end, Pa."

"Yes," he said, "what a tragedy. The end of a person."

"No, Pa," I begged him. "It doesn't have to be. She's only about forty. She could be a hundred different things in this world as time goes on. A teacher or a social worker. An ex-junkie! Sometimes it's better than having a master's in education."

"Jokes," he said. "As a writer that's your main trouble. You don't want to recognize it. Tragedy! Plain tragedy! Historical tragedy! No hope. The end."

"Oh, Pa," I said. "She could change."

"In your own life, too, you have to look it in the face." He took a couple of nitroglycerin. "Turn to five," he said, pointing to the dial on the oxygen tank. He inserted the tubes into his nostrils and breathed deep. He closed his eyes and said, "No."

I had promised the family to always let him have the last word when arguing, but in this case I had a different responsibility. That woman lives across the street. She's my knowledge and my invention. I'm sorry for her. I'm not going to leave her there in that house crying. (Actually neither would Life, which unlike me has no pity.)

Therefore: She did change. Of course her son never came home again. But right now, she's the receptionist in a storefront community clinic in the East Village. Most of the customers are young people, some old friends. The head doctor has said to her, "If we only had three people in this clinic with your experiences . . ."

"The doctor said that?" My father took the oxygen tubes out of his nostrils and said, "Jokes. Jokes again."

"No, Pa, it could really happen that way, it's a funny world nowadays."

"No," he said. "Truth first. She will slide back. A person must have character. She does not."

"No, Pa," I said. "That's it. She's got a job. Forget it. She's in that storefront working."

"How long will it be?" he asked. "Tragedy! You too. When will you look it in the face?"

EDWARD ALBEE

The Sandbox (1959)

A Brief Play, in Memory of My Grandmother (1876–1959)

The Players:

THE YOUNG MAN..........25	A good-looking, well-built boy in a bathing suit.
MOMMY.......................55	A well-dressed, imposing woman.
DADDY..........................60	A small man; gray, thin.
GRANDMA 86	A tiny, wizened woman with bright eyes.
THE MUSICIAN	No particular age, but young would be nice.

Note:

When, in the course of the play, MOMMY and DADDY call each other by these names, there should be no suggestion of regionalism. These names are of empty affection and point up the pre-senility and vacuity of their characters.

The Scene:

A bare stage, with only the following: Near the footlights, far stage-right, two simple chairs set side by side, facing the audience; near the footlights, far stage-left, a chair facing stage-right with a music stand before it; farther back, and stage-center, slightly elevated and raked, a large child's sandbox with a toy pail and shovel; the background is the sky, which alters from brightest day to deepest night.

At the beginning, it is brightest day; the YOUNG MAN is alone on stage, to the rear of the sandbox, and to one side. He is doing calisthenics; he does calisthenics until quite at the very end of the play. These calisthenics, employing the arms only, should suggest the beating and fluttering of wings. The YOUNG MAN is, after all, the Angel of Death.

MOMMY *and* DADDY *enter from stage-left,* MOMMY *first.*

MOMMY

(*Motioning to* DADDY) Well, here we are; this is the beach.

DADDY

(*Whining*) I'm cold.

247

MOMMY

(*Dismissing him with a little laugh*) Don't be silly; it's as warm as toast. Look at that nice young man over there: *he* doesn't think it's cold. (*Waves to the* YOUNG MAN) Hello.

YOUNG MAN

(*With an endearing smile*) Hi!

MOMMY

(*Looking about*) This will do perfectly . . . don't you think so, Daddy? There's sand there . . . and the water beyond. What do you think, Daddy?

DADDY

(*Vaguely*) Whatever you say, Mommy.

MOMMY

(*With the same little laugh*) Well, of course . . . whatever I say. Then, it's settled, is it?

DADDY

(*Shrugs*) She's *your* mother, not mine.

MOMMY

I know she's my mother. What do you take me for? (*A pause*) All right, now; let's get on with it. (*She shouts into the wings, stage-left*) You! Out there! You can come in now.
   (*The* MUSICIAN *enters, seats himself in the chair, stage-left, places music on the music stand, is ready to play.* MOMMY *nods approvingly*)

MOMMY

Very nice; very nice. Are you ready, Daddy? Let's go get Grandma.

DADDY

Whatever you say, Mommy.

MOMMY

(*Leading the way out, stage-left*) Of course, whatever I say. (*To the* MUSICIAN) You can begin now.
   (*The* MUSICIAN *begins playing;* MOMMY *and* DADDY *exit; the* MUSICIAN, *all the while playing, nods to the* YOUNG MAN)

EDWARD ALBEE

YOUNG MAN

(*With the same endearing smile*) Hi!
(*After a moment,* MOMMY *and* DADDY *re-enter, carrying* GRANDMA. *She is borne in by their hands under her armpits; she is quite rigid; her legs are drawn up; her feet do not touch the ground; the expression on her ancient face is that of puzzlement and fear*)

DADDY

Where do we put her?

MOMMY

(*The same little laugh*) Wherever I say, of course. Let me see . . . well . . . all right, over there . . . in the sandbox. (*Pause*) Well, what are you waiting for, Daddy? . . . The sandbox!
(*Together they carry* GRANDMA *over to the sandbox and more or less dump her in*)

GRANDMA

(*Righting herself to a sitting position; her voice a cross between a baby's laugh and cry*) Ahhhhhh! Graaaaa!

DADDY

(*Dusting himself*) What do we do now?

MOMMY

(*To the* MUSICIAN) You can stop now.
(*The* MUSICIAN *stops*)
(*Back to* DADDY) What do you mean, what do we do now? We go over there and sit down, of course. (*To the* YOUNG MAN) Hello there.

YOUNG MAN

(*Again smiling*) Hi!
(MOMMY *and* DADDY *move to the chairs, stage-right, and sit down. A pause*)

GRANDMA

(*Same as before*) Ahhhhhh! Ah-haaaaaa! Graaaaaa!

DADDY

Do you think . . . do you think she's . . . comfortable?

MOMMY

(*Impatiently*) How would I know?

DADDY

(*Pause*) What do we do now?

MOMMY

(*As if remembering*) We . . . wait. We . . . sit here . . . and we wait . . . that's what we do.

DADDY

(*After a pause*) Shall we talk to each other?

MOMMY

(*With that little laugh; picking something off her dress*) Well, *you* can talk, if you want to . . . if you can think of anything to *say* . . . if you can think of anything *new*.

DADDY

(*Thinks*) No . . . I suppose not.

MOMMY

(*With a triumphant laugh*) Of course not!

GRANDMA

(*Banging a toy shovel against the pail*) Haaaaaa! Ah-haaaaaa!

MOMMY

(*Out over the audience*) Be quiet, Grandma . . . just be quiet, and wait.
    (GRANDMA *throws a shovelful of sand at* MOMMY)

MOMMY

(*Still out over the audience*) She's throwing sand at me! You stop that, Grandma; you stop throwing sand at Mommy! (*To* DADDY) She's throwing sand at me.
    (DADDY *looks around at* GRANDMA, *who screams at him*)

GRANDMA

GRAAAAAA!

MOMMY

Don't look at her. Just . . . sit here . . . be very still . . . and wait. (*To the* MUSICIAN) You . . . uh . . . you go ahead and do whatever it is you do.
    (*The* MUSICIAN *plays*)

EDWARD ALBEE

(MOMMY *and* DADDY *are fixed, staring out beyond the audience.* GRANDMA *looks at them, looks at the* MUSICIAN, *looks at the sandbox, throws down the shovel*)

GRANDMA

Ah-haaaaaa! Graaaaaa! (*Looks for reaction; gets none. Now . . . directly to the audience*) Honestly! What a way to treat an old woman! Drag her out of the house . . . stick her in a car . . . bring her out here from the city . . . dump her in a pile of sand . . . and leave her here to set. I'm eighty-six years old! I was married when I was seventeen. To a farmer. He died when I was thirty. (*To the* MUSICIAN) Will you stop that, please?

(*The* MUSICIAN *stops playing*)

I'm a feeble old woman . . . how do you expect anybody to hear me over that peep! peep! peep! (*To herself*) There's no respect around here. (*To the* YOUNG MAN) There's no respect around here!

YOUNG MAN

(*Same smile*) Hi!

GRANDMA

(*After a pause, a mild double-take, continues, to the audience*) My husband died when I was thirty (*indicates* MOMMY), and I had to raise that big cow over there all by my lonesome. You can imagine what *that was like*. Lordy! (*To the* YOUNG MAN) Where'd they get *you*?

YOUNG MAN

Oh . . . I've been around for a while.

GRANDMA

I'll bet you have! Heh, heh, heh. Will you look at you!

YOUNG MAN

(*Flexing his muscles*) Isn't that something? (*Continues his calisthenics*)

GRANDMA

Boy, oh boy; I'll say. Pretty good.

YOUNG MAN

(*Sweetly*) I'll say.

GRANDMA

Where ya from?

YOUNG MAN

Southern California.

GRANDMA

(*Nodding*) Figgers; figgers. What's your name, honey?

YOUNG MAN

I don't know. . . .

GRANDMA

(*To the audience*) Bright, too!

YOUNG MAN

I mean . . . I mean, they haven't given me one yet . . . the studio . . .

GRANDMA

(*Giving him the once-over*) You don't say . . . you don't say. Well . . . uh, I've got to talk some more . . . don't you go 'way.

YOUNG MAN

Oh, no.

GRANDMA

(*Turning her attention back to the audience*) Fine; fine. (*Then, once more, back to the* YOUNG MAN) You're . . . you're an actor, hunh?

YOUNG MAN

(*Beaming*) Yes. I am.

GRANDMA

(*To the audience again; shrugs*) I'm smart that way. *Anyhow,* I had to raise . . . *that* over there all by my lonesome; and what's next to her there . . . that's what she married. Rich? I tell you . . . money, money, money. They took me off the *farm* . . . which was real decent of them . . . and they moved me into the big town house with *them* . . . fixed a nice place for me under the stove . . . gave me an army blanket . . . and my own dish . . . my very own dish! So, what have I got to complain about? Nothing, of course. I'm not complaining. (*She looks up at the sky, shouts to someone off stage*) Shouldn't it be getting dark now, dear?
(*The lights dim; night comes on. The* MUSICIAN *begins to play; it becomes deepest night. There are spots on all the players, including the* YOUNG MAN, *who is, of course, continuing his calisthenics*)

EDWARD ALBEE

DADDY

(*Stirring*) It's nighttime.

MOMMY

Shhhh. Be still . . . wait.

DADDY

(*Whining*) It's so hot.

MOMMY

Shhhhhh. Be still . . . wait.

GRANDMA

(*To herself*) That's better. Night. (*To the* MUSICIAN) Honey, do you play all through this part?
(*The* MUSICIAN *nods*)
Well, keep it nice and soft; that's a good boy.
(*The* MUSICIAN *nods again; plays softly*)
That's nice.
(*There is an off-stage rumble*)

DADDY

(*Starting*) What was that?

MOMMY

(*Beginning to weep*) It was nothing.

DADDY

It was . . . it was . . . thunder . . . or a wave breaking . . . or something.

MOMMY

(*Whispering, through her tears*) It was an off-stage rumble . . . and you know what *that* means. . . .

DADDY

I forget. . . .

MOMMY

(*Barely able to talk*) It means the time has come for poor Grandma . . . and I can't bear it!

DADDY

(*Vacantly*) I . . . I suppose you've got to be brave.

GRANDMA

(*Mocking*) That's right, kid; be brave. You'll bear up; you'll get over it.
    (*Another off-stage rumble . . . louder*)

MOMMY

Ohhhhhhhhhh . . . poor Grandma . . . poor Grandma. . . .

GRANDMA

(*To* MOMMY) I'm fine! I'm all right! It hasn't happened yet!
    (*A violent off-stage rumble. All the lights go out, save the spot on the*
    YOUNG MAN; *the* MUSICIAN *stops playing*)

MOMMY

Ohhhhhhhhhh. . . . Ohhhhhhhhhh. . . .
    (*Silence*)

GRANDMA

Don't put the lights up yet . . . I'm not ready; I'm not quite ready. (*Silence*)
All right, dear . . . I'm about done.
    (*The lights come up again, to brightest day; the* MUSICIAN *begins to*
    play. GRANDMA *is discovered, still in the sandbox, lying on her side,*
    propped up on an elbow, half covered, busily shoveling sand over
    herself)

GRANDMA

(*Muttering*) I don't know how I'm supposed to do anything with this goddam
toy shovel. . . .

DADDY

Mommy! It's daylight!

MOMMY

(*Brightly*) So it is! Well! Our long night is over. We must put away our tears,
take off our mourning . . . and face the future. It's our duty.

GRANDMA

(*Still shoveling; mimicking*) . . . take off our mourning . . . face the future. . . . Lordy!
    (MOMMY *and* DADDY *rise, stretch.* MOMMY *waves to the* YOUNG
    MAN)

YOUNG MAN

(*With that smile*) Hi!

EDWARD ALBEE

(GRANDMA *plays dead.* (!) MOMMY *and* DADDY *go over to look at her; she is a little more than half buried in the sand; the toy shovel is in her hands, which are crossed on her breast*)

MOMMY

(*Before the sandbox; shaking her head*) Lovely! It's . . . it's hard to be sad . . . she looks . . . so happy. (*With pride and conviction*) It pays to do things well. (*To the* MUSICIAN) All right, you can stop now, if you want to. I mean, stay around for a swim, or something; it's all right with us. (*She sighs heavily*) Well, Daddy . . . off we go.

DADDY

Brave Mommy!

MOMMY

Brave Daddy!
    (*They exit stage-left*)

GRANDMA

(*After they leave; lying quite still*) It pays to do things well. . . . Boy, oh Boy! (*She tries to sit up*) . . . well, kids . . . (*but she finds she can't*) . . . I . . . I can't get up. I . . . I can't move. . . .
    (*The* YOUNG MAN *stops his calisthenics, nods to the* MUSICIAN, *walks over to* GRANDMA, *kneels down by the sandbox*)

GRANDMA

I . . . I can't move. . . .

YOUNG MAN

Shhhhh . . . be very still. . . .

GRANDMA

I . . . I can't move

YOUNG MAN

Uh . . . ma'am; I . . . I have a line here.

GRANDMA

Oh, I'm sorry, sweetie; you go right ahead.

YOUNG MAN

I am . . . uh . . .

GRANDMA

Take your time, dear.

YOUNG MAN

(*Prepares; delivers the line like a real amateur*) I am the Angel of Death. I am . . . uh . . . I am come for you.

GRANDMA

What . . . wha . . . (*Then, with resignation*) . . . ohhhh . . . ohhhh, I see. (The YOUNG MAN *bends over, kisses* GRANDMA *gently on the forehead*)

GRANDMA

(*Her eyes closed, her hands folded on her breast again, the shovel between her hands, a sweet smile on her face*)
Well . . . that was very nice, dear. . . .

YOUNG MAN

(*Still kneeling*) Shhhhhh . . . be still. . . .

GRANDMA

What I meant was . . . you did that very well, dear. . . .

YOUNG MAN

(*Blushing*) . . . oh . . .

GRANDMA

No; I mean it. You've got that . . . you've got a quality.

YOUNG MAN

(*With his endearing smile*) Oh . . . thank you; thank you very much . . . ma'am.

GRANDMA

(*Slowly; softly—as the* YOUNG MAN *puts his hands on top of* GRANDMA'S)
You're . . . you're welcome . . . dear.
(*Tableau. The* MUSICIAN *continues to play as the curtain slowly comes down*)

CURTAIN

The 90th Year

for Lore Segal

High in the jacaranda shines the gilded thread
of a small bird's curlicue of song—too high
for her to see or hear.
                 I've learned
not to say, these last years,
'O, look!—O, listen, Mother!'
as I used to.

            (It was she
who taught me to look;
to name the flowers when I was still close to the ground,
my face level with theirs;
or to watch the sublime metamorphoses
unfold and unfold
over the walled back gardens of our street . . .

It had not been given her
to know the flesh as good in itself,
as the flesh of a fruit is good. To her
the human body has been a husk,
a shell in which souls were prisoned.
Yet, from within it, with how much gazing
her life has paid tribute to the world's body!
How tears of pleasure
would choke her, when a perfect voice,
deep or high, clove to its note unfaltering!)

She has swept the crackling seedpods,
the litter of mauve blossoms, off the cement path,
tipped them into the rubbish bucket.
She's made her bed, washed up the breakfast dishes,
wiped the hotplate. I've taken the butter and milkjug
back to the fridge next door—but it's not my place,

257

visiting here, to usurp the tasks
that weave the day's pattern.
Now she is leaning forward in her chair,
       by the lamp lit in the daylight,
rereading *War and Peace*.
                When I look up
from her wellworn copy of *The Divine Milieu*,
which she wants me to read, I see her hand
loose on the black stem of the magnifying glass,
she is dozing.
'I am so tired,' she has written to me, 'of appreciating
the gift of life.'

The Stroke

Later he'll say Death stepped right up
to shake his hand, then squeezed
until he sank to his knees. (*Get up,
nigger. Get up and try again.*)

Much later he'll admit he'd been afraid,
curled tight in the center of the rug, sunlight
striking one cheek and plaited raffia
scratching the other. He'll leave out

the part about daydream's aromatic fields
and the strap-worn flanks of the mule
he followed through them. When his wife asks
how did it feel, he won't mention

that the sun shone like the summer
she was pregnant with their first, and
that she craved watermelon which he smuggled
home wrapped in a newspaper, and how

the bus driver smirked as his nickel
clicked through—no, he'll say
it was like being kicked by a mule.
Right now, though, pinned to the bull's-eye,

he knows it was Lem all along:
Lem's knuckles tapping his chest in passing,
Lem's heart, for safekeeping,
he shores up in his arms.

Strokes

The left side of her world is gone—
the rest sustained by memory
and a realization: There are still the children.

Going down our porch steps her pastor
calls back: "We are proud of her recovery,
and there is a chiropractor up in Galesburg. . . . "

The birthdays of the old require such candles.

Grandmother's Stroke

Her eyes stare back like posters
and her tongue, the sharpest in the family,
is slack between her teeth.
I talk a long time, making things up,
hoping my voice is at least familiar.
After a while she blinks hard once
and flaps her right hand against the bed.
It's minutes before I understand.
When I give her the pencil she writes DEATH
NOT MENTIONED TO THE DYING ISN'T TASTEFUL
OR KIND in a big, childish scrawl—
laying down the law.

Sequel

It was right after Burt and Francine died that I began the saga of Joey Moxey the clown.

Tillie was too young for details, I thought, so I spared her—and myself. Burt had taken his wife to Warsaw where he had been invited to perform some of his music. Though she couldn't go, Tillie had been part of their excitement. When they brought her to stay with me she couldn't wait to trace her parents' journey on the map. She stumbled over her suitcases in her impatience, and there amidst the clutter we both followed her small finger over the rumpled countries from the bed to the floor.

Never. Tillie grasped the concept right away. She repeated it to fix it in her mind. I saw the pain enter, briefly scorching her bright, solemn eyes. They closed deliberately and it was buried. She plucked at a bandaid on her ankle. They'll never come back now. Something went wrong with the plane and it fell down. She was seated on the edge of the table I had been sanding. Her face and limbs were scrawny, intense, her hair gritty, like blonde static. The smell of sawdust was still in the air. I pulled the plug out and wrapped the cord around the sander. I could not endure any more machinery noise that day.

Never.

It struck me that a child's world is made up of such categorical imperatives. Experiences are unique. Laws are absolute. You cannot have any candy. At Tillie's age it meant you can never have candy. You must go to your room meant you must go there forever. My adult world by then had perverted nature, admittedly relativity, forgiveness, recompense. I had grown soft.

In order to come to terms with what I had rediscovered—the uncompromising absurdity of the universe, I began to create the character of the clown. I told myself I owed it to my granddaughter, Tillie, to keep everything intact. Events were like pieces in a jigsaw puzzle, I said to her. By themselves they might look . . . well, weird. But they all fit together.

The truth is I had myself to persuade. Burt, my only son was dead, and all the music the world would ever get from him ended. God knows it could have done with more.

At first the adventures of Joey Moxey were ordinary enough. He was your typical clown: bald with a fringe of long hair around his head, red nose, baggy clothes, big feet. The feet were so big that in Joey's case one shoe also served as a sportscar. Naturally he made his entrance by driving his shoe into the arena and when he stopped dozens of clowns tumbled out to the astonishment and delight of the children in the audience. They loved Joey Moxey and there was no better place in the world than under the enormous circus tent.

Joey had many adventures and he picked up a variety of friends in his travels, including a bird who made her nest on his head and flew out every time he took off his hat, Tina the cat, Oogak the jungle boy, and last but not least, Sadie Donut, a policewoman who followed him everywhere, presenting him with innumerable speeding tickets and parking tickets because she was so much in love with him. Their adventures would end in breathtaking escapes and Joey would hurry back to the circus tent just in time for the show to begin.

It was not long before my imagination ran out and it was up to Tillie to suggest subjects for the stories. Tell me about Joey Moxey falling off his bike, Tillie would say on a day she had had a catastrophic fall off her bike. And my story would begin, "It just so happened Joey Moxey did fall off his bike . . . " And in the hundreds of nights that followed, it just so happened Joey Moxey fell off a wall, spilled ketchup on his new clothes, got chased by a dog, bit by a cat, frightened by a snake, knocked over by a wave, awakened by a nightmare . . .

Tell me about Joey Moxey flying a plane, Tillie once said, and without hesitation, I launched into the fantastic adventure. "It just so happened, Joey Moxey did fly a plane once . . . " And I told how the clown and the President were the only two celebrities on board the maiden flight of a gigantic new supersonic plane when it developed engine trouble. The engine made such indescribable noises that the pilot fainted with fright. Joey Moxey took over. The control tower kept radioing instructions, but because this was such a new plane, no one knew exactly how it worked. Control tower would tell him to push a button on the elaborate instrument panel and when Joey pushed what he thought was the right button a wheel would fall off. Control tower would suggest something else, a lever perhaps, or a knob, or an overhead handle, and every time he followed the instructions another piece of the plane would disappear.

Things were getting precarious, and the complicated plane was getting smaller. But somehow the remarkable clown managed to bring it down with the quivering President on board who for his part managed to recover in time to make an inspiring speech to the gathered crowd of reporters and television cameramen. Joey Moxey was nowhere to be seen, of course, for he had slipped away to begin the show.

I was rather pleased with that story when I leaned down to kiss Tillie goodnight. Her eyes were somber, her face wet with tears. "You're never serious," she whispered angrily, and I lay there beside her, wondering at my need to deceive her, until she fell asleep.

Burt had inherited my stark baldness. I had shaved my head until the sixties when I adopted his long-haired style for the fringe around my skull. We were an amusing pair then, and friends were always telling us how much we looked alike. But it wasn't until that night that I realized how much we had in common with the remarkable clown.

When Burt and Francine were killed I worried briefly that Francine's folks would seek custody of Tillie. Not that I would have contested it. I loved Tillie, wanted only the best for her, and could recognize the arguments on their behalf. The Oaks were a married pair as solid as their name. Whereas I lived alone, Sarah and I having parted long ago. Duncan Oaks had already "put money away" for retirement while I had never really considered retirement, it always having been my natural life-style.

But I underestimated Duncan's and Mattie's determination to follow their own rainbow to its end—a condo in Florida, surrounded by water and golf courses, with assured re-sale potential. "This is no environment to bring up a little girl," Duncan crooned petulantly. I agreed. Besides, he complained, they had worked hard all their lives, sacrificed, deprived themselves. They deserved this. In agitated voices made scratchy by the long-distance wires they told me of the tickets they had bought for tours, boat trips, chartered planes, vacation clubs. I agreed with their good judgment. Tillie should stay with me.

Tillie stayed with me. She followed me everywhere. For awhile I worried about her attachment to me. Every time we were near each other she had to hug me, every time we passed we had to kiss. Tillie's kiss was a darting wetness, a sparrow sound. Was I somehow the living ghost of her father, the death and rebirth? *But I was never serious.* Was I the embodiment of the spirit of Joey Moxey, the clown? The question formed in Tillie's eyes, glowed like hot sand. And the answer? Perhaps it was there for a moment, a brief shadowy scowl. Then gone. Her eyes again caught streaks of sunlight, as did her hair which scattered about her in curls as though charged with electricity.

"Joey Moxey can be more than a clown," Tillie reproached me. "Joey Moxey is happy being a clown," I insisted. Her voice cracked with feeling. Tillie talked so often with an adult's sense of the world that I was taken by surprise whenever she broke down and wept over simple childish things.

I knew it was not considered healthy for Tillie to come home after school and stay with me rather than find friends to play with. These were dangerous signs of social maladjustment. But for Tillie, these moments of maladjustment seemed her happiest ones. She had inherited not so much my love of solitude, but my penchant for intimate experience.

Not surprisingly she was exquisitely musical. She asked to learn the cello, Burt's instrument, and I managed to find a small size second-hand one and fix it up for her. I could never understand music. In Burt's case it was like an underground spring which broke open some time in his childhood and never stopped bubbling. He was a furious worker. Even before his teens Burt was practicing long hours in his room. When it was silent it meant he was composing. There was nothing we needed to do to encourage such onrushing talent, but keep out of the way. When Burt grew older, his music seemed to grow firmer, more self-assured. Like his voice. And like his voice it deepened, became gentle, more resonant.

Where all this came from I'll never know. Sarah's only distinct talent and obsession was for alcohol, and I was lazy, frankly and peacefully so. I once played the piano, but let it drift when my parents decided lessons were too expensive. I'm a good, but rather slow-moving sort of furniture maker.

Tillie, though she could hardly have known Burt as a man, having barely known him as a father, seemed destined to follow his career. When she came home from school she joined me with her cello, whether outside in the backyard under the fruit trees, in the workshop or in the kitchen. She even played as I sat on the toilet.

The night of the day Tillie fell and gashed her wrist which required stitches and prevented her from practicing the cello I told her it just so happened Joey Moxey had cut his hand before a concert, but he carried it off any way by hiding Tina the cat inside his cello and having her sing Bach's sarabande for the unaccompanied cello, which happened to be Tillie's favorite piece at the time. The audience loved it, Joey made it to the circus on time. And Tillie, bandaged arm on the pillow, fell asleep.

Naturally, it was not possible for Tillie to avoid alienating her schoolmates. They did not like this lonely creature who found so many levels of meaning in child's play. They were suspicious of her laughter. It expressed a pleasure in too many things at once. And yet, serious as she was, she did not take the important things seriously enough. This was my fault. I had trouble keeping up with the laundry, much less with the styles, and instead of brightly colored variations on women's-lib junior pant suits, Tillie more often than not wore plain, faded dresses.

And her knowledge of boy's anatomy disconcerted them. I told her that it was a matter of principle never to strike in the vulnerable area unless the boy fought unfairly. To her credit Tillie reserved this weapon for just such occasions. Once however, she temporarily disabled a teacher, and I had to pay a visit to Principal Rodney's office.

Tillie was exercising her right of free expression, I said. (She had remained seated for the Pledge of Allegiance the day after the President was pictured smiling with another Latin American dictator.) The teacher who hauled her up by the hair was committing assault and battery. Principal Rodney assured me things were quite the other way as measured by the outcome.

They gave her more room from then on, but it did not stop laughing at her, teachers as well as children. It just so happened that everyone laughed at Joey Moxey too when he was little, I said. Which is why he decided to become a clown. Instead of feeling sorry for himself, he came to love his unique gift. Unhappy people fear their uniqueness; happy people love their uniqueness. This, too, I think Tillie understood.

She was standing on the bathtub swinging her brown lunch bag while I was sitting on the toilet. How many times I found myself issuing proclamations from that throne. My bowels, which all my life scarcely had been more noticeable than my breathing or my heartbeat, had become rebellious of late. I had reached the Serutan age.

Fortified with the lessons of Joey Moxey, Tillie went off to school. The lessons barely held to the end of the school day when Tillie would come racing home, her eyes moist, her cheeks drained, more often than not to greet me where she had left me, on the toilet. This was good for a bedtime story, of course. It just so happened that Joey Moxey was sitting on the throne when the King and Queen of England decided to pay him a surprise royal visit with all their lords and ladies . . .

Tillie and I talked quite thoroughly about things, probably more than the things deserved. But we enjoyed talking. She would set up her cello as I warmed the chocolate milk. Out of this would come a discussion of motion. The vibration of the cello string, the melodic movement of sound, the stirring of the molecules of chocolate milk as it became warm. We imagined ourselves as molecules of chocolate milk, part of a delicious storm of other chocolate molecules. Would we recognize each other as we flew by? Would we see each other again? Would we remember each other as we grew old?

She helped me with my work. I showed her how to drive 20d nails into three-inch thick planks. It took sensitive hammering. The wood was hard and full of knots—one had to *find* the hole—and a clumsy swat would curl the nail.

Or sometimes she would sit beside me as I worked on my plastic bottle sculpture. There was a time when I had first begun that I would take plastic bottles and with great enthusiasm cut them and twist them and melt them into all sorts of peculiar shapes. It was my rococo period. As I grew older I began to adopt a more classical approach. Michelangelo once said he tried to *free* the sculpture from the block of stone. And so did I with plastic bottles. Each bottle I discovered had all the elements of its sculpture within it.

Tillie would stop playing and watch quietly as I held a bottle in my hand, turning it over and examining it. Suddenly, almost as though a dressmaker had drawn a pattern, the pieces would declare themselves. With a linoleum cutter I would slice the bottle along the lines and assemble them. Tillie was always delighted. You see, I said, what people saw as the purpose of the bottle—what they bought it for in a store—that was really not its purpose, but only its transitional state. Its real purpose was to stand there along with all the other plastic bottle spirits scattered through our house and back yard.

"Why don't you sell them?" Tillie asked.

"Because no one would buy them," I answered.

"Why wouldn't anyone buy them?"

"Because I wouldn't sell them."

"Why wouldn't you sell them?"

"Because no one would buy them."

Tillie slapped her cello furiously. "Must you always talk like a clown?"

But she laughed when I nodded yes.

Tillie was always clinging to me, yet she was never possessive. When she came home from school she would find a customer in my workshop now and then, a fashionably dressed woman on a spree or a decorator looking for some odd piece among my sprawling chairs and strange tables. Tillie would listen with delight to the conversation. I would catch her eyes glowing on me. She knew I was charming our guest. If I really liked the woman I would pour her some beer in a hollow-stem champagne glass and hold it up high as I passed it to her. The bubbles glittered in the sunlight. The women were invariably delighted. I made them feel comfortable. I was easily pleased.

And if Tillie saw them at breakfast the next morning she greeted them cheerfully and hugged them too before going off to school.

Once she wandered into the bedroom while my houseguest was still in bed. I was shaving. Fascinated, Tillie climbed up on the sink and followed my stroking closely. The houseguest looked up somewhat uncertainly, a condition that was not alleviated very much by the conversation that followed.

"When I grow up, do you think I should shave," Tillie asked, "or should I let my beard grow?"

"It all depends, Tillie," I answered without hesitation. "Whatever you think looks best on you."

We laughed and wrestled on the bed, and Joey Moxey decided to let his beard grow until it was so long he tripped on it as he ran and when he tried to untangle himself it got caught between his toes and in the carburetor of his shoe. Eventually it so locked him up into a ball of fuzz that Sadie Donut had to roll him, dust, dirt, sticky wads of chewing gum and all, into a trough of hair remover. Which is why Joey Moxey had no hair except for the fringe around his head. But this only made Sadie Donut love him more, for to her he seemed handsomer than ever.

But that night, Tillie came home from school, her eyes burning with rage. "It's not true. Girls don't grow beards!"

I nodded solemnly.

"You're never *serious*," Tillie protested. "How do you expect to *amount* to anything?"

As she ran off to fetch her cello, I wondered what moment in Tillie's school had first shined light on the phrase "amount to anything."

The next day I spurted blood into the toilet bowl.

Dr. Chernock had a polished brass nameplate, British magazines in the waiting room and a long silver instrument with which he peered inside me. I heard him groan impatiently—"Oh, Ah . . . " as he struggled with some invisible and apparently unappreciative part of my body. Then suddenly he issued a triumphant sigh. "Eureka, I found it." He snapped off his rubber gloves and reassembled his French cuffs. It was cancer, he said.

That night, it just so happened Joey Moxey was subject to the same curious procedure. A very famous scientific institute was interested in doing research on the famous clown to find out what made him so funny. They kept him in the research institute subjecting him to all sorts of elaborate chemical analyses while Nobel-prize winning scientists paraded back and forth between his bed and mahogany panelled conference rooms. Until at last, one of the scientists, while peering in the most unlikely place through his long silver tube, cried, "Eureka! I found it!"

When it came time to kiss her goodnight, Tillie kept her head buried under the pillow.

The next day, Dr. Chernock admitted me to the hospital. He assured me he looked forward to ridding me of this annoyance. Tillie stayed with a neighbor.

The night before surgery Tillie took her bedtime story in my bed for a change. It just so happened Joey Moxey was in the hospital with a runny nose. It was a bad runny nose, of course, and soon the great clown ran out of Kleenex. He called for the nurse, but she was too busy to come, so Joey had to shift for himself. Out of bed he stumbled and into the next room where he helped himself to a handful of Kleenex. The patient in the room awoke from a deep sleep just in time to see the weirdest sight he had ever seen: a clown blowing his nose with all his might. Poor Joey. He had to blow so hard that his red ball of a nose collapsed and only gradually swelled up again with a long eerie whistle.

You can imagine what this did to the patient's nerves. He lay there absolutely transfixed until this apparition's nose finally stopped growing and the long eerie whistle came to an end.

No sooner was Joey Moxey gone than the terrified patient rang for the nurse. And no sooner did the nurse hear the patient's ridiculous story than she decided he must have been awakened by a nightmare and presented him with an enormous sleeping pill. Zonk went the patient. Out cold. Meanwhile, in and out of all the rooms went Joey in his never-ending lust for more Kleenex. And from every room came the same frightened ringing for the nurse. The nurse could not understand why all her patients were suddenly having such wild nightmares, but she had no doubt how to deal with the problem. Every one of the patients got the same treatment. And every one of them went Zonk. Out cold.

The next morning when the doctor arrived he found all his patients absolutely stretched out, snoring, unarousable. Except for poor Joey Moxey who was sitting up in bed, still blowing his nose. When the nurse saw him she began to think she was having her own nightmare.

Tillie tried, but she couldn't help it—soon she was laughing uncontrollably, particularly at the sound effects, and when I kissed her goodnight from the bed I felt the tears—this time of happiness: though they flashed with the memory of sorrow.

The surgery was over quickly.

I had heard stories about patients being totally aware during an operation despite the anesthesia. But for these stories I would assume I had been visited by my own bad dreams. I remember visions, starkly colored and vibrating with sound, which must have taken place during the depths of my unconsciousness or during my fitful awakening in the recovery room. I remember faces appearing suddenly, hands groping toward my wrist, other hands moving like mountains, burying me in their darkness. Somewhere within all this unreal universe I heard something very real, the great hollow groan of disappointment as Dr. Chernock looked inside and saw that it was too late.

When the surgeon appeared again at my bedside his mood was much changed. He seemed resentful. Gone were optimism and gracious enthusiasm, the powers he had brought to bear on his patients' behalf. These, and the magic of the scalpel were what he had counted on to drive away the evil cancers. I had let him down, demeaned him. His mood told me all, though in specific words, Dr. Chernock told me nothing.

That night Joey Moxey was visited in the hospital by all his friends and they put on a show for the patients. My voice faded and Tillie finished the story for me. She said everyone in the hospital loved the performance except for one person. Guess who. The nurse. She was bored by it and fell fast asleep. It hurt so much when I laughed that I begged Tillie to stop. She kissed me goodnight and left.

The next day Dr. Chernock told me I could leave soon and recuperate at home. He suggested that I find another doctor. He was a specialist, a surgeon, and his services would no longer be necessary.

That night it just so happened Joey Moxey's runny nose got worse and worse and to everyone's disappointment he died.

For an instant Tillie's eyes flared at me.

All of Joey's friends gathered to see what should be done. Sadie Donut led the discussion. They wondered whether they should bury him or cremate him. After hardly any debate they agreed that the clown would have wanted them to find out whichever was cheaper and be done with it. They reminisced, of course, about all the wonderful adventures they had had with him. No doubt about it, there would never be another Joey Moxey. But Sadie Donut pointed out that Joey would have been the first to say that about them, too. She for one would continue to have adventures even without Joey Moxey, and she was sure everyone else would do the same. But, she said, wouldn't Joey Moxey want them most of all to continue being friends, meeting, and sharing with each other all the things that happened?

That night as Tillie and I kissed, the tears that flashed between us were hers and mine.

The next night, Tillie began the saga of Sadie Donut.

Appropriate Affect

Grandma Frannie was a tall, slim woman, stooped now, who had been pretty before all her children were born. She still had a beautiful smile, with all her own teeth. It was sweet and sad, perhaps even reproachful, and she had used it for years to shame the family into orderly compliance. She had met Henry Winter before she finished library school, and brought to her marriage all the passion she had once lavished on the Dewey decimal system. In passion, she was disappointed. Henry was a rigid and unimaginative man, though a dutiful lover. She was pregnant within two months of the wedding, and within five years she had four daughters, Maggie, Laura, Frieda and Martha.

No one escaped the bright beam of Grandma Frannie's love. At eighty-six, she still sent birthday presents to every grandchild and great-grandchild. She remembered who was married to whom, and even who was living with whom, what his name was, and what he did. Although it didn't really matter what anyone did. Her love leapt all hurdles. Her oldest grandson, Martin, who had a coming out party within a month of moving to San Francisco, had dedicated his first volume of poetry to Frannie. His mother cried when he told her he'd sent Frannie a copy, but Frannie kept it in plain view, on the coffee table in the living room. When Martin's mother saw it there, she didn't comment. She figured Frannie probably didn't even know what it was about. And the Christmas after Fred showed up at a family Thanksgiving party with a black stripper, Frannie sent a card that brought love "to that pretty Tanya" and a gift (small, because she wasn't family) from the church bazaar.

"Christ," said Louisa, Frieda's youngest and a graduate student in psychology, "you can't be a black sheep in this family even if you want." It was true. The steady pressure of Grandma's love reduced them all, eventually, to gray normality. Even Julian, who was in prison in Joliet, Illinois, for forgery, wrote her regularly.

Frannie and Henry lived in Connecticut in a large frame house built on a hill. It had once overlooked an abandoned orchard where wizened little apples grew. Ten years before, a developer had leveled the field and built row on row of identical two-story gray town houses with fake mansard roofs.

Henry and Frannie's house was a faded salmon pink that was gently peeling, and here and there a shutter had fallen off and never been replaced. It was darkened by overgrown cedars in the front yard which reached above the roof for sunlight. The front porch listed slightly, but Bob Hancock, Laura's son-in-law, had jumped up and down on it and it held. It was pronounced safe for Frannie and Henry for the time being.

All the children wanted them to move to the retirement community nearby, but Henry couldn't bear to think of it. He loved the ornate woodwork and soot-streaked wallpaper, the dark furniture inherited from his mother, and the threadbare Oriental rugs.

One Sunday afternoon, an hour or so after their return from the Congregational church, Henry was watching football on television. Frannie came into the living room to tell him that dinner was ready. It was in the middle of the third quarter and that irritated Henry. Because he was slightly deaf and had the television on loud, he didn't hear her coming and that irritated him even more. She stepped suddenly into his line of vision and turned the set off. She shouted, "Dinner, Henry," at him, and smiled her warm, browbeaten smile.

Henry stood up. "There's no need to shout," he said. "What's more, I'm not ready for dinner and I won't be for a good long while. The Sabbath was made for man, madam, not man for the Sabbath." And he walked right over to the TV set and turned it back on.

She said something to him, but he ignored her, so she started her long, slow shuffle back to the kitchen.

Henry turned the set off about forty-five minutes later and started toward the kitchen himself. His walk was brisker and more steady than Frannie's. He stopped abruptly when he rounded the doorway to the dining room. Frannie's legs were sticking straight out from behind the highboy on the floor. He felt a numbed panic as he approached her. She was sitting up, wedged in the corner between the highboy and the wall. Her face was white and agonized. Her mouth had dropped open and her eyes were closed.

"My dear!" Henry said, bending over her stiffly from the waist. He saw her lips move slightly as though she were trying to talk. Her left arm rested uselessly on the floor and her right was somehow bent behind her. Henry reached down and tried to lift her up, but he only managed to slide her forward slightly. Her head lolled back and smacked the wall. Henry cried out. He straightened and started into the kitchen. Halfway to the telephone, with his arms already lifting to take off the receiver and dial, he turned and went back to her. He bent down again.

"I'll be right back, my darling," he said very loudly and clearly, as though she were the deaf one. She made no sign that she'd heard. He went back and placed the call.

No one answered when the ambulance driver rang the bell, so the men walked in with the stretcher. They looked around the dark, empty front hall and then heard a murmuring voice from the room on their right, the dining room. Henry had pulled a chair over next to Frances, and he was sitting in it, holding her hand across his knees and patting it, talking softly to her.

When the ambulance driver was only a few steps away, Henry saw him and stopped talking. He stood up. "Sir, my name is Henry Winter and this is my wife," he said. He began to explain the circumstances under which he'd found her, but the men were already lifting her onto the stretcher and strapping her in, giving loud instructions to each other.

"You coming in the ambulance, Pop?" the driver asked as he picked up his end of the stretcher.

"What say?" asked Henry, turning his head so his good ear was nearer the driver.

"Are you coming with us?" the driver yelled.

"Ah! Much obliged, but I'll follow in my car," said Henry, and he went to get his hat and coat.

"Christ!" the driver said a minute later as they hoisted Frannie into the truck. "Can you imagine them letting an old guy like that have a license?"

In the days following Frannie's stroke, different children, grandchildren and great-grandchildren came and went in the house. As though it were an old country hotel getting ready for the season, rooms that had been shut up for years were opened, mouse droppings and dead insects were swept up and mattresses turned over. Frannie's daughters ransacked the bedding box and clucked to each other about the down puffs and heavy linen sheets with hand stitching that you would think Mother might have handed down by now.

For the first three days they took turns going in one at a time to sit by Frannie in intensive care. They got permission to have a member of the family stay by her straight through the night. The third night it was her granddaughter Charlotte's turn.

The overhead lights were off in the hospital room, but a white plastic nipple plugged into the wall socket next to Frannie's bed glowed like a child's night light and Charlotte could see the shape of her grandmother's skinny body under the bedclothes. She didn't like to look at Gram's face, so embryonic and naked without her glasses, her hair uncombed for three days and her mouth slack. Instead she looked at the sac of IV fluid with its plastic umbilicus running into Gram's bruised arm. Or she held Gram's freckled hand, which lay alongside the mound of bones under the sheets; or she slept; or wept. She rubbed her hands up and down her slightly thickening waist and cried as she thought of life and death; of Gram about to die, and of the baby, her third, taking life inside her own body.

She had tried to talk about this to her younger sister, Louisa, the afternoon before at Frannie and Henry's house, but Louisa had been irritable. Louisa was always irritable when Charlotte cried. "Oh, spare us, why don't you," she'd said, chopping onions for stew. Her knife whacked the board rapidly, like a burst of gunfire. "Next you'll be going on about reincarnation."

Charlotte blew her nose loudly into a Kleenex, and wiped her lower lids carefully so the mascara wouldn't smear. Grandma Frannie stirred slightly and swung her head toward Charlotte. Her mouth closed with a smacking sound and opened again. Charlotte leaned toward the bed, grabbing the steel railings that boxed her grandmother in.

"Gram?" she whispered. She cleared her throat. "Gram?" Her grandmother's eyes snapped open and stared wildly for a second. Then the lids seemed to grow heavy and they drooped again.

Charlotte stood up and put one hand on her grandmother's shoulder. The other hand rested on her own belly. At her touch, her grandmother's eyes opened again and she frowned and seemed to try to fix Charlotte in focus with the anxious intensity of a newborn.

"Gram? Do you hear me?" Charlotte said. "Do you hear me?"

After a few seconds' pause, Grandma Frannie nodded, a slow swaying of her frizzy head.

"Do you know me?" asked Charlotte. Gram shut her lips and tightened them and frowned hard at Charlotte.

"It's Charlotte, Grandma," she said, and started to weep again. Her right hand was furiously rubbing her belly. She was already thinking of how she would tell the others of this moment. She leaned over and put her face close to her grandmother's.

"It's Charlotte, Grandma. Do you know me?"

Again her grandmother moved her head slightly, up and down. Her lips quivered with some private effort.

"Oh, Grandma, I wanted you to know. I'm going to have a baby." Tears ran down Charlotte's face and plopped onto the neatly folded sheet covering her grandmother's chest. "I'm going to have another baby, Gram."

There was no change in the intense frown on Grandma Frannie's face, but her mouth opened. Charlotte leaned closer still and Grandma Frannie's breath was horrible in her face. Frannie's lips worked and her breathing was shallow and fast.

"The. Nasty. Man," she whispered.

Charlotte reported to the doctors and the family that Grandma Frannie had waked in the night and had spoken. When they asked, as they did eagerly and repeatedly, what she had said, Charlotte would only say that she hadn't been herself. Her cousin Elinore thought Charlotte was being "a bit of a snot" not to tell, trying to rivet all that attention on herself. Charlotte felt everyone's irritation with her all the next day. Frannie was fluttering delicately in and out of consciousness and muttered only incoherent phrases as the nurses changed her bedding or inserted another IV. But Charlotte still tearfully refused to tell what it was Grandma had said to her, although she insisted that Grandma had spoken clearly. "God, you'd think it was her mantra," Louisa said.

After Charlotte heard Grandma Frannie speak, the family came by twos and threes for several days. Slowly Frannie began to recognize them, calling out their names as they walked in. Sometimes she couldn't seem to say the name and then she'd spell it aloud, carefully and often correctly. It was a small hospital, and the doctors and nurses came to know the family as they sat in little clusters in the lounge or cafeteria, waiting for a turn to see Frannie.

In the evening at the house, there were always nine or ten around the dinner table. Henry felt an almost unbearable joy sometimes when he was called in to the extended table covered with a white linen cloth. The china and glassware glittered. The tureens and platters that had come down from his parents were heaped with food like creamed onions and scalloped potatoes, food Henry hadn't eaten at home in years, except at Thanksgiving or Christmas.

They talked animatedly at the table of what Gram had said or done that day. Everyone had a favorite story he liked to tell. Frannie had asked Elinore to get the bedpan, but called it a perambulator. She had clearly asked Maggie if she was going to die and cried when Maggie told her she would not, that she was getting better. She rambled on and on to Emily, her youngest grandchild, who was down from Smith for the weekend. She talked about apple trees and she had said, "I think of all those trees gone, don't you know, the apples, all cut down. Well, that's the way. All those trees." Emily had sat in the darkened room and stroked her hand. "Why would they do a thing like that?" Grandma Frannie had asked, and Emily had said, honestly, that she didn't know. Then Grandma Frannie had said, "Those assholes!" but Emily was sure she had meant to say "apples," so she didn't repeat that part.

Henry told over and over how he had found her and called for the ambulance. He didn't tell the whole truth. He said, "My dearest was in the kitchen making dinner. I sat in the corner of the living room, you see, watching football—it was, I believe, the Los Angeles Rams that day, but I could be wrong—and when the game was over, I walked back towards the kitchen to inquire about dinner, and as I came around the corner, what do you think I saw?" He would wait here however long it took some listener to ask, "What?"

"*There* was my darling sitting on the floor with her legs protruding out from behind the highboy that Auntie gave us for a wedding present." He would go on, detailing every step of the process of getting Frannie to the hospital, and making himself sound very heroic.

The group staying at the house shrank and stabilized somewhat after it became clear that Frannie was going to survive. Maggie stayed on with Henry to take care of him, and Charlotte, who lived nearby, often came for part of the day while her children were in school. Sometimes she returned later with them and her husband, to have dinner with Maggie and Henry.

Frequently, one of the other children or grandchildren would arrive for a day or two. Michael stopped in one night with his entire band, Moonshot, and a few of their girlfriends on the way to a gig in the Berkshires. Maggie told everyone later, "Who knows who was with whom. I just told them where the bedrooms were and shut my eyes."

Grandma Frannie made extraordinary progress. She was having therapy with a walker and physically she had recovered almost completely, except for a dragging in her left leg. Most of her powers of speech had returned. But she still had trouble with an occasional word and when she was tired she would lose track of where she was and to whom she was speaking and drift off to other places and times. Like a baby, she napped three or four times a day.

One afternoon, Henry went in alone to visit her. She was asleep. Her mouth puffed out with each exhalation and she snored faintly. Henry stood in the open doorway and tried to engage some of the passing hospital staff in conversation. His loud voice woke Frannie up.

"Henry!" she called to him.

He turned. "Oh, my dear, now you're awake, and looking so well today, so very well." He leaned over and kissed her cheek.

"Graphics," she said.

"Eh?"

She bit her lip and looked angry. "Now I didn't mean that," she said. "Fetch me my . . . you know." She pointed to her nose. The marks of her glasses were like permanent bluish stains on either side of the bridge. "They're somewhere or other in that coffin there," and she gestured at the stand by her bed.

Henry opened the drawer and got her glasses out. He started to help her put them on, but she waved his hands away and hooked them over her ears herself.

"My love," Henry began, seating himself by her bed.

But she cut him off. "Where *were* you?" she asked.

"Why, my dear, I just arrived, but you were asleep so I stood by the door. . . ."

"Not likely!" she snapped, and behind her glasses her eyes glinted malevolently at him.

"Very well, my love," he said in an injured tone, resolved to be patient. The doctors had told him it was a miracle she had survived at all, and besides, Henry couldn't forget the shame of his behavior to her in the moments before her stroke. Worse yet, he found himself hoping she would never recover fully enough to recall it herself, to blame him or tell the children.

"I heard you down there in that other room," Frannie said, slowly and carefully.

"Now, Frannie, you must stay calm."

She shut her eyes and seemed for a moment to relax or to be asleep. Then her eyes opened and she smiled. "Yes, I'm not well. Not a bit well."

"But you're getting better."

Her lips labored, as though choosing the exact position they needed to be in to form the next word. "The children were here."

"That's right, dear."

"Maggie. And Frieda. And Martha. And that other."

"Laura? She couldn't come. She wasn't here."

"Not Laura," she said irritably. "Not one of mine. That other."

"Louisa? Charlotte?"

"Yes! That one." She smiled in satisfaction. A moment later she said, "Did I tell you the children were here?"

"Yes, you just did, my love. You just said that." And he laughed loudly at her.

Her eyes narrowed behind the bifocals. Her mouth tensed into an angry line. A nurse walked in briskly.

"Ah, here comes that . . . " She stopped.

"It's Nurse Gorman, Mrs. Winter. Just checking your blood pressure again."

"Again? You have nothing superior to do?" Something funny in her sentence made Frannie shake her head angrily.

"I just wanted to get another reading 'cause it's been a few hours, honey." She pumped up the band around Frannie's skinny arm, squeezing the loose flesh close to the bone. "Your wife is my favorite patient, Mr. Winter. She's a doll."

"Eh?" said Henry.

"Your wife is doing well," yelled the nurse. She was tall and wore glasses and very red lipstick.

"Oh, I know, yes, thanks," said Henry.

After the nurse left, Frannie closed her eyes for a while and seemed to sleep again. Henry looked at a copy of *Newsweek* he'd picked up in the lobby.

"Oh, you're still here." She labored over the words.

"Yes, my love," he said, and patted her hand.

"Why don't you just go down there. If you want to. Go right on down. To your little nurse."

Henry frowned.

"I heard you down there. Yes. The children, probably. Thought it was just me again. Making that noise. But I knew just what it was with that Mrs. Sheffield." She said this very slowly and precisely. "Fuck-ing Mrs. Sheffield."

Henry started and withdrew his hand.

"Always that. Mrs. Sheffield. When I wanted some other nurse, but oh, no, you had to have her. Again. Sneaking off down the hall. Did you think I couldn't hear? You? I knew just what it was. I heard you."

"You're upset, Frances. You—you should sleep."

"Yes. Sleep. Don't you wish. I saw you looking at her. As soon as I sleep you'll go off. Down the hall again. Why couldn't we have some other nurse? I didn't want Mrs. Sheffield again." Her voice had become plaintive.

Henry stood up.

Frances began to cry. Her face crumpled into bitter lines. "I don't want her. There's too many children here, and you. Always sneaking around with her, making those noises down the hall. Yes, go. Go on. I know where you're . . . you're going."

Henry drove home slowly. He didn't notice the line of cars forming behind him and he didn't hear the honking. The sun was low and pink in the Connecticut sky. He was remembering Mrs. Sheffield, whose eyes had bulged out slightly so that the whites showed all the way around the iris and made Henry think of nipples sitting round and staring in the middle of her breasts. She was quiet and solemn as she performed her duties after Maggie's birth and she wouldn't sit with him at meals. He had known what he wanted from her when he wrote to hire her again for the second child. After that she had come and stayed with them at each birth, and Frannie, he thought, had never known. Mrs. Sheffield was small and plump, with dark hair, and he had been right, her nipples did sit exactly in the middle of her small breasts, unlike his wife's, which drooped down and leaked milk at his mouth's pull for years on end.

When he got home, Henry called the doctor and explained that he thought his presence was distressing to his wife, and with his permission Henry wouldn't come in for a bit. The doctor was surprised that Henry thought he needed permission to stay away.

And now each person who visited Frannie came to a point in telling how she was doing where he or she would fall silent and then say in a perplexed tone that Grandma Frannie was still not really herself. In little groups of two and three they discussed her and they agreed that they wouldn't have believed Grandma Frannie even knew the meaning of half the words she was using. She told Charlotte's husband that Henry didn't know the first thing about fucking. She said "fucking." "In and out," she said. "That was his big idea. I hope you take a little more time and care. And if you don't know what's up," she said, "there's no shame in asking."

She told Maggie that she had thought she would die when they were all little. She said she'd spent fifteen years "up to my elbows in runny yellow shit. Not one of you children turned out a well-formed stool until you were doing it on your own."

Maggie had blushed and spoken to her as though she were a child. "Be nice, Mother," she'd said, nervously smiling.

"Oh, nice, nice!" said Grandma Frannie. "I know very well how to be nice."

Like Henry, the children and grandchildren began to think of reasons why they couldn't visit. Maggie still went once a day, but most of the time the others stayed away. Late one night Maggie called her husband long-distance in Pennsylvania. She stood in her flannel nightgown in the hall and sobbed softly into the phone so Henry wouldn't hear her. "I can't imagine where she ever heard that kind of language. I almost wished she'd died rather than end up like this."

A few weeks after this, when Frannie began to get better, the doctors called it the return of "appropriate affect." Maggie sent out a family letter saying: "Mother's coming around. She's practically back to normal except for forgetting a few words and we're planning on a homecoming party soon."

And later: "Mother seems just about okay now. Sends her love to everyone and asks about you all. She can't remember who visited and who didn't, but she's talking normally now, thank goodness. For those who can come, we'll bring her home February 16 in the early afternoon and the doctor says a very short party would be all right."

Snow had fallen the night of the fifteenth, but the sixteenth was bright and cold. Frannie's daughters and granddaughters took charge of lunch. One of the sons-in-law put the extra leaf in the table again and took three of the smaller children out to shovel the walk. They ran in and out all morning, bringing cold air and snow into the front hall. "Here, here," Henry said crossly. "In or out. I'm not paying to heat all outdoors."

Someone brought a towel and left it by the front door to mop up the puddles of melting snow. Charlotte's husband lugged two high chairs up from the basement, washed off the dust and cobwebs, and set them at corners of the table.

The chime of the metal shovel ringing on concrete outside, the banging of the front door, the good smells from the kitchen, the table gleaming with silver, made it seem like a dozen Christmases they'd shared in the past. But there was a subdued anxiousness among the adults and several tense abbreviated conversations. Maggie said over and over to people, "Really, she's quite all right now." Henry was surly and spent the morning watching TV or scolding his great-grandchildren.

At one o'clock, Bob Hancock's car swung up the driveway. His oldest boy, Nick, jumped out from the far side and extracted a walker from the back seat. He brought it around to the door Bob was opening at the foot of the walk. Frannie rose slowly out of the car and Nick put the walker down in front of his great-grandmother. The children who were outside danced around her and their muffled shouts brought the family in the house to the windows. "She's home! She's home!" they cried. Henry rose and went to the window.

Slowly, with Nick at one elbow and Bob at the other, Frannie made her way across the shoveled, sanded walk. Her entourage of great-grandchildren in bright nylon snowsuits leapt around her. She was watching her feet, so Henry couldn't see her face. Charlotte had gone to the hospital two days before to give her a permanent, and her hair was immobilized in rigid waves on her head, though the wind made her coat flap.

She turned at the bottom of the porch stairs and Bob came to face her. Holding each other's hands like partners in some old court dance, they stepped sideways up the stairs. Then the children burst open the front door, yelling and stomping the snow off their feet and taking advantage of the excitement to dance around in the front hall without having to remove their boots. Frannie shuffled in and looked around at her family gathered in an irregular circle in the hallway. Charlotte fished a Kleenex out of her maternity smock and several others wiped at their eyes.

"Where's Henry?" Frannie asked. Henry felt a slight constriction in his chest, but he pushed past his children and grandchildren and stood before her. "Here I am, my darling," he said. She looked at him a moment. Then she smiled her sad smile and raised her face to be kissed. Gratefully, he put his lips to hers.

The children yelled and danced, the adults broke into applause. Henry said softly, "It's wonderful to see you yourself again, Frances."

Grandma Frannie looked at him and then at her clapping family. She raised her hands slightly as though to ward off the noise, and for a moment her face registered confusion. But the applause continued.

Then she seemed to realize what they wanted from her. Unassisted and shaky, she stepped forward and smiled again. Slowly she bowed her head, as though to receive the homage due a long and difficult performance.

Spelling

In the store, in the old days, Flo used to say she could tell when some woman was going off the track. Special headgear or footwear were often the first giveaways. Galoshes flopping open on a summer day. Rubber boots they slopped around in, or men's workboots. They might say it was on account of corns, but Flo knew better. It was deliberate, it was meant to tell. Next might come the old felt hat, the torn raincoat worn in all weathers, the trousers held up at the waist with twine, the dim shredded scarves, the layers of ravelling sweaters.

Mothers and daughters often the same way. It was always in them. Waves of craziness, always rising, irresistible as giggles, from some place deep inside, gradually getting the better of them.

They used to come telling Flo their stories. Flo would string them along. "Is that so?" she would say. "Isn't that a shame?"

My vegetable grater is gone and I know who took it.

There is a man comes and looks at me when I take my clothes off at night. I pull the blind down and he looks through the crack.

Two hills of new potatoes stolen. A jar of whole peaches. Some nice ducks' eggs.

One of those women they took to the County Home at last. The first thing they did, Flo said, was give her a bath. The next thing they did was cut off her hair, which had grown out like a haystack. They expected to find anything in it, a dead bird or maybe a nest of baby mouse skeletons. They did find burrs and leaves and a bee that must have got caught and buzzed itself to death. When they had cut down far enough they found a cloth hat. It had rotted on her head and the hair had just pushed up through it, like grass through wire.

Flo had got into the habit of keeping the table set for the next meal, to save trouble. The plastic cloth was gummy, the outline of the plate and saucer plain on it as the outline of pictures on a greasy wall. The refrigerator was full of sulfurous scraps, dark crusts, furry oddments. Rose got to work cleaning, scraping, scalding. Sometimes Flo came lumbering through on her two canes. She might ignore Rose's presence altogether, she might tip the jug of maple syrup up against her mouth and drink it like wine. She loved sweet things now, craved them. Brown sugar by the spoonful, maple syrup, tinned puddings, jelly, globs of sweetness to slide down her throat. She had given up smoking, probably for fear of fire.

Another time she said, "What are you doing in there behind the counter? You ask me what you want, and I'll get it." She thought the kitchen was the store.

"I'm *Rose*," Rose said in a loud, slow voice. "We're in the *kitchen*. I'm cleaning up the *kitchen*."

The old arrangement of the kitchen: mysterious, personal, eccentric. Big pan in the oven, medium-sized pan under the potato pot on the corner shelf, little pan hanging on the nail by the sink. Colander under the sink. Dishrags, newspaper clippings, scissors, muffin tins, hanging on various nails. Piles of bills and letters on the sewing machine, on the telephone shelf. You would think someone had set them down a day or two ago, but they were years old. Rose had come across some letters written by herself, in a forced and spritely style. False messengers; false connections, with a lost period of her life.

"Rose is away," Flo said. She had a habit now of sticking her bottom lip out, when she was displeased or perplexed. "Rose got married."

The second morning Rose got up and found that a gigantic stirring-up had occurred in the kitchen, as if someone had wielded a big shaky spoon. The big pan was lodged behind the refrigerator; the egg lifter was in with the towels, the bread knife was in the flour bin and the roasting pan wedged in the pipes under the sink. Rose made Flo's breakfast porridge and Flo said, "You're that woman they were sending to look after me."

"Yes."

"You aren't from around here?"

"No."

"I haven't got money to pay you. They sent you, they can pay you."

Flo spread brown sugar over her porridge until the porridge was entirely covered, then patted the sugar smooth with her spoon.

After breakfast she spied the cutting board, which Rose had been using when she cut bread for her own toast. "What is this thing doing here getting in our road?" said Flo authoritatively, picking it up and marching off—as well as anybody with two canes could march—to hide it somewhere, in the piano bench or under the back steps.

Years ago, Flo had had a little glassed-in side porch built on to the house. From there she could watch the road just as she used to watch from behind the counter of the store (the store window was now boarded up, the old advertising signs painted over). The road wasn't the main road out of Hanratty through West Hanratty to the Lake anymore; there was a highway bypass. And it was paved, now, with wide gutters, new mercury vapor street lights. The old bridge was gone and a new, wide bridge, much less emphatic, had taken its place. The change from Hanratty to West Hanratty was hardly noticeable. West Hanratty had got itself spruced up with paint and aluminum siding; Flo's place was about the only eyesore left.

What were the things Flo put up to look at, in her little porch, where she had been sitting for years now with her joints and arteries hardening?

A calendar with a picture of a puppy and a kitten on it. Faces turned toward each other so that the noses touched, and the space between the two bodies made a heart.

A photograph, in color, of Princess Anne as a child.

A Blue Mountain pottery vase, gift from Brian and Phoebe, with three yellow plastic roses in it, vase and roses bearing several seasons' sifting of dust.

Six shells from the Pacific coast, sent home by Rose but not gathered by her, as Flo believed, or had once believed. Bought on a vacation in the state of Washington. They were an impulse item in a plastic bag by the cashier's desk in a tourist restaurant.

THE LORD IS MY SHEPHERD, in black cutout scroll with a sprinkling of glitter. Free gift from a dairy.

Newspaper photograph of seven coffins in a row. Two large and five small. Parents and children, all shot by the father in the middle of the night, for reasons nobody knew, in a farmhouse out in the country. That house was not easy to find but Flo had seen it. Neighbors took her, on a Sunday drive, in the days when she was using only one cane. They had to ask directions at a gas station on the highway, and again at a crossroads store. They were told that many people had asked the same questions, had been equally determined. Though Flo had to admit there was nothing much to see. A house like any other. The chimney, the windows, the shingles, the door. Something that could have been a dish towel, or a diaper, that nobody had felt like taking in, left to rot on the line.

Rose had not been back to see Flo for nearly two years. She had been busy, she had been traveling with small companies, financed by grants, putting on plays or scenes from plays, or giving readings, in high school auditoriums and community halls, all over the country. It was part of her job to go on local television chatting about these productions, trying to drum up interest, telling amusing stories about things that had happened during the tour. There was nothing shameful about any of this, but sometimes Rose was deeply, unaccountably ashamed. She did not let her confusion show. When she talked in public she was frank and charming; she had a puzzled, diffident way of leading into her anecdotes, as if she were just now remembering, had not told them a hundred times already. Back in her hotel room, she often shivered and moaned, as if she were having an attack of fever. She blamed it on exhaustion, or her approaching menopause. She couldn't remember any of the people she had met, the charming, interesting people who had invited her to dinner and to whom, over drinks in various cities, she had told intimate things about her life.

Neglect in Flo's house had turned a final corner, since Rose saw it last. The rooms were plugged up with rags and papers and dirt. Pull a blind to let some light in, and the blind comes apart in your hand. Shake a curtain and the curtain falls to rags, letting loose a choking dust. Put a hand into a drawer and it sinks into something soft and dark and rubbishy.

We hate to write bad news but it looks like she has got past where she can look after herself. We try to look in on her but we are not so young ourselves anymore so it looks like maybe the time has come.

The same letter, more or less, had been written to Rose and to her half brother, Brian, who was an engineer, living in Toronto. Rose had just come back from her tour. She had assumed that Brian and his wife, Phoebe, whom she saw seldom, were keeping in touch with Flo. After all, Flo was Brian's mother, Rose's stepmother. And it turned out that they had been keeping in touch, or so they thought. Brian had recently been in South America but Phoebe had been phoning Flo every Sunday night. Flo had little to say but she had never talked to Phoebe anyway; she had said she was fine, everything was fine, she had offered some information about the weather. Rose had observed Flo on the telephone, since she came home, and she saw how Phoebe could have been deceived. Flo spoke normally, she said hello, fine, that was a big storm we had last night, yes, the lights were out here for hours. If you didn't live in the neighborhood you wouldn't realize there hadn't been any storm.

It wasn't that Rose had entirely forgotten Flo in those two years. She had fits of worry about her. It was just that for some time now she had been between fits. One time the fit had come over her in the middle of a January storm, she had driven two hundred miles through blizzards, past ditched cars, and when she finally parked on Flo's street, finally tramped up the walk Flo had not been able to shovel, she was full of relief for herself and concern for Flo, a general turmoil of feelings both anxious and pleasurable. Flo opened the door and gave a bark of warning.

"You can't park there!"

"What?"

"Can't park there!"

Flo said there was a new bylaw; no parking on the streets during the winter months.

"You'll have to shovel out a place."

Of course Rose had an explosion.

"If you say one more word right now I'll get in the car and drive back."

"Well you can't park—"

"One more word!"

"Why do you have to stand here and argue with the cold blasting into the house?"

Rose stepped inside. Home.

That was one of the stories she told about Flo. She did it well; her own exhaustion and sense of virtue; Flo's bark, her waving cane, her fierce unwillingness to be the object of anybody's rescue.

After she read the letter Rose had phoned Phoebe, and Phoebe had asked her to come to dinner, so they could talk. Rose resolved to behave well. She had an idea that Brian and Phoebe moved in a permanent cloud of disapproval of her. She thought that they disapproved of her success, limited and precarious and provincial though it might be, and that they disapproved of her even more when she failed. She also knew it was not likely they would have her on their minds so much, or feel anything so definite.

She put on a plain skirt and an old blouse, but at the last minute changed into a long dress, made of thin red and gold cotton from India, the very thing that would justify their saying that Rose was always so theatrical.

Nevertheless she made up her mind as she usually did that she would speak in a low voice, stick to facts, not get into any stale and silly arguments with Brian. And as usual most of the sense seemed to fly out of her head as soon as she entered their house, was subjected to their calm routines, felt the flow of satisfaction, self-satisfaction, perfectly justified self-satisfaction, that emanated from the very bowls and draperies. She was nervous, when Phoebe asked her about her tour, and Phoebe was a bit nervous too, because Brian sat silent, not exactly frowning but indicating that the frivolity of the subject did not please him. In Rose's presence Brian had said more than once that he had no use for people in her line of work. But he had no use for a good many people. Actors, artists, journalists, rich people (he would never admit to being one himself), the entire Arts faculty of universities. Whole classes and categories, down the drain. Convicted of woolly-mindedness, and showy behavior; inaccurate talk, many excesses. Rose did not know if he spoke the truth or if this was something he had to say in front of her. He offered the bait of his low-voiced contempt; she rose to it; they had fights, she had left his house in tears. And underneath all this, Rose felt, they loved each other. But they could never stop the old, old competition; who is the better person, who has chosen the better work? What were they looking for? Each other's good opinion, which perhaps they meant to grant, in full, but not yet. Phoebe, who was a calm and dutiful woman with a great talent for normalizing things (the very opposite of their family talent for blowing things up), would serve food and pour coffee and regard them with a polite puzzlement; their contest, their vulnerability, their hurt, perhaps seemed as odd to her as the antics of comic-strip characters who stick their fingers into light sockets.

"I always wished Flo could have come back for another visit with us," Phoebe said. Flo had come once, and asked to be taken home after three days. But afterward it seemed to be a pleasure to her, to sit and list the things Brian and Phoebe owned, the features of their house. Brian and Phoebe lived quite unostentatiously, in Don Mills, and the things Flo dwelt on—the door chimes, the automatic garage doors, the swimming pool— were among the ordinary suburban acquisitions. Rose had said as much to Flo who believed that she, Rose, was jealous.

"You wouldn't turn them down if you was offered."

"Yes I would."

That was true, Rose believed it was true, but how could she ever explain it to Flo or anybody in Hanratty? If you stay in Hanratty and do not get rich it is all right because you are living out your life as was intended, but if you go away and do not get rich, or, like Rose, do not remain rich, then what was the point?

After dinner Rose and Brian and Phoebe sat in the backyard beside the pool, where the youngest of Brian and Phoebe's four daughters was riding an inflated dragon. Everything had gone amicably, so far. It had been decided that Rose would go to Hanratty, that she would make arrangements to get Flo into the Wawanash County Home. Brian had already made inquiries about it, or his secretary had, and he said that it seemed not only cheaper but better run, with more facilities, than any private nursing home.

"She'll probably meet old friends there," Phoebe said.

Rose's docility, her good behavior, was partly based on a vision she had been building up all evening, and would never reveal to Brian and Phoebe. She pictured herself going to Hanratty and looking after Flo, living with her, taking care of her for as long as was necessary. She thought how she would clean and paint Flo's kitchen, patch the shingles over the leaky spots (that was one of the things the letter had mentioned), plant flowers in the pots, and make nourishing soup. She wasn't so far gone as to imagine Flo fitting comfortably into this picture, settling down to a life of gratitude. But the crankier Flo got, the milder and more patient Rose would become, and who, then, could accuse her of egotism and frivolity?

This vision did not survive the first two days of being home.

"Would you like a pudding?" Rose said.

"Oh, I don't care."

The elaborate carelessness some people will show, the gleam of hope, on being offered a drink.

Rose made a trifle. Berries, peaches, custard, cake, whipped cream and sweet sherry.

Flo ate half the bowlful. She dipped in greedily, not bothering to transfer a portion to a smaller bowl.

"That was lovely," she said. Rose had never heard such an admission of grateful pleasure from her. "Lovely," said Flo and sat remembering, appreciating, belching a little. The suave dreamy custard, the nipping berries, robust peaches, luxury of sherry-soaked cake, munificence of whipped cream.

Rose thought that she had never done anything in her life that came as near pleasing Flo as this did.

"I'll make another soon."

Flo recovered herself. "Oh well. You do what you like."

Rose drove out to the County Home. She was conducted through it. She tried to tell Flo about it when she came back.

"Whose home?" said Flo.

"No, the *County* home."

Rose mentioned some people she had seen there. Flo would not admit to knowing any of them. Rose spoke of the view and the pleasant rooms. Flo looked angry; her face darkened and she stuck out her lip. Rose handed her a mobile she had bought for fifty cents in the County Home Crafts Center. Cutout birds of blue and yellow paper were bobbing and dancing, on undetectable currents of air.

"Stick it up your arse," said Flo.

Rose put the mobile up in the porch and said she had seen the trays coming up, with supper on them.

"They go to the dining room if they're able, and if they're not they have trays in their rooms. I saw what they were having.

"Roast beef, well done, mashed potatoes and green beans, the frozen not the canned kind. Or an omelette. You could have a mushroom omelette or a chicken omelette or a plain omelette, if you liked."

"What was for dessert?"

"Ice cream. You could have sauce on it."

"What kind of sauce was there?"

"Chocolate. Butterscotch. Walnut."

"I can't eat walnuts."

"There was marshmallow too."

Out at the Home the old people were arranged in tiers. On the first floor were the bright and tidy ones. They walked around, usually with the help of canes. They visited each other, played cards. They had singsongs and hobbies. In the Crafts Center they painted pictures, hooked rugs, made quilts. If they were not able to do things like that they could make rag dolls, mobiles like the one Rose bought, poodles and snowmen which were constructed of Styrofoam balls, with sequins for eyes; they also made silhouette pictures by placing thumbtacks on traced outlines: knights on horseback, battleships, airplanes, castles.

They organized concerts; they held dances; they had checker tournaments.

"Some of them say they are the happiest here they have ever been in their lives."

Up one floor there was more television watching, there were more wheelchairs. There were those whose heads drooped, whose tongues lolled, whose limbs shook uncontrollably. Nevertheless sociability was still flourishing, also rationality, with occasional blanks and absences.

On the third floor you might get some surprises.

Some of them up there had given up speaking.

Some had given up moving, except for odd jerks and tosses of the head, flailing of the arms, that seemed to be without purpose or control.

Nearly all had given up worrying about whether they were wet or dry.

Bodies were fed and wiped, taken up and tied in chairs, untied and put to bed. Taking in oxygen, giving out carbon dioxide, they continued to participate in the life of the world.

Crouched in her crib, diapered, dark as a nut, with three tufts of hair like dandelion floss sprouting from her head, an old woman was making loud shaky noises.

"Hello Aunty," the nurse said. "You're spelling today. It's lovely weather outside." She bent to the old woman's ear. "Can you spell weather?"

This nurse showed her gums when she smiled, which was all the time; she had an air of nearly demented hilarity.

"Weather," said the old woman. She strained forward, grunting, to get the word. Rose thought she might be going to have a bowel movement. "W-E-A-T-H-E-R."

That reminded her.

"Whether. W-H-E-T-H-E-R."

So far so good.

"Now you say something to her," the nurse said to Rose.

The words in Rose's mind were for a moment all obscene or despairing. But without prompting came another.

"Forest. F-O-R-E-S-T."

"Celebrate," said Rose suddenly.

"C-E-L-E-B-R-A-T-E."

You had to listen very hard to make out what the old woman was saying, because she had lost much of the power to shape sounds. What she said seemed to come not from her mouth or her throat, but from deep in her lungs and belly.

"Isn't she a wonder," the nurse said. "She can't see and that's the only way we can tell she can hear. Like if you say, 'Here's your dinner,' she won't pay any attention to it, but she might start spelling *dinner.*

"Dinner," she said, to illustrate, and the old woman picked it up. "D-I-N-N . . . " Sometimes a long wait, a long wait between letters. It seemed she had only the thinnest thread to follow, meandering through that emptiness or confusion that nobody on this side can do more than guess at. But she didn't lose it, she followed it through to the end, however tricky the word might be, or cumbersome. Finished. Then she was sitting waiting; waiting, in the middle of her sightless eventless day, till up from somewhere popped another word. She would encompass it, bend all her energy to master it. Rose wondered what the words were like, when she held them in her mind. Did they carry their usual meaning, or any meaning at all? Were they like words in dreams or in the minds of young children, each one marvelous and distinct and alive as a new animal? This one limp and clear, like a jellyfish, that one hard and mean and secretive, like a horned snail. They could be austere and comical as top hats, or smooth and lively and flattering as ribbons. A parade of private visitors, not over yet.

Something woke Rose early the next morning. She was sleeping in the little porch, the only place in Flo's house where the smell was bearable. The sky was milky and brightening. The trees across the river—due to be cut down soon, to make room for a trailer park—were hunched against the dawn sky like shaggy dark animals, like buffalo. Rose had been dreaming. She had been having a dream obviously connected with her tour of the Home the day before.

Someone was taking her through a large building where there were people in cages. Everything was dim and cobwebby at first, and Rose was protesting that it seemed a poor arrangement. But as she went on the cages got larger and more elaborate, they were like enormous wicker birdcages, Victorian birdcages, fancifully shaped and decorated. Food was being offered to the people in the cages and Rose examined it, saw that it was choice; chocolate mousse, trifle, Black Forest cake. Then in one of the cages Rose spotted Flo, who was handsomely seated on a thronelike chair, spelling out words in a clear authoritative voice (what the words were, Rose, wakening, could not remember) and looking pleased with herself, for showing powers she had kept secret till now.

Rose listened to hear Flo breathing, stirring, in her rubble-lined room. She heard nothing. What if Flo had died? Suppose she had died at the very moment she was making her radiant, satisfied appearance in Rose's dream? Rose hurried out of bed, ran barefoot to Flo's room. The bed there was empty. She went into the kitchen and found Flo sitting at the table, dressed to go out, wearing the navy blue summer coat and matching turban hat she had worn to Brian's and Phoebe's wedding. The coat was rumpled and in need of cleaning, the turban was crooked.

"Now I'm ready for to go," Flo said.

"Go where?"

"Out there," said Flo, jerking her head. "Out to the whattayacallit. The Poorhouse."

"The Home," said Rose. "You don't have to go today."

"They hired you to take me, now you get a move on and take me," Flo said.

"I'm not hired. I'm Rose. I'll make you a cup of tea."

"You can make it. I won't drink it."

She made Rose think of a woman who had started in labor. Such was her concentration, her determination, her urgency. Rose thought Flo felt her death moving in her like a child, getting ready to tear her. So she gave up arguing, she got dressed, hastily packed a bag for Flo, got her to the car and drove her out to the Home, but in the matter of Flo's quickly tearing and relieving death she was mistaken.

Some time before this, Rose had been in a play, on national television. *The Trojan Women.* She had no lines, and in fact she was in the play simply to do a favor for a friend, who had got a better part elsewhere. The director thought to liven all the weeping and mourning by having the Trojan women go bare-breasted. One breast apiece, they showed, the right in the case of royal personages such as Hecuba and Helen; the left, in case of ordinary virgins or wives, such as Rose. Rose didn't think herself enhanced by this exposure—she was getting on, after all, her bosom tended to flop—but she got used to the idea. She didn't count on the sensation they would create. She didn't think many people would be watching. She forgot about those parts of the country where people can't exercise their preference for quiz shows, police-car chases, American situation comedies, and are compelled to put up with talks on public affairs and tours of art galleries and ambitious offerings of drama. She did not think they would be so amazed, either, now that every magazine rack in every town was serving up slices and cutlets of bare flesh. How could such outrage fasten on the Trojan ladies' sad-eyed collection, puckered with cold then running with sweat under the lights, badly and chalkily made-up, all looking rather foolish without their mates, rather pitiful and unnatural, like tumors?

Flo took to pen and paper over that, forced her still swollen fingers, crippled almost out of use with arthritis, to write the word *Shame.* She wrote that if Rose's father had not been dead long ago he would now wish that he was. That was true. Rose read the letter, or part of it, out loud to some friends she was having for dinner. She read it for comic effect, and dramatic effect, to show the gulf that lay behind her, though she did realize, if she thought about it, that such a gulf was nothing special. Most of her friends, who seemed to her ordinarily hard-working, anxious, and hopeful people, could lay claim to being disowned or prayed for, in some disappointed home.

Halfway through she had to stop reading. It wasn't that she thought how shabby it was, to be exposing and making fun of Flo this way. She had done it often enough before; it was no news to her that it was shabby. What stopped her was, in fact, that gulf; she had a fresh and overwhelming realization of it, and it was nothing to laugh about. These reproaches of Flo's made as much sense as a protest about raising umbrellas, a warning against eating raisins. But they were painfully, truly, meant; they were all a hard life had to offer. Shame on a bare breast.

Another time, Rose was getting an award. So were several other people. A reception was being held, in a Toronto hotel. Flo had been sent an invitation, but Rose had never thought that she would come. She had thought she should give someone's name, when the organizers asked about relatives, and she could hardly name Brian and Phoebe. Of course it was possible that she did, secretly, want Flo to come, wanted to show Flo, intimidate her, finally remove herself from Flo's shade. That would be a natural thing to want to do.

Flo came down on the train, unannounced. She got to the hotel. She was arthritic then, but still moving without a cane. She had always been decently, soberly, cheaply, dressed, but now it seemed she had spent money and asked advice. She was wearing a mauve and purple checked pants suit, and beads like strings of white and yellow popcorn. Her hair was covered by a thick gray-blue wig, pulled low on her forehead like a woollen cap. From the vee of the jacket, and its too-short sleeves, her neck and wrists stuck out brown and warty as if covered with bark. When she saw Rose she stood still. She seemed to be waiting—not just for Rose to go over to her but for her feelings about the scene in front of her to crystallize.

Soon they did.

"Look at the nigger!" said Flo in a loud voice, before Rose was anywhere near her. Her tone was one of simple, gratified astonishment, as if she had been peering down the Grand Canyon or seen oranges growing on a tree.

She meant George, who was getting one of the awards. He turned around, to see if someone was feeding him a comic line. And Flo did look like a comic character, except that her bewilderment, her authenticity, were quite daunting. Did she note the stir she had caused? Possibly. After that one outburst she clammed up, would not speak again except in the most grudging monosyllables, would not eat any food or drink any drink offered her, would not sit down, but stood astonished and unflinching in the middle of that gathering of the bearded and beaded, the unisexual and the unashamedly un-Anglo-Saxon, until it was time for her to be taken to her train and sent home.

Rose found that wig under the bed, during the horrifying cleanup that followed Flo's removal. She took it out to the Home, along with some clothes she had washed or had dry-cleaned, and some stockings, talcum powder, cologne, that she had bought. Sometimes Flo seemed to think Rose was a doctor, and she said, "I don't want no woman doctor, you can just clear out." But when she saw Rose carrying the wig she said, "Rose! What is that you got in your hands, is it a dead gray squirrel?"

"No," said Rose, "it's a wig."

"What?"

"A wig," said Rose, and Flo began to laugh. Rose laughed too. The wig did look like a dead cat or squirrel, even though she had washed and brushed it; it was a disturbing-looking object.

"My God, Rose, I thought what is she doing bringing me a dead squirrel! If I put it on somebody'd be sure to take a shot at me."

Rose stuck it on her own head, to continue the comedy, and Flo laughed so that she rocked back and forth in her crib.

When she got her breath Flo said, "What am I doing with these damn sides up on my bed? Are you and Brian behaving yourselves? Don't fight, it gets on your father's nerves. Do you know how many gallstones they took out of me? Fifteen! One as big as a pullet's egg. I got them somewhere. I'm going to take them home." She pulled at the sheets searching. "They were in a bottle."

"I've got them already," said Rose. "I took them home."

"Did you? Did you show your father?"

"Yes."

"Oh, well, that's where they are then," said Flo, and she lay down and closed her eyes.

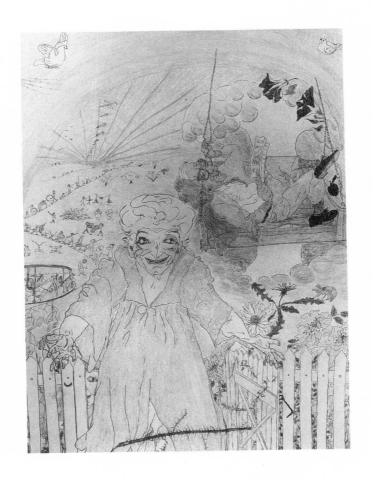

AGING AND THE COMMUNITY

Introduction

William Faulkner's "A Rose for Emily" is narrated by a voice who speaks for "our whole town" and who sees the old woman as "a tradition, a duty, and a care: a sort of hereditary obligation upon the town." Small communities everywhere have their elderly citizens, many of whom have lived in the same houses for decades—the houses becoming like their inhabitants. When these old people have acquired the community's respect and concern, a neighborly network checks on them—with companionship for their loneliness and with food and medical help for their needs. When the community does not approve of its elderly, it can abuse them with unkind gossip, with pointed avoidances, and with intrusions on their privacy in ways that force them to accommodate the community's will. In small towns, the advantages and disadvantages of everyone knowing each other go hand in hand into every situation. The community develops a collective personality that can be generous and loving as well as cold and manipulative.

Aging in the city presents different kinds of problems. The elderly can much more easily disappear in the anonymity of many busy people minding their own business. While the city allows the individual much more privacy and independence in one sense, it is also an environment in which the individual can be radically isolated—"lost in the lonely crowd"—unnoticed and ignored. The large community counts on its legal system and various institutions to take care of the elderly. They become abstract generalities rather than real individual people; and many of these real people fall through the cracks. In Harold Pinter's *Black and White*, for instance, two homeless old women spend their dreary nights and days riding the city's buses, giving them the illusion that they have somewhere to go. In his play *The Caretaker*, an old tramp desperately claims squatter's rights possession of part of an old apartment where he has been allowed as a temporary "guest." The aged homeless haunt the bus stations and airport terminals.

Another problem for the aging in a city is the irony of no one to talk to— a swarm of strangers all around, none of whom want to listen to some old person's complaints. In fact, if an elderly person tries to start a conversation with someone who does not know him, he is seen as rude or senile. In

Chekhov's story, "Misery," the old cabdriver cannot "find among those thousands someone who will listen to him. . . . The crowds flit by heedless of him and his misery." Such painful isolation can be healed by someone who is willing to listen and to observe carefully, as Selzer's doctor in "Toenails" or the neighborly woman in Williams's "Ancient Gentility." But such sensitivity and willingness to get involved are rare.

The community provides several institutions designed to meet the needs of the elderly. While some retirement centers may be ideal places for companionship and interest, most "old folks homes" resemble warehouses, storing their contents until they die. Often the community concern stops once the aging people are out of sight, except for the occasional church choir that goes to sing for them or the Girl Scouts who earn points towards a badge by doing their charitable service. Eudora Welty's "A Visit of Charity" presents the startling contrast between the attitudes of the charity dispensers and those on the receiving end. Most of the community tends to think of aging as a disease—unpleasant, unattractive and disturbing—something to be put out of sight and out of mind. *The Gin Game* recognizes the impact of this community avoidance on the aging residents of the old folks home. The problem is not new in the twentieth century. The psalmist cries out, "Cast me not off in the time of old age; forsake me not when my strength faileth."

Emperor of the Air

Let me tell you who I am. I'm sixty-nine years old, live in the same house I was raised in, and have been the high school biology and astronomy teacher in this town so long that I have taught the grandson of one of my former students. I wear my father's wristwatch, which tells me it is past four-thirty in the morning, and though I have thought otherwise, I now think that hope is the essence of all good men.

My wife, Vera, and I have no children. This has enabled us to do a great many things in our lives: we have stood on the Great Wall of China, toured the Pyramid of Cheops, sunned in Lapland at midnight. Vera, who is near my age, is off on the Appalachian Trail. She has been gone two weeks and expects to be gone one more, on a trip on which a group of men and women, some of them half her age, are walking all the way through three states. Age, it seems, has left my wife alone. She ice-skates and hikes and will swim nude in a mountain lake. She does these things without me, however, for now my life has slowed. Last fall, as I pushed a lawnmower around our yard, I felt a squeezing in my chest and a burst of pain in my shoulder, and I spent a week in a semiprivate hospital room. A heart attack. Myocardial infarction, minor. I will no longer run for a train, and in my shirt pocket I keep a small vial of nitroglycerine pills. In slow supermarket lines or traffic snarls I tell myself that impatience is not worth dying over, and last week, as I stood at the window and watched my neighbor, Mr. Pike, cross the yard toward our front door carrying a chain saw, I told myself that he was nothing but a doomed and hopeless man.

I had found the insects in my elm a couple of days before, the slim red line running from the ground up the long trunk and vanishing into the lower boughs. I brought out a magnifying glass to examine them—their shiny arthroderms, torsos elongated like drops of red liquid; their tiny legs, jointed and wiry, climbing the fissured bark. The morning I found them, Mr. Pike came over from next door and stood on our porch. "There's vermin in your elm," he said.

"I know," I said. "Come in."

"It's a shame, but I'll be frank: there's other trees on this block. I've got my own three elms to think of."

Mr. Pike is a builder, a thick and unpleasant man with whom I have rarely spoken. Though I had seen him at high school athletic events, the judgmental tilt to his jaw always suggested to me that he was merely watching for the players' mistakes. He is short, with thick arms and a thick neck and a son, Kurt, in whose bellicose shouts I can already begin to hear the thickness of his father. Mr. Pike owns or partly owns a construction company that erected a line of low prefabricated houses on the outskirts of town, on a plot I remember from my youth as having been razed by fire. Once, a plumber who was working on our basement pipes told me that Mr. Pike was a poor craftsman, a man who valued money over quality. The plumber, a man my age who kept his tools in a wooden chest, shook his head when he told me that Mr. Pike used plastic pipes in the houses he had built. "They'll last ten years," the plumber told me. "Then the seams will go and the walls and ceilings will start to fill with water." I myself had had little to do with Mr. Pike until he told me he wanted my elm cut down to protect the three saplings in his yard. Our houses are separated by a tall stand of rhododendron and ivy, so we don't see each other's private lives as most neighbors do. When we talked on the street, we spoke only about a football score or the incessant rain, and I had not been on his property since shortly after he moved in, when I had gone over to introduce myself and he had shown me the spot where, underneath his rolling back lawn, he planned to build a bomb shelter.

Last week he stood on my porch with the chain saw in his hands. "I've got young elms," he said. "I can't let them be infested."

"My tree is over two hundred years old."

"It's a shame," he said, showing me the saw, "but I'll be frank. I just wanted you to know I could have it cut down as soon as you give the word."

All week I had a hard time sleeping. I read Dickens in bed, heated cups of milk, but nothing worked. The elm was dying. Vera was gone, and I lay in bed thinking of the insects, of their miniature jaws carrying away heartwood. It was late summer, the nights were still warm, and sometimes I went outside in my nightclothes and looked up at the sky. I teach astronomy, as I have said, and though sometimes I try to see the stars as milky dots or pearls, they are forever arranged in my eye according to the astronomic charts. I stood by the elm and looked up at Ursa Minor and Lyra, at Cygnus and Corona Borealis. I went back inside, read, peeled an orange. I sat at the window and thought about the insects, and every morning at five a boy who had once taken my astronomy class rode by on his bicycle, whistling the national anthem, and threw the newspaper onto our porch.

Sometimes I heard them, chewing the heart of my splendid elm.

The day after I first found the insects I called a man at the tree nursery. He described them for me, the bodies like red droplets, the wiry legs; he told me their genus and species.

"Will they kill the tree?"

"They could."

"We can poison them, can't we?"

"Probably not," he said. He told me that once they were visible outside the bark they had already invaded the tree too thoroughly for pesticide. "To kill them," he said, "we would end up killing the tree."

"Does that mean the tree is dead?"

"No," he said. "It depends on the colony of insects. Sometimes they invade a tree but don't kill it, don't even weaken it. They eat the wood, but sometimes they eat it so slowly that the tree can replace it."

When Mr. Pike came over the next day, I told him this. "You're asking me to kill a two-hundred-and-fifty-year-old tree that otherwise wouldn't die for a long time."

"The tree's over eighty feet tall," he said.

"So!"

"It stands fifty-two feet from my house."

"Mr. Pike, it's older than the Liberty Bell."

"I don't want to be unpleasant," he said, "but a storm could blow twenty-eight feet of that tree through the wall of my house."

"How long have you lived in that house?"

He looked at me, picked at his tooth. "You know."

"Four years," I said. "I was living here when a czar ruled Russia. An elm grows one quarter inch in width each year, when it's still growing. That tree is four feet thick, and it has yet to chip the paint on either your house or mine."

"It's sick," he said. "It's a sick tree. It could fall."

"Could," I said. "It *could* fall."

"It very well *might* fall."

We looked at each other for a moment. Then he averted his eyes, and with his right hand adjusted something on his watch. I looked at his wrist. The watch had a shiny metal band, with the hours, minutes, seconds, blinking in the display.

The next day he was back on my porch.

"We can plant another one," he said.

"What?"

"We can plant another tree. After we cut the elm, we can plant a new one."

"Do you have any idea how long it would take to grow a tree like that one?"

"You can buy trees half-grown. They bring them in on a truck and replant them."

"Even a half-grown tree would take a century to reach the size of the elm. A century."

He looked at me. Then he shrugged, turned around, and went back down the steps. I sat down in the open doorway. A century. What would be left of the earth in a century? I didn't think I was a sentimental man, and I don't weep at plays or movies, but certain moments have always been peculiarly moving for me, and the mention of a century was one. There have been others. Standing out of the way on a fall evening, as couples and families converge on the concert hall from the radiating footpaths, has always filled me with a longing, though I don't know for what. I have taught the life of the simple hydra that is drawn, for no reasons it could ever understand, toward the bright surface of the water, and the spectacle of a thousand human beings organizing themselves into a single room to hear the quartets of Beethoven is as moving to me as birth or death. I feel the same way during the passage in an automobile across a cantilever span above the Mississippi, mother of rivers. These moments overwhelm me, and sitting on the porch that day as Mr. Pike retreated up the footpath, paused at the elm, and then went back into his house, I felt my life open up and present itself to me.

When he had gone back into his house I went out to the elm and studied the insects, which emerged from a spot in the grass and disappeared above my sight, in the lowest branches. Their line was dense and unbroken. I went inside and found yesterday's newspaper, which I rolled up and brought back out. With it I slapped up and down the trunk until the line was in chaos. I slapped until the newspaper was wet and tearing; with my fingernails I squashed stragglers between the narrow crags of bark. I stamped the sod where they emerged, dug my shoe tip into their underground tunnels. When my breathing became painful, I stopped and sat on the ground. I closed my eyes until the pulse in my neck was calm, and I sat there, mildly triumphant, master at last. After a while I looked up again at the tree and found the line perfectly restored.

That afternoon I mixed a strong insect poison, which I brought outside and painted around the bottom of the trunk. Mr. Pike came out onto his steps to watch. He walked down, stood on the sidewalk behind me, made little chuckling noises. "There's no poison that'll work," he whispered.

But that evening, when I came outside, the insects were gone. The trunk was bare. I ran my finger around the circumference. I rang Mr. Pike's doorbell and we went out and stood by the tree together. He felt in the notches of the bark, scratched bits of earth from the base. "I'll be damned," he said.

When I was a boy in this town, the summers were hot and the forest to the north and east often dried to the point where the undergrowth, not fit to compete with the deciduous trees for groundwater, turned crackling brown. The shrubbery became as fragile as straw, and the summer I was sixteen the forest ignited. A sheet of flame raced and bellowed day and night as loud as a fleet of propeller planes. Whole families gathered in the street and evacuation plans were made, street routes drawn out beneath the night sky, which, despite the ten miles' distance to the fire, shone with orange light. My father had a wireless with which he communicated to the fire lines. He stayed up all night and promised that he would wake the neighbors if the wind changed or the fire otherwise turned toward town. That night the wind held, and by morning a firebreak the width of a street had been cut. My father took me down to see it the next day, a ribbon of cleared land as bare as if it had been drawn with a razor. Trees had been felled, the underbrush sickled down and removed. We stood at the edge of the cleared land, the town behind us, and watched the fire. Then we got into my father's Plymouth and drove as close as we were allowed. A fireman near the flames had been asphyxiated, someone said, when the cone of fire had turned abruptly and sucked up all the oxygen in the air. My father explained to me how a flame breathed oxygen like a man. We got out of the car. The heat curled the hair on our arms and turned the ends of our eyelashes white.

My father was a pharmacist and had taken me to the fire out of curiosity. Anything scientific interested him. He kept tide tables and collected the details of nature—butterflies and moths, seeds, wildflowers—and stored them in glass-fronted cases, which he leaned against the stone wall of our cellar. One summer he taught me the constellations of the Northern Hemisphere. We went outside at night, and as the summer progressed he showed me how to find Perseus and Boötes and Andromeda, how some of the brightest stars illuminated Lyra and Aquila, how, though the constellations proceed with the seasons, Polaris remains most fixed and is thus the set point of a mariner's navigation. He taught me the night sky, and I find now that this is rare knowledge. Later, when I taught astronomy, my students rarely cared about the silicon or iron on the sun, but when I spoke of Cepheus or Lacerta, they were silent and attended my words. At a party now I can always find a drinking husband who will come outside with me and sip cognac while I point out the stars and say their names.

That day, as I stood and watched the fire, I thought the flames were as loud and powerful as the sea, and that evening, when we were home, I went out to the front yard and climbed the elm to watch the forest burn. Climbing the elm was forbidden me, because the lowest limbs even then were well above my reach and because my father believed that anybody lucky enough to make it up into the lower boughs would almost certainly fall on the way down. But I knew how to climb it anyway. I had done it before, when my parents were gone. I had never made it as far as the first limbs, but I had learned the knobs and handholds on which, with balance and strength, I could climb to within a single jump of the boughs. The jump frightened me, however, and I had never attempted it. To reach the boughs one had to gather strength and leap upward into the air, propelled only by the purchase of feet and hands on the small juttings of bark. It was a terrible risk. I could no more imagine myself making this leap than I could imagine diving head-long from a coastal cliff into the sea. I was an adventurous youth, as I was later an adventurous man, but all my adventures had a quality about them of safety and planned success. This is still true. In Ethiopia I have photo-graphed a lioness with her cubs; along the Barrier Reef I have dived among barracuda and scorpion fish—but these things have never frightened me. In my life I have done few things that have frightened me.

That night, though, I made the leap into the lower boughs of the elm. My parents were inside the house, and I made my way upward until I crawled out of the leaves onto a narrow top branch and looked around me at a world that on two sides was entirely red and orange with flame. After a time I came back down and went inside to sleep, but that night the wind changed. My father woke us, and we gathered outside on the street with all the other fam-ilies on our block. People carried blankets filled with the treasures of their lives. One woman wore a fur coat, though the air was suffused with ash and was as warm as an afternoon. My father stood on the hood of a car and spoke. He had heard through the radio that the fire had leaped the break, that a house on the eastern edge of town was in full flame, and, as we all could feel, that the wind was strong and blowing straight west. He told the families to finish loading their cars and leave as soon as possible. Though the fire was still across town, he said, the air was filling with smoke so rapidly that breathing would soon be difficult. He got down off the car and we went in-side to gather things together. We had an RCA radio in our living room and a set of Swiss china in my mother's cupboard, but my father instead loaded a box with the *Encyclopaedia Britannica* and carried up from the basement the heavy glass cases that contained his species chart of the North American butterflies. We carried these things outside to the Plymouth. When we re-turned, my mother was standing in the doorway.

"This is my home," she said.

"We're in a hurry," said my father.

"This is my home, this is my children's home. I'm not leaving."

My father stood on the porch looking at her. "Stay here," he said to me. Then he took my mother's arm and they went into the house. I stood on the steps outside, and when my father came out again in a few minutes, he was alone, just as when we drove west that night and slept with the rest of our neighborhood on army cots in the high school gym in the next town, we were alone. My mother had stayed behind.

Nothing important came of this. That night the wind calmed and the burning house was extinguished; the next day a heavy rain wet the fire and it was put out. Everybody came home, and the settled ash was swept from the houses and walkways into black piles in the street. I mention the inci-dent now only because it points out, I think, what I have always lacked: I inherited none of my mother's moral stubbornness. In spite of my age, still, arriving on foot at a crosswalk where the light is red but no cars are in sight, I'm thrown into confusion. My decisions never seem to engage the certainty that I had hoped to enjoy late in my life. But I was adamant and angry when Mr. Pike came to my door. The elm was ancient and exquisite: we could not let it die.

Now, though, the tree was safe. I examined it in the morning, in the afternoon, in the evening, and with a lantern at night. The bark was clear. I slept.

The next morning Mr. Pike was at my door.

"Good morning, neighbor," I said.

"They're back."

"They can't be."

"They are. Look," he said, and walked out to the tree. He pointed up to the first bough.

"You probably can't see them," he said, "but I can. They're up there, a whole line of them."

"They couldn't be."

"They sure are. Listen," he said, "I don't want to be unpleasant, but I'll be frank."

That evening he left a note in our mail slot. It said that he had contacted the authorities, who had agreed to enforce the cutting of the tree if I didn't do it myself. I read the note in the kitchen. Vera had been cooking some Indian chicken before she left for the Appalachian Trail, and on the counter was a big jar filled with flour and spices that she shook pieces of chicken in. I read Mr. Pike's note again. Then I got a fishing knife and a flashlight from the closet, emptied Vera's jar, and went outside with these things to the elm. The street was quiet. I made a few calculations, and then with the knife cut the bark. Nothing. I had to do it only a couple more times, however, before I hit the mark and, sure enough, the tree sprouted insects. Tiny red bugs shot crazily from the slit in the bark. I touched my finger there and they spread in an instant all over my hand and up my arm. I had to shake them off. Then I opened the jar, laid the fishing knife out from the opening like a bridge, and touched the blade to the slit in the tree. They scrambled up the knife and began to fill the jar as fast as a trickling spring. After a few minutes I pulled out the knife, closed the lid, and went back into the house.

Mr. Pike is my neighbor, and so I felt a certain remorse. What I contemplated, however, was not going to kill the elms. It was going to save them. If Mr. Pike's trees were infested, they would still more than likely live, and he would no longer want mine chopped down. This is the nature of the world. In the dark house, feeling half like a criminal and half like a man of mercy, my heart arrhythmic in anticipation, I went upstairs to prepare. I put on black pants and a black shirt. I dabbed shoe polish on my cheeks, my neck, my wrists, the backs of my hands. Over my white hair I stretched a tight black cap. Then I walked downstairs. I picked up the jar and the flashlight and went outside into the night.

I have always enjoyed gestures—never failing to bow, for example, when I finished dancing with a woman—but one attribute I have acquired with age is the ability to predict when I am about to act foolishly. As I slid calmly into the shadowy cavern behind our side yard rhododendron and paused to catch my breath, I thought that perhaps I had better go back inside and get into my bed. But then I decided to go through with it. As I stood there in the shadow of the swaying rhododendron, waiting to pass into the back yard of my neighbor, I thought of Hannibal and Napoleon and MacArthur. I tested my flashlight and shook the jar, which made a soft colliding sound as if it were filled with rice. A light was on in the Pikes' living room, but the alley between our houses was dark. I passed through.

The Pikes' yard is large, larger than ours, and slopes twice within its length, so that the lawn that night seemed like a dark, furrowed flag stretching back to the three elms. I paused at the border of the driveway, where the grass began, and looked out at the young trees outlined by the lighted houses behind them. In what strange ways, I thought, do our lives turn. Then I got down on my hands and knees. Staying along the fence that separates our yards, I crawled toward the back of the Pikes' lawn. In my life I have not crawled a lot. With Vera I have gone spelunking in the limestone caves of southern Minnesota, but there the crawling was obligate, and as we made our way along the narrow, wet channel into the heart of the rock, I felt a strange grace in my knees and elbows. The channel was hideously narrow, and my life depended on the sureness of my limbs. Now, in the Pikes' yard, my knees felt arthritic and torn. I made my way along the driveway toward the young elms against the back fence. The grass was wet and the water dampened my trousers. I was hurrying as best I could across the open lawn, the insect-filled jar in my hand, the flashlight in my pocket, when I put my palm on something cement. I stopped and looked down. In the dim light I saw what looked like the hatch door on a submarine. Round, the size of a manhole, marked with a fluorescent cross—oh, Mr. Pike, I didn't think you'd do it. I put down the jar and felt for the handle in the dark, and when I found it I braced myself and turned. I certainly didn't expect it to give, but it did, circling once, twice, around in my grasp and loosening like the lid of a bottle. I pulled the hatch and up it came. Then I picked up the insects, felt with my feet for the ladder inside, and went down.

I still planned to deposit the insects on his trees, but something about crime is contagious. I knew that what I was doing was foolish and that it increased the risk of being caught, but as I descended the ladder into Mr. Pike's bomb shelter, I could barely distinguish fear from elation. At the bottom of the ladder I switched on the flashlight. The room was round, the ceiling and floor were concrete, and against the wall stood a cabinet of metal shelves filled with canned foods. On one shelf were a dictionary and some magazines. Oh, Mr. Pike. I thought of his sapling elms, of the roots making their steady, blind way through the earth; I thought of his houses ten years from now, when the pipes cracked and the ceilings began to pool with water. What a hopeless man he seemed to me then, how small and afraid.

I stood thinking about him, and after a moment I heard a door close in the house. I climbed the ladder and peeked out under the hatch. There on the porch stood Kurt and Mr. Pike. As I watched, they came down off the steps, walked over and stood on the grass near me. I could see the watch blinking on Mr. Pike's wrist. I lowered my head. They were silent, and I wondered what Mr. Pike would do if he found me in his bomb shelter. He was thickly built, as I have said, but I didn't think he was a violent man. One afternoon I had watched as Kurt slammed the front door of their house and ran down the steps onto the lawn, where he stopped and threw an object— an ashtray, I think it was—right through the front window of the house. When the glass shattered, he ran, and Mr. Pike soon appeared on the front steps. The reason I say that he is not a violent man is that I saw something beyond anger, perhaps a certain doom, in his posture as he went back inside that afternoon and began cleaning up the glass with a broom. I watched him through the broken front window of their house.

How would I explain to him, though, the bottle of mad insects I now held? I could have run then, I suppose, made a break up and out of the shelter while their backs were turned. I could have been out the driveway and across the street without their recognizing me. But there was, of course, my heart. I moved back down the ladder. As I descended and began to think about a place to hide my insects, I heard Mr. Pike speak. I climbed back up the ladder. When I looked out under the hatch, I saw the two of them, backs toward me, pointing at the sky. Mr. Pike was sighting something with his finger, and Kurt followed. Then I realized that he was pointing out the constellations, but that he didn't know what they were and was making up their names as he spoke. His voice was not fanciful. It was direct and scientific, and he was lying to his son about what he knew. "These," he said, "these are the Mermaid's Tail, and south you can see the three peaks of Mount Olympus, and then the sword that belongs to the Emperor of the Air. I looked where he was pointing. It was late summer, near midnight, and what he had described was actually Cygnus's bright tail and the outstretched neck of Pegasus.

Presently he ceased speaking, and after a time they walked back across the lawn and went into the house. The light in the kitchen went on, then off. I stepped from my hiding place. I suppose I could have continued with my mission, but the air was calm, it was a perfect and still night, and my plan,

I felt, had been interrupted. In my hand the jar felt large and dangerous. I crept back across the lawn, staying in the shadows of the ivy and rhododendron along the fence, until I was in the driveway between our two houses. In the side window of the Pikes' house a light was on. I paused at a point where the angle allowed me a view through the glass, down the hallway, and through an open door into the living room. Mr. Pike and Kurt were sitting together on a brown couch against the far wall of the room, watching television. I came up close to the window and peered through. Though I knew this was foolish, that any neighbor, any man walking his dog at night, would have thought me a burglar in my black clothing, I stayed and watched. The light was on inside, it was dark around me, and I knew I could look in without being seen. Mr. Pike had his hand on Kurt's shoulder. Every so often when they laughed at something on the screen, he moved his hand up and tousled Kurt's hair, and the sight of this suddenly made me feel the way I do on the bridge across the Mississippi River. When he put his hand on Kurt's hair again, I moved out of the shadows and went back to my own house.

I wanted to run, or kick a ball, or shout a soliloquy into the night. I could have stepped up on a car hood then and lured the Pikes, the paper boy, all the neighbors, out into the night. I could have spoken about the laboratory of a biology teacher, about the rows of specimen jars. How could one not hope here? At three weeks the human embryo has gill arches on its neck, like a fish; at six weeks, amphibians' webs still connect its blunt fingers. Miracles. This is true everywhere in nature. The evolution of five hundred million years is mimicked in each gestation: birds that in the egg look like fish; fish that emerge like their spineless, leaflike ancestors. What it is to study life! Anybody who had seen a cell divide could have invented religion.

I sat down on the porch steps and looked at the elm. After a while I stood up and went inside. With turpentine I cleaned the shoe polish from my face, and then I went upstairs. I got into bed. For an hour or two I lay there, sleepless, hot, my thoughts racing, before I gave up and went to the bedroom window. The jar, which I had brought up with me, stood on the sill, and I saw that the insects were either asleep or dead. I opened the window then and emptied them down onto the lawn, and at that moment, as they rained away into the night, glinting and cascading, I thought of asking Vera for a child. I knew it was not possible, but I considered it anyway. Standing there at the window, I thought of Vera, ageless, in forest boots and shorts, perspiring through a flannel blouse as she dipped drinking water from an Appalachian stream. What had we, she and I? The night was calm, dark. Above me Polaris blinked.

I tried going to sleep again. I lay in bed for a time, and then gave up and went downstairs. I ate some crackers. I drank two glasses of bourbon. I sat at the window and looked out at the front yard. Then I got up and went outside and looked up at the stars, and I tried to see them for their beauty and mystery. I thought of billions of tons of exploding gases, hydrogen and helium, red giants, supernovas. In places they were as dense as clouds. I thought of magnesium and silicon and iron. I tried to see them out of their constellatory order, but it was like trying to look at a word without reading it, and I stood there in the night unable to scramble the patterns. Some clouds had blown in and begun to cover Auriga and Taurus. I was watching them begin to spread and refract moonlight when I heard the paper boy whistling the national anthem. When he reached me, I was standing by the elm, still in my nightclothes, unshaven, a little drunk.

"I want you to do something for me," I said.

"Sir?"

"I'm an old man and I want you to do something for me. Put down your bicycle," I said. "Put down your bicycle and look up at the stars."

The Very Old

The very old are forever
hurting themselves,

burning their fingers
on skillets, falling

loosely as trees
and breaking their hips

with muffled explosions of bone.
Down the block

they are wheeled in
out of our sight

for years at a time.
To make conversation,

the neighbors ask
if they are still alive.

Then, early one morning
through our kitchen windows

we see them again,
first one and then another,

out in their gardens
on crutches and canes,

perennial,
checking their gauges for rain.

Near the Old People's Home

The people on the avenue at noon,
Sharing the sparrows and the wintry sun,
The turned-off fountain with its basin drained
And cement benches etched with checkerboards,

Are old and poor, most every one of them
Wearing some decoration of his damage,
Bandage or crutch or cane; and some are blind,
Or nearly, tap-tapping along with white wands.

When they open their mouths, there are no teeth.
All the same, they keep on talking to themselves
Even while bending to hawk up spit or blood
In gutters that will be there when they are gone.

Some have the habit of getting hit by cars
Three times a year; the ambulance comes up
And away they go, mumbling even in shock
The many secret names they have for God.

He Makes a House Call

Six, seven years ago
when you began to begin to faint
I painted your leg with iodine

threaded the artery
with the needle and then the tube
pumped your heart with dye enough

to see the valve
almost closed with stone.
We were both under pressure.

Today, in your garden,
kneeling under the sticky fig tree
for tomatoes

I keep remembering your blood.
Seven, it was. I was just
beginning to learn the heart

inside out.
Afterward, your surgery
and the precise valve of steel

and plastic that still pops and clicks
inside like a ping-pong ball.
I should try

chewing tobacco sometimes
if only to see how it tastes.
There is a trace of it at the corner

of your leathery smile
which insists that I see inside
the house: someone named Bill I'm supposed

to know; the royal plastic soldier
whose body fills with whiskey
and marches on a music box

How Dry I Am;
the illuminated 3-D Christ who turns
into Mary from different angles;

the watery basement
the pills you take, the ivy
that may grow around the ceiling

if it must. Here, you
are in charge—of figs, beans,
tomatoes, life.

At the hospital, a thousand times
I have heard your heart valve open, close.
I know how clumsy it is.

But health is whatever works
and for as long. I keep thinking
of seven years without a faint

on my way to the car
loaded with vegetables
I keep thinking of seven years ago

when you bled in my hands like a saint.

Ancient Gentility

In those days I was about the only doctor they would have on Guinea Hill. Nowadays some of the kids I delivered then may be practising medicine in the neighborhood. But in those days I had them all. I got to love those people, they were all right. Italian peasants from the region just south of Naples, most of them, living in small jerry-built houses—doing whatever they could find to do for a living and getting by, somehow.

Among the others, there was a little frame building, or box, you might almost say, which had always interested me but into which I had never gone. It stood in the center of the usual small garden patch and sometimes there would be an old man at the gate, just standing there, with a big curved and silver-capped pipe in his mouth, puffing away at his leisure.

Sure enough, one day I landed in that house also.

I had been seeing a child at the Petrello's or Albino's or whoever it was when, as often happened, the woman of the house stopped me with a smile at the door just as I was leaving.

Doc, I want you to visit the old people next door. The old lady's sick. She don't want to call nobody, but you go just the same. I'll fix it up with you sometime. Will you do it—for me?

Would I! It was a June morning. I had only to go twenty feet or so up the street—with a view of all New York City spread out before me over the meadows just beginning to turn green—and push back the low gate to the little vegetable garden.

The old man opened the house door for me before I could knock. He smiled and bowed his head several times out of respect for a physician and pointed upstairs. He couldn't speak a word of English and I knew practically no Italian, so he let it go at that.

He was wonderful. A gentle, kindly creature, big as the house itself, almost, with long pure white hair and big white moustache. Every movement he made showed a sort of ancient gentility. Finally he said a few words as if to let me know he was sorry he couldn't talk English and pointed upstairs again.

Where I stood at that moment it was just one room, everything combined: you cooked in one corner, ate close by, and sat yourself down to talk

312

with your friends and relatives over beyond. Everything was immaculately clean and smelt just tinged with that faint odor of garlic, peppers and olive oil which one gets to expect in all these peasant houses.

There was one other room, immediately above. To it there ascended a removable ladder. At this moment the trap was open and the ladder in place. I went up. The old man remained below.

What a thrill I got! There was an enormous bed that almost filled the place, it seemed, perhaps a chair or two besides, but no other furniture, and in the bed sinking into the feather mattress and covered with a great feather quilt was the woman I had been summoned to attend.

Her face was dry and seamed with wrinkles, as old peasant faces will finally become, but it had the same patient smile upon it as shone from that of her old husband. White hair framing her face with silvery abundance, she didn't look at all sick to me.

She said a few words, smiling the while, by which I understood that after all it wasn't much and that she knew she didn't need a doctor and would have been up long since—or words to that effect—if the others hadn't insisted. After listening to her heart and palpating her abdomen I told her she could get up if she wanted to, and as I backed down the ladder after saying good-bye, she had already begun to do so.

The old man was waiting for me as I arrived below.

We walked to the door together, I trying to explain to him what I had found and he bowing and saying a word or two of Italian in reply. I could make out that he was thanking me for my trouble and that he was sorry he had no money, and so forth and so on.

At the gate we paused in one of those embarrassed moments which sometimes arrive during any conversation between relative strangers who wish to make a good impression on each other. Then as we stood there, slightly ill at ease, I saw him reach into his vest pocket and take something into his hand which he held out toward me.

It was a small silver box, about an inch and a quarter along the sides and half an inch thick. On the cover of it was the embossed figure of a woman reclining among flowers. I took it in my hand but couldn't imagine what he wanted me to do with it. He couldn't be giving it to me?

Seeing that I was puzzled, he reached for it, ever so gently, and I returned it to him. As he took it in his hand he opened it. It seemed to contain a sort of brown powder. Then I saw him pick some of it up between the thumb and finger of his right hand, place it at the base of his left thumb and . . .

Why snuff! Of course. I was delighted.

As he whiffed the powder into one generous nostril and then the other, he handed the box back to me—in all, one of the most gracious, kindly proceedings I had ever taken part in.

Imitating him as best I could, I shared his snuff with him, and that was about the end of me for a moment or two. I couldn't stop sneezing. I suppose I had gone at it a little too vigorously. Finally, with tears in my eyes, I felt the old man standing there, smiling, an experience the like of which I shall never, in all probability, have again in my life on this mundane sphere.

To Hell with Dying

"*To hell with dying*," my father would say. "These children want Mr. Sweet!"

Mr. Sweet was a diabetic and an alcoholic and a guitar player and lived down the road from us on a neglected cotton farm. My older brothers and sisters got the most benefit from Mr. Sweet, for when they were growing up he had quite a few years ahead of him and so was capable of being called back from the brink of death any number of times—whenever the voice of my father reached him as he lay expiring. "To hell with dying, man," my father would say, pushing the wife away from the bedside (in tears although she knew the death was not necessarily the last one unless Mr. Sweet really wanted it to be). "These children want Mr. Sweet!" And they did want him, for at a signal from Father they would come crowding around the bed and throw themselves on the covers, and whoever was the smallest at the time would kiss him all over his wrinkled brown face and begin to tickle him so that he would laugh all down in his stomach, and his moustache, which was long and sort of straggly, would shake like Spanish moss and was also that color.

Mr. Sweet had been ambitious as a boy, wanted to be a doctor or lawyer or sailor, only to find that black men fare better if they are not. Since he could become none of these things he turned to fishing as his one earnest career and playing the guitar as his sole claim to doing anything extraordinarily well. His son, the only one that he and his wife, Miss Mary, had, was shiftless as the day is long and spent money as if he were trying to see the bottom of the mint, which Mr. Sweet would tell him was the clear brown palm of his hand. Miss Mary loved her "baby," however, and worked hard to get him the "li'l necessaries" of life, which turned out mostly to be women.

Mr. Sweet was a tall, thinnish man with thick kinky hair going dead white. He was dark brown, his eyes were very squinty and sort of bluish, and he chewed Brown Mule tobacco. He was constantly on the verge of being blind drunk, for he brewed his own liquor and was not in the least a stingy sort of man, and was always very melancholy and sad, though frequently when he was "feelin' good" he'd dance around the yard with us, usually keeling over just as my mother came to see what the commotion was.

Toward all of us children he was very kind, and had the grace to be shy with us, which is unusual in grown-ups. He had great respect for my mother for she never held his drunkenness against him and would let us play with him even when he was about to fall in the fireplace from drink. Although Mr. Sweet would sometimes lose complete or nearly complete control of his head and neck so that he would loll in his chair, his mind remained strangely acute and his speech not too affected. His ability to be drunk and sober at the same time made him an ideal playmate, for he was as weak as we were and we could usually best him in wrestling, all the while keeping a fairly coherent conversation going.

We never felt anything of Mr. Sweet's age when we played with him. We loved his wrinkles and would draw some on our brows to be like him, and his white hair was my special treasure and he knew it and would never come to visit us just after he had had his hair cut off at the barbershop. Once he came to our house for something, probably to see my father about fertilizer for his crops because, although he never paid the slightest attention to his crops, he liked to know what things would be best to use on them if he ever did. Anyhow, he had not come with his hair since he had just had it shaved off at the barbershop. He wore a huge straw hat to keep off the sun and also to keep his head away from me. But as soon as I saw him I ran up and demanded that he take me up and kiss me with his funny mustache, which smelled so strongly of tobacco. Looking forward to burying my small fingers into his woolly hair I threw away his hat only to find he had done something to his hair, that it was no longer there! I let out a squall which made my mother think that Mr. Sweet had finally dropped me in the well or something and from that day I've been wary of men in hats. However, not long after, Mr. Sweet showed up with his hair grown out and just as white and kinky and impenetrable as it ever was.

Mr. Sweet used to call me his princess, and I believed it. He made me feel pretty at five and six, simply outrageously devastating at the blazing age of eight and a half. When he came to our house with his guitar the whole family would stop whatever they were doing and sit around him and listen to him play. He liked to play "Sweet Georgia Brown," that was what he called me sometimes, and also he liked to play "Caldonia" and all sorts of sweet, sad, wonderful songs which he sometimes made up. It was from one of those songs that I learned that he had had to marry Miss Mary when he had in fact loved somebody else (now living in Chi-ca-go, or De-stroy, Michigan). He was not sure that Joe Lee, her "baby," was also his baby. Sometimes he would cry and that was an indication that he was about to die again. And so we would all get prepared, for we were sure to be called upon.

I was seven the first time I remember actually participating in one of Mr. Sweet's "revivals"—my parents told me I had participated before, I had been the one chosen to kiss him and tickle him long before I knew the rite of Mr. Sweet's rehabilitation. He had come to our house, it was a few years after his wife's death, and was very sad, and also, typically, very drunk. He sat on the floor next to me and my older brother, the rest of the children were grown up and lived elsewhere, and began to play his guitar and cry. I held his woolly head in my arms and wished I could have been old enough to have been the woman he loved so much and that I had not been lost years and years ago.

When he was leaving, my mother said to us that we'd better sleep light for we'd probably have to go over to Mr. Sweet's before daylight. And we did. For soon after we had gone to bed one of the neighbors knocked on our door and called my father and said that Mr. Sweet was sinking fast and if he wanted to get in a word before the crossover he'd better shake a leg and get over to Mr. Sweet's house. All the neighbors knew to come to our house if something was wrong with Mr. Sweet, but they did not know how we always managed to make him well, or at least stop him from dying, when he was often so near death. As soon as we heard the cry we got up, my brother and I and my mother and father, and put on our clothes. We hurried out of the house and down the road, for we were always afraid that we might someday be too late and Mr. Sweet would get tired of dallying.

When we got to the house, a very poor shack really, we found the front room full of neighbors and relatives and a man met us at the door and said that it was all very sad that old Mr. Sweet Little (for Little was his family name, although we mostly ignored it) was about to kick the bucket. He advised my parents not to take my brother and me into the "death room," seeing we were so young and all, but we were so much more accustomed to the death room than he that we ignored him and dashed in without giving his warning a second thought. I was almost in tears, for these deaths upset me fearfully, and the thought of how much depended on me and my brother (who was such a ham most of the time) made me very nervous.

The doctor was bending over the bed and turned back to tell us for at least the tenth time in the history of my family that, alas, old Mr. Sweet Little was dying and that the children had best not see the face of implacable death (I didn't know what "implacable" was, but whatever it was, Mr. Sweet was not!). My father pushed him rather abruptly out of the way saying, as he always did and very loudly, for he was saying it to Mr. Sweet, "To hell with dying, man, these children want Mr. Sweet"—which was my cue to throw myself upon the bed and kiss Mr. Sweet all around the whiskers and under the eyes and around the collar of his nightshirt where he smelled so strongly of all sorts of things, mostly liniment.

I was very good at bringing him around, for as soon as I saw that he was struggling to open his eyes I knew he was going to be all right, and so could finish my revival sure of success. As soon as his eyes were open he would begin to smile and that way I knew that I had surely won. Once, though, I got a tremendous scare, for he could not open his eyes and later I learned that he had had a stroke and that one side of his face was stiff and hard to get into motion. When he began to smile I could tickle him in earnest because I was sure that nothing would get in the way of his laughter, although once he began to cough so hard that he almost threw me off his stomach, but that was when I was very small, little more than a baby, and my bushy hair had gotten in his nose.

When we were sure he would listen to us we would ask him why he was in bed and when he was coming to see us again and could we play with his guitar, which more than likely would be leaning against the bed. His eyes would get all misty and he would sometimes cry out loud, but we never let it embarrass us, for he knew that we loved him and that we sometimes cried too for no reason. My parents would leave the room to just the three of us; Mr. Sweet, by that time, would be propped up in bed with a number of pillows behind his head and with me sitting and lying on his shoulder and along his chest. Even when he had trouble breathing he would not ask me to get down. Looking into my eyes he would shake his white head and run a scratchy old finger all around my hairline, which was rather low down, nearly to my eyebrows, and made some people say I looked like a baby monkey.

My brother was very generous in all this, he let me do all the revivaling— he had done it for years before I was born and so was glad to be able to pass it on to someone new. What he would do while I talked to Mr. Sweet was pretend to play the guitar, in fact pretend that he was a young version of Mr. Sweet, and it always made Mr. Sweet glad to think that someone wanted to be like him—of course, we did not know this then, we played the thing by ear, and whatever he seemed to like, we did. We were desperately afraid that he was just going to take off one day and leave us.

It did not occur to us that we were doing anything special; we had not learned that death was final when it did come. We thought nothing of triumphing over it so many times, and in fact became a trifle contemptuous of people who let themselves be carried away. It did not occur to us that if our own father had been dying we could not have stopped it, that Mr. Sweet was the only person over whom we had power.

When Mr. Sweet was in his eighties I was studying in the university many miles from home. I saw him whenever I went home, but he was never on the verge of dying that I could tell and I began to feel that my anxiety for his health and psychological well-being was unnecessary. By this time he had not only had a mustache but was beginning to grow a beard. He was very peaceful, fragile, gentle, and the only jarring note about him was his old guitar, which he still played in the old sad, down-home blues way.

On Mr. Sweet's ninetieth birthday I was finishing my doctorate in Massachusetts and had been making arrangements to go home for several weeks' rest. That morning I got a telegram telling me that Mr. Sweet was dying again and could I please drop everything and come home. Of course I could. My dissertation could wait and my teachers would understand when I explained to them after I got back. I ran to the phone, called the airport, and within four hours I was speeding along the dusty road to Mr. Sweet's.

The house was more dilapidated than when I was last there, but it was overgrown with yellow roses which my family had planted many years ago. The air was heavy and sweet and very peaceful. I felt strange walking through the gate and up the old rickety steps. But the strangeness left me as I caught sight of the thin body I loved so well beneath the familiar quilt coverlet. Mr. Sweet!

His eyes were closed tight and his hands, crossed over his stomach, were thin and delicate, no longer scratchy. I remembered how as a small child I had run and jumped up on him just anywhere; now I knew he would not be able to support my weight. I looked around at my parents, and was surprised to see that my father and mother also looked old and frail. My father, his own hair very gray, leaned over the quietly sleeping old man, who, incidentally, smelled still of wine and tobacco, and said, as he'd done so many times, "To hell with dying, man! My daughter is home to see Mr. Sweet!" My brother hadn't been able to come, as he was in the war in Asia. I bent down and gently stroked the closed eyes and gradually they began to open. The closed wine-stained lips twitched a little, then parted in a warm, slightly embarrassed smile. Mr. Sweet could see me and he recognized me and his eyes looked very spry and twinkly for a moment. I put my head down on the pillow next to his and we just looked at each other for a long time. Then he began to trace my peculiar hairline with a thin, smooth finger. I closed my eyes when his finger halted above my ear (he used to rejoice at the dirt in my ears when I was little), his hand stayed cupped around my neck. When I opened my eyes, sure that I had reached him in time, his were closed.

Even at twenty-four how could I believe that I had failed? that Mr. Sweet was really gone? He had never gone before. But when I looked up at my parents I saw that they were holding back tears. They had loved him dearly. He was like a piece of rare and delicate china which was always being saved from breaking and which finally fell. I looked long at the old face, the wrinkled forehead, the red lips, the hands that still reached out to me. Soon I felt my father pushing something cool into my hands. It was Mr. Sweet's guitar. He had asked him months before to give it to me; he had known that even if I came next time he would not be able to respond in the old way. He did not want me to feel that my trip had been for nothing.

The old guitar! I plucked the strings, hummed "Sweet Georgia Brown." The magic of Mr. Sweet lingered still in the smooth wooden box. Through the window I could catch the fragrant delicate scent of tender yellow roses. The man on the high old-fashioned bed with the quilt coverlet and the glowing white hair had been my first love.

Toenails

*It **is the custom*** of many doctors, I among them, to withdraw from the practice of medicine every Wednesday afternoon. This, only if there is no patient who demands the continuous presence of his physician. I urge you, when the time comes, to do it, too. Such an absence from duty ought not to win you the accusation of lèse responsibility. You will, of course, have secured the availability of a colleague to look after your patients for the few hours you will spend grooming and watering your spirit. Nor is such idleness a reproach to those who do not take time off from their labors, but who choose to scramble on without losing the pace. Loafing is not better than frenzied determination. It is but an alternate mode of living.

Long ago I made a vow that I would never again delve away the month of July in the depths of the human body. In July it would be my own cadaver that engaged me. There is a danger in becoming too absorbed in Anatomy. At the end of eleven months of dissection, you stand in fair risk of suffering a kind of rapture of the deep, wherein you drift, tumbling among the coils of intestine in a state of helpless enchantment. Only a month's vacation can save you. It is wrongheaded to think of total submersion in the study and practice of Medicine. That is going too far. And going too far is for saints. I know medical students well enough to exclude you from that slender community.

Nor must you be a priest who does nothing but preserve the souls of his parishioners and lets his own soul lapse. Such is the burnt-out case who early on drinks his patients down in a single radiant gulp and all too soon loses the desire to practice Medicine at all. In a year or two he is to be found lying in bed being fed oatmeal with a spoon. Like the fruit of the Amazon he is too quickly ripe and too quickly rotten.

Some doctors spend Wednesday afternoon on the golf course. Others go fishing. Still another takes a lesson on the viola da gamba. I go to the library where I join that subculture of elderly men and women who gather in the Main Reading Room to read or sleep beneath the world's newspapers, and thumb through magazines and periodicals, educating themselves in any number of esoteric ways, or just keeping up. It is not the least function of a library to provide for these people a warm, dry building with good working toilets and, ideally, a vending machine from which to buy a cup of hot broth or coffee. All of which attributes a public library shares with a neighborhood saloon, the only difference being the beer of one and the books of the other.

How brave, how reliable they are! plowing through you-name-what inclemencies to get to the library shortly after it opens. So unbroken is their attendance that, were one of them to be missing, it would arouse the direst suspicions of the others. And of me. For I have, furtively at first, then with increasing recklessness, begun to love them. They were, after all, living out my own fantasies. One day, with luck, I, too, would become a full-fledged, that is to say *daily*, member. At any given time, the tribe consists of a core of six regulars and a somewhat less constant pool of eight others of whom two or three can be counted on to appear. On very cold days, all eight of these might show up, causing a bit of a jam at the newspaper rack, and an edginess among the regulars.

Either out of loyalty to certain beloved articles of clothing, or from scantiness of wardrobe, they wear the same things every day. For the first year or two this was how I identified them. Old Stovepipe, Mrs. Fringes, Neckerchief, Galoshes—that sort of thing. In no other society does apparel so exactly fit the wearer as to form a part of his persona. Dior, Balenciaga, take heed! By the time I arrive, they have long since devoured the morning's newspapers and settled into their customary places. One or two, Galoshes, very likely, and Stovepipe, are sleeping it off. These two seem to need all the rest they can get. Mrs. Fringes, on the other hand, her hunger for information unappeasable, having finished all of the newspapers, will be well into the *Journal of Abnormal Psychology*, the case histories of which keep her riveted until closing time. As time went by, despite that we had not yet exchanged a word of conversation, I came to think of them as dear colleagues, fellow readers who, with me, were engaged in the pursuit of language. Reading was serious business. Only downstairs near the basement vending machine would animated conversation break out. Upstairs, in the Reading Room, the vow of silence was sacred.

I do not know by what criteria such selections are made, but Neckerchief is my favorite. He is a man well into his eighties with the kind of pink face that even in July looks as though it has just been brought in out of the cold. A single drop of watery discharge, like a crystal bead, hangs at the tip of his nose. His gait is stiff-legged, with tiny, quick, shuffling steps accompanied by rather wild arm-swinging in what seems an effort to gain momentum or maintain balance. For a long time I could not decide whether this manner of walking was due to arthritis of the knees or to the fact that for most of the year he wore two or more pairs of pants. Either might have been the cause of his lack of joint flexion. One day, as I held the door to the Men's Room for him, he pointed to his knees and announced, by way of explanation of his slowness:

"The hinges is rusty."

The fact was delivered with a shake of the head, a wry smile and without the least self-pity.

"No hurry," I said, and once again paid homage to Sir William Osler, who instructed his students to "listen to the patient. He is trying to tell you what is the matter with him." From that day, Neckerchief and I were friends. I learned that he lives alone in a rooming house eight blocks away, that he lives on his Social Security check, that his wife died a long time ago, that he has no children, and that the *Boston Globe* is the best damn newspaper in the library. He learned approximately the same number of facts about me. He himself had been an amateur fighter sixty years ago—most of his engagements having been spontaneous brawls of a decidedly ethnic nature. "It was the Polacks against the Yids," he told me, "and both of 'em against the Micks." He held up his fists to show the ancient fractures.

The actual neckerchief is a classic red cowboy rag folded into a triangle and tied about his neck in such a way that the widest part lies at the front, covering the upper chest as a kind of bib. Now and then a nose drop elongates, shimmers, wobbles and falls to be absorbed into the neckerchief. Meanwhile a new drop has taken the place of the old. So quickly is this newcomer born that I, for one, have never beheld him unadorned.

One day I watched as Neckerchief, having raided the magazine rack, journeyed back to his seat. In one flapping hand the *Saturday Review* rattled. As he passed, I saw that his usually placid expression was replaced by the look of someone in pain. Each step was a fresh onslaught of it. His lower lip was caught between his teeth. His forehead had been cut and stitched into lines of endurance. He was hissing. I waited for him to take his seat, which he did with a gasp of relief, then went up to him.

"The hinges?" I whispered.

"Nope. The toes."

"What's wrong with your toes?"

"The toenails is too long. I can't get at 'em. I'm walkin' on 'em."

I left the library and went to my office.

"What are you doing here?" said my nurse. "It's Wednesday afternoon. People are just supposed to die on Wednesday afternoon."

"I need the toenail cutters. I'll bring them back tomorrow."

"The last time you took something out of here I didn't see it for six months."

Neckerchief was right where I had left him. A brief survey, however, told me that he had made one trek in my absence. It was *U.S. News & World Report* on his lap. The *Saturday Review* was back in the rack. I could only guess what the exchange had cost him. I doubted that either of the magazines was worth it.

"Come down to the Men's Room," I said. "I want to cut your toenails." I showed him my toenail clippers, the heavy-duty kind that you grip with the palm, and with jaws that could bite through bone. One of the handles is a rasp. I gave him a ten-minute head start, then followed him downstairs to the Men's Room. There was no one else there.

"Sit here." I pointed to one of the booths. He sat on the toilet. I knelt and began to take off his shoes.

"Don't untie 'em," he said. "I just slide 'em on and off."

The two pairs of socks were another story, having to be peeled off. The underpair snagged on the toenails. Neckerchief winced.

"How do you get these things on?" I asked.

"A mess, ain't they? I hope they don't stink too bad for you."

The nail of each big toe was the horn of a goat. Thick as a thumb and curved, it projected down over the tip of the toe to the underside. With each step, the nail wold scrape painfully against the ground and be pressed into his flesh. There was dried blood on each big toe.

"Jesus, man!" I said. "How can you walk?" I thought of the eight blocks he covered twice a day.

I took an hour to do each big toe. The nails were too thick even for my nail cutters. They had to be chewed away little by little, then flattened out with the rasp. Now and then a fragment of nail would fly up, striking me in the face. The other eight toes were easy. Now and then, the door opened. Someone came and went to the row of urinals. Twice, someone occupied the booth next to ours. I never once looked up to see. They'll just have to wonder, I thought. But Neckerchief could tell from my face.

"It doesn't look decent," he said.

"Never mind," I told him. "I bet this isn't the strangest thing that's happened down here." I wet some toilet paper with warm water and soap, washed each toe, dried him off, and put his shoes and socks back on. He stood up and took a few steps, like someone who is testing the fit of a new pair of shoes.

"How is it?"

"It doesn't hurt," he said, and gave me a smile that I shall keep in my safety-deposit box at the bank until the day I die.

"That's a Cadillac of a toe job," said Neckerchief. "How much do I owe ya?"

"On the house," I said. "And besides, what kind of a boy do you think I am?"

The next week I did Stovepipe. He was an easy case. Then, Mrs. Fringes, who was a special problem. I had to do her in the Ladies' Room, which tied up the place for half an hour. A lot of people opened the door, took one look, and left in a hurry. Either it was hot in there or I had a temperature.

I never go to the library on Wednesday afternoon without my nail clippers in my briefcase. You just never know.

Misery

"To whom shall I tell my grief?"

The twilight of evening. Big flakes of wet snow are whirling lazily about the street lamps, which have just been lighted, and lying in a thin soft layer on roofs, horses' backs, shoulders, caps. Iona Potapov, the sledge-driver, is all white like a ghost. He sits on the box without stirring, bent as double as the living body can be bent. If a regular snowdrift fell on him it seems as though even then he would not think it necessary to shake it off. . . . His little mare is white and motionless too. Her stillness, the angularity of her lines, and the stick-like straightness of her legs make her look like a halfpenny gingerbread horse. She is probably lost in thought. Anyone who has been torn away from the plough, from the familiar gray landscapes, and cast into this slough, full of monstrous lights, of unceasing uproar and hurrying people, is bound to think.

It is a long time since Iona and his nag have budged. They came out of the yard before dinnertime and not a single fare yet. But now the shades of evening are falling on the town. The pale light of the street lamps changes to a vivid color, and the bustle of the street grows noisier.

"Sledge to Vyborgskaya!" Iona hears. "Sledge!"

Iona starts, and through his snow-plastered eyelashes sees an officer in a military overcoat with a hood over his head.

"To Vyborgskaya," repeats the officer. "Are you asleep? To Vyborgskaya!"

In token of assent Iona gives a tug at the reins which sends cakes of snow flying from the horse's back and shoulders. The officer gets into the sledge. The sledge-driver clicks to the horse, cranes his neck like a swan, rises in his seat, and more from habit than necessity brandishes his whip. The mare cranes her neck, too, crooks her stick-like legs, and hesitatingly sets off. . . .

"Where are you shoving, you devil?" Iona immediately hears shouts from the dark mass shifting to and fro before him. "Where the devil are you going? Keep to the r-right!"

"You don't know how to drive! Keep to the right," says the officer angrily.

A coachman driving a carriage swears at him; a pedestrian crossing the road and brushing the horse's nose with his shoulder looks at him angrily and shakes the snow off his sleeve. Iona fidgets on the box as though he were sitting on thorns, jerks his elbows, and turns his eyes about like one possessed, as though he did not know where he was or why he was there.

"What rascals they all are!" says the officer jocosely. "They are simply doing their best to run up against you or fall under the horse's feet. They must be doing it on purpose."

Iona looks at his fare and moves his lips. . . . Apparently he means to say something, but nothing comes but a sniff.

"What?" inquires the officer.

Iona gives a wry smile, and straining his throat, brings out huskily: "My son . . . er . . . my son died this week, sir."

"H'm! What did he die of?"

Iona turns his whole body round to his fare, and says:

"Who can tell! It must have been from fever. . . . He lay three days in the hospital and then he died. . . . God's will."

"Turn around, you devil!" comes out of the darkness. "Have you gone cracked, you old dog? Look where you are going!"

"Drive on! drive on! . . . " says the officer. "We shan't get there till to-morrow going on like this. Hurry up!"

The sledge-driver cranes his neck again, rises in his seat, and with heavy grace swings his whip. Several times he looks round at the officer, but the latter keeps his eyes shut and is apparently disinclined to listen. Putting his fare down at Vyborgskaya, Iona stops by a restaurant, and again sits huddled up on the box. . . . Again the wet snow paints him and his horse white. One hour passes, and then another. . . .

Three young men, two tall and thin, one short and hunchbacked, come up, railing at each other and loudly stamping on the pavement with their galoshes.

"Cabby, to the Police Bridge!" the hunchback cries in a cracked voice. "The three of us, . . . twenty kopecks!"

Iona tugs at the reins and clicks to his horse. Twenty kopecks is not a fair price, but he has no thoughts for that. Whether it is a rouble or whether it is five kopecks does not matter to him now so long as he has a fare. . . . The three young men, shoving each other and using bad language, go up to the sledge, and all three try to sit down at once. The question remains to be settled: Which are to sit down and which one is to stand? After a long altercation, ill-temper, and abuse, they come to the conclusion that the hunchback must stand because he is the shortest.

"Well, drive on," says the hunchback in his cracked voice, settling himself and breathing down Iona's neck. "Cut along! What a cap you've got, my friend! You wouldn't find a worse one in all Petersburg. . . . "

"He-he! . . . he-he! . . . " laughs Iona. "It's nothing to boast of!"

"Well, then, nothing to boast of, drive on! Are you going to drive like this all the way? Eh? Shall I give you one in the neck?"

"My head aches," says one of the tall ones. "At the Dukmasov's yesterday Vaska and I drank four bottles of brandy between us."

"I can't make out why you talk such stuff," says the other tall one angrily. "You lie like a brute."

"Strike me dead, it's the truth! . . . "

"It's about as true as that a louse coughs."

"He-he!" grins Iona. "Me-er-ry gentlemen!"

"Tfoo! the devil take you!" cries the hunchback indignantly. "Will you get on, you old plague, or won't you? Is that the way to drive? Give her one with the whip. Hang it all, give it her well."

Iona feels behind his back the jolting person and quivering voice of the hunchback. He hears abuse addressed to him, he sees people, and the feeling of loneliness begins little by little to be less heavy on his heart. The hunchback swears at him, till he chokes over some elaborately whimsical string of epithets and is overpowered by his cough. His tall companions begin talking of a certain Nadyezhda Petrovna. Iona looks round at them. Waiting till there is a brief pause, he looks round once more and says:

"This week . . . er . . . my . . . er . . . son died!"

"We shall all die, . . . " says the hunchback with a sigh, wiping his lips after coughing. "Come, drive on! drive on! My friends, I simply cannot stand crawling like this! When will he get us there?"

"Well, you give him a little encouragement . . . one in the neck!"

"Do you hear, you old plague? I'll make you smart. If one stands on ceremony with fellows like you one may as well walk. Do you hear, you old dragon? Or don't you care a hang what we say?"

And Iona hears rather than feels a slap on the back of his neck.

"He-he! . . . " he laughs. "Merry gentlemen. . . . God give you health!"

"Cabman, are you married?" asks one of the tall ones.

"I? He-he! Me-er-ry gentlemen. The only wife for me now is the damp earth. . . . He-ho-ho! . . . The grave is! . . . Here my son's dead and I am alive. . . . It's a strange thing, death has come in at the wrong door. . . . Instead of coming for me it went for my son. . . . "

And Iona turns round to tell them how his son died, but at that point the hunchback gives a faint sigh and announces that, thank God! they have arrived at last. After taking his twenty kopecks, Iona gazes for a long while after the revelers, who disappear into a dark entry. Again he is alone and again there is silence for him. . . . The misery which has been for a brief space eased comes back again and tears his heart more cruelly than ever. With a look of anxiety and suffering Iona's eyes stray restlessly among the crowds moving to and fro on both sides of the street: can he not find among those thousands someone who will listen to him? But the crowds flit by heedless of him and his misery. . . . His misery is immense, beyond all bounds. If Iona's heart were to burst and his misery to flow out, it would flood the whole world, it seems, but yet it is not seen. It has found a hiding-place in such an insignificant shell that one would not have found it with a candle by daylight. . . .

Iona sees a house-porter with a parcel and makes up his mind to address him.

"What time will it be, friend?" he asks.

"Going on ten. . . . Why have you stopped here? Drive on!"

Iona drives a few paces away, bends himself double, and gives himself up to his misery. He feels it is no good to appeal to people. But before five minutes have passed he draws himself up, shakes his head as though he feels a sharp pain, and tugs at the reins. . . . He can bear it no longer.

"Back to the yard!" he thinks. "To the yard!"

And his little mare, as though she knew his thoughts, falls to trotting. An hour and a half later Iona is sitting by a big dirty stove. On the stove, on the floor, and on the benches are people snoring. The air is full of smells and stuffiness. Iona looks at the sleeping figures, scratches himself, and regrets that he has come home so early. . . .

"I have not earned enough to pay for the oats, even," he thinks. "That's why I am so miserable. A man who knows how to do his work, . . . who has had enough to eat, and whose horse has had enough to eat, is always at ease. . . ."

In one of the corners a young cabman gets up, clears his throat sleepily, and makes for the waterbucket.

"Want a drink?" Iona asks him.

"Seems so."

"May it do you good. . . . But my son is dead, mate. . . . Do you hear? This week in the hospital. . . . It's a queer business. . . ."

Iona looks to see the effect produced by his words, but he sees nothing. The young man has covered his head over and is already asleep. The old man sighs and scratches himself. . . . Just as the young man had been thirsty for water, he thirsts for speech. His son will soon have been dead a week, and he has not really talked to anybody yet. . . . He wants to talk of it properly, with deliberation. . . . He wants to tell how his son was taken ill, how he suffered, what he said before he died, how he died. . . . He wants to describe the funeral, and how he went to the hospital to get his son's clothes. He still has his daughter Anisya in the country. . . . And he wants to talk about her too. . . . Yes, he has plenty to talk about now. His listener ought to sigh and lament. . . . It would be even better to talk to women. Though they are silly creatures, they blubber at the first word.

"Let's go out and have a look at the mare," Iona thinks. "There is always time for sleep. . . . You'll have sleep enough, no fear. . . ."

He puts on his coat and goes into the stables where his mare is standing. He thinks about oats, about hay, about the weather. . . . He cannot think about his son when he is alone. . . . To talk about him with someone is possible, but to think of him and picture him is insufferable anguish. . . .

"Are you munching?" Iona asks his mare, seeing her shining eyes. "There, munch away, munch away. . . . Since we have not earned enough for oats, we will eat hay. . . . Yes, . . . I have grown too old to drive. . . . My son ought to be driving, not I. . . . He was a real cabman. . . . He ought to have lived. . . . "

Iona is silent for a while, and then he goes on:

"That's how it is, old girl. . . . Kuzma Ionitch is gone. . . . He said good-by to me. . . . He went and died for no reason. . . . Now, suppose you had a little colt, and you were own mother to that little colt. . . . And all at once that same little colt went and died. . . . You'd be sorry, wouldn't you? . . . "

The little mare munches, listens, and breathes on her master's hands. Iona is carried away and tells her all about it.

A Visit of Charity

It was mid-morning—a very cold, bright day. Holding a potted plant before her, a girl of fourteen jumped off the bus in front of the Old Ladies' Home, on the outskirts of town. She wore a red coat, and her straight yellow hair was hanging down loose from the pointed white cap all the little girls were wearing that year. She stopped for a moment beside one of the prickly dark shrubs with which the city had beautified the Home, and then proceeded slowly toward the building, which was of white-washed brick and reflected the winter sunlight like a block of ice. As she walked vaguely up the steps she lifted the small pot from hand to hand; then she had to set it down and remove her mittens before she could open the heavy door.

"I'm a Campfire Girl. . . . I have to pay a visit to some old lady," she told the nurse at the desk. This was a woman in a white uniform who looked as if she were cold; she had close-cut hair which stood up on the very top of her head exactly like a sea wave. Marian, the little girl, did not tell her that this visit would give her a minimum of only three points in her score.

"Acquainted with any of our residents?" asked the nurse. She lifted one eyebrow and spoke like a man.

"With any old ladies? No—but—that is, any of them will do," Marian stammered. With her free hand she pushed her hair behind her ears, as she did when it was time to study Science.

The nurse shrugged and rose, "You have a nice *multiflora cineraria* there," she remarked as she walked ahead down the hall of closed doors to pick out an old lady.

There was loose, bulging linoleum on the floor. Marian felt as if she were walking on the waves, but the nurse paid no attention to it. There was a smell in the hall like the interior of a clock. Everything was silent until, behind one of the doors, an old lady of some kind cleared her throat like a sheep bleating. This decided the nurse. Stopping in her tracks, she first extended her arm, bent her elbow, and leaned forward from the hips—all to examine the watch strapped to her wrist; then she gave a loud double-rap on the door.

"There are two in each room," the nurse remarked over her shoulder.

"Two what?" asked Marian without thinking. The sound like a sheep's bleating almost made her turn around and run back.

One old woman was pulling the door open in short, gradual jerks, and when she saw the nurse a strange smile forced her old face dangerously awry. Marian, suddenly propelled by the strong, impatient arm of the nurse, saw next the side-face of another old woman, even older, who was lying flat in bed with a cap on and a counterpane drawn up to her chin.

"Visitor," said the nurse, and after one more shove she was off up the hall.

Marian stood tongue-tied; both hands held the potted plant. The old woman, still with that terrible, square smile (which was a smile of welcome) stamped on her bony face, was waiting. . . . Perhaps she said something. The old woman in bed said nothing at all, and she did not look around.

Suddenly Marian saw a hand, quick as a bird claw, reach up in the air and pluck the white cap off her head. At the same time, another claw to match drew her all the way into the room, and the next moment the door closed behind her.

"My, my, my," said the old lady at her side.

Marian stood enclosed by a bed, a washstand and a chair; the tiny room had altogether too much furniture. Everything smelled wet—even the bare floor. She held onto the back of the chair, which was wicker and felt soft and damp. Her heart beat more and more slowly, her hands got colder and colder, and she could not hear whether the old women were saying anything or not. She could not see them very clearly. How dark it was! The window shade was down, and the only door was shut. Marian looked at the ceiling. . . . It was like being caught in a robbers' cave, just before one was murdered.

"Did you come to be our little girl for a while?" the first robber asked.

Then something was snatched from Marian's hand—the little potted plant.

"Flowers!" screamed the old woman. She stood holding the pot in an undecided way. "Pretty flowers," she added.

Then the old woman in bed cleared her throat and spoke. "They are not pretty," she said, still without looking around, but very distinctly.

Marian suddenly pitched against the chair and sat down in it.

"Pretty flowers," the first old woman insisted. "Pretty—pretty . . . "

Marian wished she had the little pot back for just a moment—she had forgotten to look at the plant herself before giving it away. What did it look like?

"Stinkweeds," said the other old woman sharply. She had a bunchy white forehead and red eyes like a sheep. Now she turned them toward Marian. The fogginess seemed to rise in her throat again, and she bleated, "Who—are—you?"

To her surprise, Marian could not remember her name. "I'm a Campfire Girl," she said finally.

"Watch out for the germs," said the old woman like a sheep, not addressing anyone.

"One came out last month to see us," said the first old woman.

A sheep or a germ? wondered Marian dreamily, holding onto the chair.

"Did not!" cried the other old woman.

"Did so! read to us out of the Bible, and we enjoyed it!" screamed the first.

"Who enjoyed it!" said the woman in bed. Her mouth was unexpectedly small and sorrowful, like a pet's.

"We enjoyed it," insisted the other. "You enjoyed it—I enjoyed it."

"We all enjoyed it," said Marian, without realizing that she had said a word.

The first old woman had just finished putting the potted plant high, high on the top of the wardrobe, where it could hardly be seen from below. Marian wondered how she had succeeded in placing it there, how she could ever have reached so high.

"You mustn't pay any attention to old Addie," she now said to the little girl. "She's ailing today."

"Will you shut your mouth?" said the woman in bed. "I am not."

"You're a story."

"I can't stay but a minute—really, I can't," said Marian suddenly. She looked down at the wet floor and thought that if she were sick in here they would have to let her go.

With much to-do the first old woman sat down in a rocking chair—still another piece of furniture!—and began to rock. With the fingers of one hand she touched a very dirty cameo pin on her chest. "What do you do at school?" she asked.

"I don't know . . . " said Marian. She tried to think but she could not.

"Oh, but the flowers are beautiful," the old woman whispered. She seemed to rock faster and faster; Marian did not see how anyone could rock so fast.

"Ugly," said the woman in bed.

"If we bring flowers—" Marian began, and then fell silent. She had almost said that if Campfire Girls brought flowers to the Old Ladies' Home, the visit would count one extra point, and if they took a Bible with them on the bus and read it to the old ladies, it counted double. But the old woman had not listened, anyway; she was rocking and watching the other one, who watched back from the bed.

"Poor Addie is ailing. She has to take medicine—see?" she said, pointing a horny finger at a row of bottles on the table, and rocking so high that her black comfort shoes lifted off the floor like a little child's.

"I am no more sick than you are," said the woman in bed.

"Oh, yes you are!"

"I just got more sense than you have, that's all," said the other old woman, nodding her head.

"That's only the contrary way she talks when *you all* come," said the first old lady with sudden intimacy. She stopped the rocker with a neat pat of her feet and leaned toward Marian. Her hand reached over—it felt like a petunia leaf, clinging and just a little sticky.

"Will you hush! Will you hush!" cried the other one.

Marian leaned back rigidly in her chair.

"When I was a little girl like you, I went to school and all," said the old woman in the same intimate, menacing voice. "Not here—another town. . . ."

"Hush!" said the sick woman. "You never went to school. You never came and you never went. You never were anything—only here. You never were born! You don't know anything. Your head is empty, your heart and hands and your old black purse are all empty, even that little old box that you brought with you you brought empty—you showed it to me. And yet you talk, talk, talk, talk, talk all the time until I think I'm losing my mind! Who are you? You're a stranger—a perfect stranger! Don't you know you're a stranger? Is it possible that they have actually done a thing like this to any-one—sent them in a stranger to talk to, and rock, and tell away her whole long rigmarole? Do they seriously suppose that I'll be able to keep it up, day in, day out, night in, night out, living in the same room with a terrible old woman—forever?"

Marian saw the old woman's eyes grow bright and turn toward her. This old woman was looking at her with despair and calculation in her face. Her small lips suddenly dropped apart, and exposed a half circle of false teeth with tan gums.

"Come here, I want to tell you something," she whispered. "Come here."

Marian was trembling, and her heart nearly stopped beating altogether for a moment.

"That's not polite. Do you know what's really the matter with old Addie today?" She, too, looked at Marian; one of her eyelids drooped low.

"The matter?" the child repeated stupidly. "What's the matter with her?"

"Why, she's mad because it's her birthday!" said the first old woman, be-ginning to rock again and giving a little crow as though she had answered her own riddle.

"It is not, it is not!" screamed the old woman in bed. "It is not my birth-day, no one knows when that is but myself, and will you please be quiet and say nothing more, or I'll go straight out of my mind!" She turned her eyes toward Marian again, and presently she said in the soft, foggy voice, "When the worst comes to the worst, I ring this bell, and the nurse comes." One of her hands was drawn out from under the patched counterpane—a thin little hand with enormous black freckles. With a finger which would not hold still she pointed to a little bell on the table among the bottles.

"How old are you?" Marian breathed. Now she could see the old woman in bed very closely and plainly, and very abruptly, from all sides, as in dreams. She wondered about her—she wondered for a moment as though there was nothing else in the world to wonder about. It was the first time such a thing had happened to Marian.

"I won't tell!"

The old face on the pillow, where Marian was bending over it, slowly gathered and collapsed. Soft whimpers came out of the small open mouth. It was a sheep that she sounded like—a little lamb. Marian's face drew very close, the yellow hair hung forward.

"She's crying!" She turned a bright, burning face up to the first old woman.

"That's Addie for you," the old woman said spitefully.

Marian jumped up and moved toward the door. For the second time, the claw almost touched her hair, but it was not quick enough. The little girl put her cap on.

"Well, it was a real visit," said the old woman, following Marian through the doorway and all the way out into the hall. Then from behind she suddenly clutched the child with her sharp little fingers. In an affected, high-pitched whine she cried, "Oh, little girl, have you a penny to spare for a poor old woman that's not got anything of her own? We don't have a thing in the world—not a penny for candy—not a thing! Little girl, just a nickel—a penny—"

Marian pulled violently against the old hands for a moment before she was free. Then she ran down the hall, without looking behind her and without looking at the nurse, who was reading *Field & Stream* at her desk. The nurse, after another triple motion to consult her wrist watch, asked automatically the question put to visitors in all institutions: "Won't you stay and have dinner with *us?*"

Marian never replied. She pushed the heavy door open into the cold air and ran down the steps.

Under the prickly shrub she stooped and quickly, without being seen, retrieved a red apple she had hidden there.

Her yellow hair under the white cap, her scarlet coat, her bare knees all flashed in the sunlight as she ran to meet the big bus rocketing through the street.

"Wait for me!" she shouted. As though at an imperial command, the bus ground to a stop.

She jumped on and took a big bite out of the apple.

Dillinger in Hollywood

You know how they get after New Year's when the visits dry up and the TV is bust and there's steamed chicken for lunch three days in a row? It was one of those weeks, and Spurs Tatum starts in after rec therapy, before we could wheel them all out of the day room.

"Hoot Gibson held my horse," says Spurs. "I took falls for Randolph Scott. I hung from a wing in *The Perils of Pauline*. And Mr. Ford," he says, "Mr. Ford he always hired me on. You see a redskin blasted off a horse in one of Mr. Ford's pictures, like as not it's me. One-Take Tatum they called me, before the 'Spurs' thing took."

We'd heard it all before, every time there was a western or a combat picture on the TV, every time a patient come in with a broken hip or a busted rib, all through the last days when the Duke was dying in the news. Heard how Spurs had thought up most of the riding stunts they use today, how he'd been D. W. Griffith's drinking buddy, how he saved Tom Mix's life on the Sacramento River. It was hot and one of those weeks and we'd heard it all before so I don't know if it was that or the beating he'd just taken at Parcheesi that made old Casey up and say how he used to be John Dillinger.

His chart said that Casey had been a driver on the Fox lot long enough to qualify for the Industry fund. I told him I hadn't realized he'd done any stand-in work.

"The bird who done the stand-in work," says Casey, "is the one they potted at the Biograph Theater. I used to be Johnnie Dillinger. In the flesh."

He said the name with a hard g, like in "finger," and didn't so much as blink.

Now we've had our delusions at the Home, your standard fading of would-of-been actresses expecting their call from Mr. De Mille, a Tarzan whoop now and then during the full moon, and one old gent who goes around mouthing words without sound and overacting like he's on the silent picture screen. Generally it's some glorified notion of who they used to be. Up to this point Casey's only brag was he drove Joe DiMaggio to the airport when the Clipper was hitched to Monroe.

"If I remember right," says Spurs, giving me an eye that meant he thought the poor fella had slipped his tracks, "if I'm not too fuzzy on it, I believe that Mr. Dillinger, Public Enemy Number One, departed from our midst in the summer of '34."

"You should live so long," says Casey.

Now I try to give a man the benefit of a doubt. With Spurs I can tell there's a grain of fact to his brags because I was in the wrangler game myself. I was riding broncs in Santa Barbara for their Old Spanish Days and this fella hires me to stunt for some rodeo picture with Gig Young in it. He says I take a nice fall.

The pay was greener than what I saw on the circuit, so I stuck in Hollywood. See, I could always *ride* the sumbitches, my problem came to when it was time to get *off*. What I had was a new approach to tumbling from a horse. Whereas most folks out here bust their ass to get *into* pictures, I busted mine to get *out*. Some big damn gelding bucked me before I'd dug in and I landed smack on my tailbone. The doctor says to me—I'm laying on my stomach trying to remember my middle name—the doctor comes in with the X rays and he says, "I don't know how to tell you this, Son, but you're gonna have to learn to shit standing up."

If they'd known who I was *Variety* would of headlined "Son Bishop Swaps Bridle for Bedpan." Horses and hospitals were all I knew. Over the years I'd spent more time in emergency rooms than Dr. Kildare. So it was hospitals, and pretty soon I drifted into the geriatric game. Your geriatrics and horses hold a lot in common—they're high-strung, they bite and kick sometimes, and they're none of them too big on bowel control. Course if a geriatric steps on your foot it don't take a wood chisel to peel it off the floor.

It's a living.

So Spurs I can back sometimes, though I'm sure he didn't play such a starring role in the invention of the saddle. With Casey I had to bring it up at report.

"He thinks he's a dead gangster?" says Mrs. Goorwitz, who was the charge nurse that night.

"No, he thinks he's an old man in a Hollywood nursing home. He says he *used* to be John Dillinger."

"In another life?"

"Nope," I answered her, "in this one."

We had this reincarnated character in here once, claimed to have been all the even-numbered King Louies of France from the second right up to Louie the Sixteen. I asked how he ended up an assistant prop man at Warners and he said after all that commotion his spirit must of needed the rest.

"I thought he was shot," says Mrs. Goorwitz.

"At point-blank range," I tell her. "They couldn't of missed."

Mrs. Goorwitz was a bit untracked by the news. She hates anything out of its place, hates wolves, and many's the geriatric she's hounded to death for holding a book overdue from the Home library. She pulled Casey's chart and studied it. "It says here his name is Casey Mullins."

"Well that's that, isn't it?"

"Confused behavior," says Mrs. Goorwitz as she writes it into the report. "Inappropriate response. Watch carefully."

The only thing that gets watched carefully in this joint is the time-punch at two minutes till shift change, but I figured I might save Casey some headache.

"Maybe he's just lying," I tell her. "To work up a little attention."

"Did he say anything else?"

She was on the scent now and threatening to go practice medicine on somebody any minute.

"Not a whole lot," I tell her. "But if we breathe a word to the Feds he claims they'll find us off Santa Monica Pier with our little toes curled up."

"This bird Jimmy Lawrence, a very small-time character," says Casey, "he had this bum ticker. A rheumatic heart condition, congenital since birth. We dated the same girl once is how I got to know him. People start coming up to say, 'Jeez, you're the spittin' image of Johnnie Dillinger, you know that?' and this girl, this mutual friend, tells me and I get the idea."

After he let the Dillinger thing out Casey got very talkative, like he had it stewing in him a long time and finally it blows out all at once. I'd be in his room tapping the catheter bags on these two vegematics, Kantor and Wise, and it would be just me and this fella Roscoe Baggs who was a midget listening. Roscoe had been in *The Wizard of Oz* as a Munchkin and was a very deep thinker. He reads the kind of science-fiction books that don't have girls in loincloths on the cover.

"This girl has still got the yen for me," says Casey, "so she steers Lawrence to a doctor connection who tells him two months, maybe three, and it's the last roundup. The guy is demolished. So I make him this offer—I supply the dough to live it up his final days and he supplies a body to throw to the authorities. You could buy Chicago cops by the job lot back then so it was no big deal arranging the details. Hard times. Only two or three people had to know I was involved.

"Well the poor chump didn't even know how to paint the town right. And he kept moaning that he wanted us to hold off till after the Series, onnaconna he followed the Cardinals. That was the year Ripper Collins and the Dean brothers tore up the league."

"Just like Spangler," says Roscoe. "Remember, he wanted to see a man walk on the moon? Held off his cancer till he saw it on television and the next day he went downstairs."

Downstairs is where the morgue and the kitchen are located.

"One step for mankind," says Roscoe, "and check-out time for Spangler. You got to admire that kind of control."

"Another hoax," says Casey. "They staged the whole thing in a little studio up the coast. I know a guy in video."

I told Casey I'd read where Dillinger started to run when he saw the cops outside the picture show. And how his sister had identified the remains the next day.

"He turned chickenshit on me, Son. We hadn't told him the exact date, and there he is, coming out from the movies with a broad on each arm and all of a sudden the party's over. What would you do, you were him? And as for Sis," says Casey, "she always done what she could to help me out."

"The day after the planting we send in a truck, dig the coffin out, pour in concrete and lay it back in. Anybody wants another peek at the stiff they got to drill a mine shaft."

It sounded reasonable, sort of. And when the shrink who comes through twice a year stopped to ask about his Dillinger fixation Casey just told him to scram. Said if he wanted his brains scrambled he'd stick his head in the microwave.

I did some reading and everything he said checked out pretty close. Only I couldn't connect Casey with a guy who'd pull a stunt like that on the Lawrence fella. He was one of the nice ones, Casey—never bitched much ever with his diabetes and his infected feet and his rotting kidneys and his finger curling up. A stand-up character.

The finger was curling up independent from the others on his right hand. His trigger finger, bent like he was about to squeeze off a round.

"It's like the *Tell-Tale Heart*," says Roscoe one day. I'm picking up dinner trays in the rooms and Roscoe is working on four chocolate puddings. They had put one on Casey's tray by mistake and I didn't have the time to spoon the other two down Kantor and Wise.

"The what?" asks Casey.

"It's a story. This guy kills an old man and stuffs him under the floor-boards. When the police come to investigate he thinks he hears the old man's heart beating under the boards and he cracks and gives himself away."

"So what's that got to do with my finger?"

"Maybe your finger is trying to blow the whistle on your life of crime. Psychosomatic."

"Oh." Casey mauled it over in his mind for a minute. "I get it. We had a guy in the can, kilt his wife. Poisoned her. At first everybody figured she'd just got sick and died, happened all the time in those days. But then he starts complaining to the cops about the neighborhood kids—says they're writing nasty stuff on the sidewalk in front of his place: 'Old Man Walsh croaked his wife with rat bait,' stuff like that. So the cops send a guy

to check it out on his night rounds. The cop's passing by and out comes
Walsh, sleepwalking, with a piece of chalk in his hand. Wrote his own ticket
to the slammer, right there on the sidewalk, onnaconna he had a leaky
conscience."

It had been bothering me so I took the opening to ask. "Do you ever feel
bad? About things you done back then?"

Casey shrugged and looked away from me and then looked back. "Nah,"
he says, "What am I, mental? This guy Walsh, he was AWOL."

AWOL is what we call the senile ones. Off base and not coming back.

"Hey Roscoe," says Casey, "why'd this telltale character kill the old man
in the first place?"

"Because this old man had a big eye. He wanted to kill the big eye."

Just then Spurs wheels in looking to vulture a loose dessert.

"I wonder," says Casey, "what he would of done to a fat head?"

It seemed to make him feel better, talking about his life as Dillinger. Kept
him up and alert even when his health took a big slide.

"Only reason I'm still percolating," he'd say, "is I still got my pride. They
beat that into me my first stretch."

I told him I'd never heard of beating pride into somebody.

"They beat on you one way or the other," he says. "The pride comes in
how you stand up to it."

I went on the graveyard shift and after two o'clock check I'd go down to
chew the fat with Casey. Roscoe slept like the dead and the two veggies were
on automatic pilot so it didn't make any difference how loud we were. Casey
was a hurtin' cowboy and his meds weren't up to knocking him out at night.
We'd play cards by the light from the corridor sometimes or sometimes he'd
cut up old scores for me. He told me about one where their advance man
posed as a Hollywood location scout for a gangster movie. When they come
out of the bank holding hostages the next day, sniping at the local shields,
the townspeople just smiled and looked around for cameras.

He didn't have much to say on his years driving for Fox. He only hung
on because of what he called the "fringe benefits," which mostly had to do
with women.

"Used to be a disease with me," he'd say. "I'd go two days without a tum-
ble and my eyeballs would start to swoll up, my brains would start pushing
out my ears. Shut me out for three days and I'd hump anything, just anything. Like some dope fiend."

When I asked how he'd dealt with that while he was in the slammer he
clammed up.

He was still able to wheel himself around a bit when Norma took up with
him. Norma had bad veins and was in a chair herself. She'd been in the si-

lents in her teens, getting rescued from fates worse than death. Her mother was ninety and shared a room with her. The old vulture just sat, deaf as a post, glaring at Norma for not being Mary Pickford. Norma had been one of the backgammon crowd till word spread that Casey thought he was John Dillinger. She studied him for a week, keeping her distance, eavesdropping on his sparring matches with Spurs Tatum, watching how he moved and how he talked. Then one day as the singalong is breaking up she wheels up beside him. Norma's voice had gone deeper and deeper with the years and she filled in at bass on "What a Friend We Have in Jesus."

"All I do is dream of you," she sings to Casey, "the whole night through."

"That used to be my favorite song," he says.

"I know," says Norma.

It gives me the fantods sometimes, the way they'd look at each other like they known one another forever. Norma had been one of those caught up by the press on Dillinger when he had his year in the headlines. A woman near thirty years old keeping a scrapbook. She had picked up some work as an extra after her silent days were over, but it never came to much. She still had a shoe box full of postcards her mother had sent out every year to agents and flacks and producers—a grainy blowup of Norma in a toga or a buckskin shift or a French peasant outfit. Norma Nader in *Cimarron*. Norma Nader in *The Pride and the Passion*. Norma Nader in *The Greatest Story Ever Told*. They were the only credits she got in the talkies, those postcards, but her mother kept the heat on. I'd find Norma out in the corridor at night, wheels locked, watching the light coming out from her room.

"Is she in bed yet?" she'd ask, and I'd go down and peek in on Old Lady Nader.

"She's still awake, Norma."

"She always stood up till I come home, no matter what hour. I come in the door and it's not 'Where you been?' or 'Who'd you see?' but 'Any work today?' She had spies at all the studios so I could never lie about making rounds. Once I had an offer for a secretary job, good pay, steady, and I had to tell them sorry, I got to be an actress."

Casey had his Dillinger routine down pretty well, but with Norma along he was unstoppable.

"Johnnie," she'd say, "you member that time in St. Paul they caught you in the alleyway?" or "Johnnie, remember how Nelson and Van Meter were always at each other's throats?"—just like she'd been there. And Casey he'd nod and say he remembered or correct some little detail, reminding her like any old couple sharing memories.

I'd come on at eleven and they'd be in the day room with only the TV for light, Casey squirming in his chair, hurting, and Norma waiting for her mother to go to sleep, holding Casey's hand against the pain. We had another old pair like them, a couple old bachelors were crazy for chess. One game could take them two, three days. Personally, I'd rather watch paint dry.

Usually some time around one o'clock Norma would call and we'd wheel them back to their rooms. I'd park Casey by the window so he could watch the traffic on Cahuenga.

By the time I got back on day shift Casey needed a push when he wanted to get anywhere. He could still feed himself and hit the pee-jug nine times out of ten, though we were checking his output to see what was left of his kidneys. This one morning we had square egg for breakfast, which is the powdered variety cooked up in cake pans and cut into little bars like brownies. If they don't get the coloring just right they'll come up greenish and they wiggle on your fork just like jello. Even the blind patients won't touch them. Usually our only taker is this character Mao, who we call after his resemblance to the late Chinese head Red. Mao is a mongoloid in his mid-thirties whose favorite dishes are square egg and thermometers. Already that morning a new candy striper had given him an oral instead of a rectal and he'd chomped it clear in half. Now she was fluttering around looking for Mr. Hellman's other slipper.

"I looked in his stand and under his bed," she says to me, "and all I could find is the right one."

"He doesn't have a left one," I tell her.

"Why not?"

"He doesn't have a left leg."

"Oh." The candy stripers are good for morale but they take a lot of looking after.

"Next time peek under the covers first."

"Well I started to," she says, "but he was flipping his—you know—his *thing* at me."

"Don't you worry, honey," says Spurs Tatum. "Worst comes to worst I'd lay odds you could outrun the old goat."

"When they give us this shit in the state pen," says Casey so's everybody in the day room could hear him, "we'd plaster the walls with it."

The candy striper waggles her finger at him. "If you don't care for your breakfast, Mr. Mullins, I'm sure somebody else would appreciate it."

"No dice," says Casey. "I want to see it put down the trash barrel where it can't do no harm. And the name's Dillinger."

"I'm sure you don't mind if somebody shares what you don't want. I mean what are we here for?" Lately we've been getting candy stripers with a more Christian outlook.

"What we're *here* for," says Casey, "is to die. To die. And some of us," he says looking to Spurs, "aren't doing much of a job of it."

Casey was on the rag that morning, with a bad case of the runs his new meds give him and a wobbling pile of square egg staring up at him. So when the candy striper reaches to give his portion over to Mao, Casey pushes his tray over onto the floor.

"You birds keep swallowin' this shit," he calls out to the others, "they'll keep sending it up."

Mao was well known for his oatmeal tossing. You'd get two spoonfuls down him and he'd decide to chuck the whole bowl acrost the room. Or wing it straight up so big globs stuck to the ceiling. The old-timers liked to sit against the back wall of the day room afternoons and bet on which glob would loosen and fall first. So when Mao picked up on Casey and made like a catapult with his plate there was chunks sent scattering clear to the bingo tables.

"Food riot!" yells Roscoe, flicking egg off his fork, aiming for old oatmeal stains on the ceiling. "Every man for himself!" he yells and then goes into "Ding-Dong the Witch Is Dead."

I didn't think the old farts had it in them. It was like being inside a popcorn popper, yellow hunks of egg flying every whichway, squishing, bouncing, coffee sloshing, toast frisbeeing, plates smashing, orange juice showering while Mrs. Shapiro, stone blind and AWOL for years is yelling "Boys, don't fight! Don't fight, your father will get crazy!"

The rec therapist is a togetherness freak. They sing together, they make place mats together, they have oral history sessions together. So somebody starts throwing food the rest of them are bound to pitch in. When there was nothing left to toss they calmed down. We decided to wheel them all back to their rooms before we cleaned out the day room.

"I'm hungry," says Spurs. "Crazy sumbitch made me lose my breakfast. Senile bastard."

"Shove it, cowboy," says Casey. "In my day we'd of used you for a toothpick."

"In *my* day we'd of stuck you in the bughouse. Dillinger my ass."

Casey didn't say a thing but Norma wheeled up between them, a big smear of grape jelly on her check.

"John Dillinger," she said, "was the only one in the whole lousy country was his own man, the only one that told them all to go hang and went his own way. Have some respect."

I never learned if she really thought he was Dillinger or if they just shared the same interest like the chess players or the crowd that still reads the trade papers together. When Norma went AWOL it was like her mother called her in from the playground. She left us quick, fading in and out for two weeks till she give up all the way and just sat in her chair in her room, staring back at her mother.

"I'm sorry," she'd say from time to time. No word on why or what for, just stare at Old Lady Nader and say, "I'm sorry."

Casey tried to pull her out of it at first. But it's like when we have a cardiac arrest and we pull the curtain around the bed—even if you're right in the room you can't see through to know what's happening.

"You remember me?" he'd say. "You remember about Johnnie Dillinger?"

"Usually she'd just look at him blank. One time she said, "I seen a movie about him once."

For a while Casey would have us wheel him into Norma's room and he'd talk at her some but she didn't know who he was. Finally it made him so low he stopped visiting. Acted like she'd gone downstairs.

"You lose your mind," he'd say, "the rest of you ain't worth spit."

Mrs. Goorwitz got on his case then and tried to locate relatives. None to be found. What with the way people move around out here that's not so unusual. Casey's chart was nothing but a medical record starting in 1937. Next Mrs. Goorwitz loosed the social worker on him, Friendly Phil, who ought to be selling health food or real estate somewhere. Casey wasn't buying any.

"So what if I am crazy?" he'd say to Phil. "Delusional, schizo, whatever you wanna call it. I can't do squat one way or the other. What difference does it make if I was Dillinger or Norma was Pearl White or Roscoe was the King of Poland? You're all just a bag a bones in the end."

He went into a funk, Casey, after Norma faded—went into a silence that lasted a good month. Not even Spurs could get his goat enough to argue. He spent a good part of the day trying to keep himself clean.

"I'm on the cycle," he whispered to me one day. "I'm riding the down side."

The geriatric racket is a collection of cycles. Linen goes on beds, gets dirtied, down the chute, washed, dried and back onto the beds. Patients are checked in downstairs, up to the beds, maintained a while and then down to the slabs with them. Casey even found a new cycle, a thing in the paper about scientists who had learned how to make cow flops back into cow food.

"I don't want to make accusations here," says Casey one day, pointing to his lunch, "but what does *that* look like to you?"

The day came when Casey lost his control, racked up six incontinents on the report in one week. His health was shot but I tried to talk Mrs. Goorwitz out of it when she handed me the kit. He had a thing about it, Casey.

"A man that can't control his bowels," he'd say, "is not a man."

He knew what was up when I started to draw the curtain. Roscoe scowled at me from across the room and rolled over to face the wall. Kantor and Wise lay there like house plants. It was midnight and they'd given Casey some heavy meds with his dinner. He looked at me like I come to snuff him with a pillow over the face. He was too weak to raise his arms so I didn't have to put the restraints on.

"It has to be, Casey," I told him. "Or else you'll be wettin all over yourself."

I washed my hands with the soap from the kit.

"If they ask why I done it, the banks and all," he whispers, "tell them I was just bored. Just bored crapless."

I took the gloves out of their cellophane and managed to wriggle into them without touching my fingers to their outside. I washed Casey and laid the fenestrated sheet over so only his thing stuck through. If the stories about Dillinger's size are true, Casey was qualified. The girls on the evening shift called it "The Snake." I swabbed the tip of it, unwrapped the catheter tube, and coated it with K-Y.

"You been white to me, Son," says Casey. "I don't put no blame on you."

"I'm sorry."

"Don't ever say that," says Casey. "Don't ever say you're sorry. Do it or don't do it but don't apologize."

I pushed the catheter tube down till it blocked at his sphincter, wiggled it and it slipped past. It was the narrowest gauge but still it's a surprise that you can fit one into a man. I stuck the syringe into the irrigation branch and shot the saline up till the bulb was inflated in his bladder. I gave a tug to see if it was anchored. Casey was crying, looking away from me. His eyes had gone fuzzy, the way fish do after you beach them. I hooked the plastic tubing and the piss-bag to the catheter.

"I used to be somebody," said Casey.

I had a long weekend, and when I came back on I didn't get a chance to talk with him. Mrs. Goorwitz said in report how he'd been moved to Intensive Care. On my first check I found him looking like the pictures of the Biograph shooting—blood everywhere, hard yellow light. Something had popped inside and he'd bled out the mouth. He had pulled the catheter out, bulb and all, and he was bleeding down there. We put sheets on the floor and rolled him sideways across the bed on his belly so he drained out onto them. It takes a half hour or so.

I traced him back through the medical plan at Fox and ran into nothing but dead ends. Usually I forget about them once they go downstairs but Casey had gotten his hooks in. There at Fox I found an old fella in custodial who remembered him.

"Always taking the limos for joyrides," he said. "It's a wonder he didn't get his ass fired."

I brought up the subject at the nurses' station one night—how maybe he could of been—and they asked me how much sleep I'd been getting. So I don't know one way or the other. Roscoe, he's sure, he's positive, but Roscoe also thinks our every move is being watched by aliens with oversized IQs. I figure if they're so smart they got better things to occupy their time.

One day I'm tube-feeding some vegomatic when out in the corridor I hear Spurs Tatum giving his brag to a couple recent admissions that come in with their feet falling off.

"Hoot Gibson held my horse," says Spurs. "I took falls for Randy Scott. John Wayne blew me off a stagecoach. And once," he says, "I played Parcheesi with John Herbert Dillinger."

Idiots First

The thick ticking of the tin clock stopped. Mendel, dozing in the dark, awoke in fright. The pain returned as he listened. He drew on his cold embittered clothing, and wasted minutes sitting at the edge of the bed.

"Isaac," he ultimately sighed.

In the kitchen, Isaac, his astonished mouth open, held six peanuts in his palm. He placed each on the table. "One . . . two . . . nine."

He gathered each peanut and appeared in the doorway. Mendel, in loose hat and long overcoat, still sat on the bed. Isaac watched with small eyes and ears, thick hair graying the sides of his head.

"Schlaf," he nasally said.

"No," muttered Mendel. As if stifling he rose. "Come, Isaac."

He wound his old watch though the sight of the stopped clock nauseated him.

Isaac wanted to hold it to his ear.

"No, it's late." Mendel put the watch carefully away. In the drawer he found the little paper bag of crumpled ones and fives and slipped it into his overcoat pocket. He helped Isaac on with his coat.

Isaac looked at one dark window, then at the other. Mendel stared at both blank windows.

They went slowly down the darkly lit stairs, Mendel first, Isaac watching the moving shadows on the wall. To one long shadow he offered a peanut.

"Hungrig."

In the vestibule the old man gazed through the thin glass. The November night was cold and bleak. Opening the door he cautiously thrust his head out. Though he saw nothing he quickly shut the door.

"Ginzburg, that he came to see me yesterday," he whispered in Isaac's ear.

Isaac sucked air.

"You know who I mean?"

Isaac combed his chin with his fingers.

"That's the one, with the black whiskers. Don't talk to him or go with him if he asks you."

Isaac moaned.

"Young people he don't bother so much," Mendel said in afterthought.

It was suppertime and the street was empty but the store windows dimly lit their way to the corner. They crossed the deserted street and went on. Isaac, with a happy cry, pointed to the three golden balls. Mendel smiled but was exhausted when they got to the pawnshop.

The pawnbroker, a red-bearded man with black horn-rimmed glasses, was eating a whitefish at the rear of the store. He craned his head, saw them, and settled back to sip his tea.

In five minutes he came forward, patting his shapeless lips with a large white handkerchief.

Mendel, breathing heavily, handed him the worn gold watch. The pawnbroker, raising his glasses, screwed in his eyepiece. He turned the watch over once. "Eight dollars."

The dying man wet his cracked lips. "I must have thirty-five."

"So go to Rothschild."

"Cost me myself sixty."

"In 1905." The pawnbroker handed back the watch. It had stopped ticking. Mendel wound it slowly. It ticked hollowly.

"Isaac must go to my uncle that he lives in California."

"It's a free country," said the pawnbroker.

Isaac, watching a banjo, snickered.

"What's the matter with him?" the pawnbroker asked.

"So let be eight dollars," muttered Mendel, "but where will I get the rest till tonight?"

"How much for my hat and coat?" he asked.

"No sale." The pawnbroker went behind the cage and wrote out a ticket. He locked the watch in a small drawer but Mendel still heard it ticking.

In the street he slipped the eight dollars into the paper bag, then searched in his pockets for a scrap of writing. Finding it, he strained to read the address by the light of the street lamp.

As they trudged to the subway, Mendel pointed to the sprinkled sky.

"Isaac, look how many stars are tonight."

"Eggs," said Isaac.

"First we will go to Mr. Fishbein, after we will eat."

They got off the train in upper Manhattan and had to walk several blocks before they located Fishbein's house.

"A regular palace," Mendel murmured, looking forward to a moment's warmth.

Isaac stared uneasily at the heavy door of the house.

Mendel rang. The servant, a man with long sideburns, came to the door and said Mr. and Mrs. Fishbein were dining and could see no one.

"He should eat in peace but we will wait till he finishes."

"Come back tomorrow morning. Tomorrow morning Mr. Fishbein will talk to you. He don't do business or charity at this time of the night."

"Charity I am not interested—"

"Come back tomorrow."

"Tell him it's life or death—"

"Whose life or death?"

"So if not his, then mine."

"Don't be such a big smart aleck."

"Look me in my face," said Mendel, "and tell me if I got time till tomorrow morning?"

The servant stared at him, then at Isaac, and reluctantly let them in.

The foyer was a vast high-ceilinged room with many oil paintings on the walls, voluminous silken draperies, a thick flowered rug at foot, and a marble staircase.

Mr. Fishbein, a paunchy bald-headed man with hairy nostrils and small patent leather feet, ran lightly down the stairs, a large napkin tucked under a tuxedo coat button. He stopped on the fifth step from the bottom and examined his visitors.

"Who comes on Friday night to a man that he has guests, to spoil him his supper?"

"Excuse me that I bother you, Mr. Fishbein," Mendel said. "If I didn't come now I couldn't come tomorrow."

"Without more preliminaries, please state your business. I'm a hungry man."

"Hungrig," wailed Isaac.

Fishbein adjusted his pince-nez. "What's the matter with him?"

"This is my son Isaac. He is like this all his life."

Isaac mewled.

"I am sending him to California."

"Mr. Fishbein don't contribute to personal pleasure trips."

"I am a sick man and he must go tonight on the train to my Uncle Leo."

"I never give to unorganized charity," Fishbein said, "but if you are hungry I will invite you downstairs in my kitchen. We having tonight chicken with stuffed derma."

"All I ask is thirty-five dollars for the train ticket to my uncle in California. I have already the rest."

"Who is your uncle? How old a man?"

"Eighty-one years, a long life to him."

Fishbein burst into laughter. "Eighty-one years and you are sending him this halfwit."

Mendel, flailing both arms, cried, "Please, without names."

Fishbein politely conceded.

"Where is open the door there we go in the house," the sick man said. "If you will kindly give me thirty-five dollars, God will bless you. What is thirty-five dollars to Mr. Fishbein? Nothing. To me, for my boy, is everything."

Fishbein drew himself up to his tallest height.

"Private contributions I don't make—only to institutions. This is my fixed policy."

Mendel sank to his creaking knees on the rug.

"Please, Mr. Fishbein, if not thirty-five, give maybe twenty."

"Levison," Fishbein angrily called.

The servant with the long sideburns appeared at the top of the stairs.

"Show this party where is the door—unless he wishes to partake food before leaving the premises."

"For what I've got chicken won't cure it," Mendel said.

"This way if you please," said Levison, descending.

Isaac assisted his father up.

"Take him to an institution," Fishbein advised over the marble balustrade. He ran quickly up the stairs and they went at once outside, buffeted by winds.

The walk to the subway was tedious. The wind blew mournfully. Mendel, breathless, glanced furtively at shadows. Isaac, clutching his peanuts in his frozen fist, clung to his father's side. They entered a small park to rest for a minute on a stone bench under a leafless two-branched tree. The thick right branch was raised, the thin left one hung down. A very pale moon rose slowly. So did a stranger as they approached the bench.

"Gut yuntif," he said hoarsely.

Mendel, drained of blood, waved his wasted arms. Isaac yowled sickly. Then a bell chimed and it was only ten. Mendel let out a piercing anguished cry as the bearded stranger disappeared into the bushes. A policeman came running, and though he beat the bushes with his nightstick, could turn up nothing. Mendel and Isaac hurried out of the little park. When Mendel glanced back the dead tree had its thin arm raised, the thick one down. He moaned.

They boarded a trolley, stopping at the home of a former friend, but he had died years ago. On the same block they went into a cafeteria and ordered two fried eggs for Isaac. The tables were crowded except where a heavy-set man sat eating soup with kasha. After one look at him they left in haste, although Isaac wept.

Mendel had another address on a slip of paper but the house was too far away, in Queens, so they stood in a doorway shivering.

What can I do, he frantically thought, in one short hour?

He remembered the furniture in the house. It was junk but might bring a few dollars. "Come, Isaac." They went once more to the pawnbroker's to talk to him, but the shop was dark and an iron gate—rings and gold watches glinting through it—was drawn tight across his place of business.

They huddled behind a telephone pole, both freezing. Isaac whimpered.

"See the big moon, Isaac. The whole sky is white."

He pointed but Isaac wouldn't look.

Mendel dreamed for a minute of the sky lit up, long sheets of light in all directions. Under the sky, in California, sat Uncle Leo drinking tea with lemon. Mendel felt warm but woke up cold.

Across the street stood an ancient brick synagogue.

He pounded on the huge door but no one appeared. He waited till he had breath and desperately knocked again. At last there were footsteps within, and the synagogue door creaked open on its massive brass hinges.

A darkly dressed sexton, holding a dripping candle, glared at them.

"Who knocks this time of night with so much noise on the synagogue door?"

Mendel told the sexton his troubles. "Please, I would like to speak to the rabbi."

"The rabbi is an old man. He sleeps now. His wife won't let you see him. Go home and come back tomorrow."

"To tomorrow I said goodbye already. I am a dying man."

Though the sexton seemed doubtful he pointed to an old wooden house next door. "In there he lives." He disappeared into the synagogue with his lit candle casting shadows around him.

Mendel, with Isaac clutching his sleeve, went up the wooden steps and rang the bell. After five minutes a big-faced, gray-haired bulky woman came out on the porch with a torn robe thrown over her nightdress. She emphatically said the rabbi was sleeping and could not be waked.

But as she was insisting, the rabbi himself tottered to the door. He listened a minute and said, "Who wants to see me let them come in."

They entered a cluttered room. The rabbi was an old skinny man with bent shoulders and a wisp of white beard. He wore a flannel nightgown and black skullcap; his feet were bare.

"Vey is mir," his wife muttered. "Put on shoes or tomorrow comes sure pneumonia." She was a woman with a big belly, years younger than her husband. Staring at Isaac, she turned away.

Mendel apologetically related his errand. "All I need more is thirty-five dollars."

"Thirty-five?" said the rabbi's wife. "Why not thirty-five thousand? Who has so much money? My husband is a poor rabbi. The doctors take away every penny."

"Dear friend," said the rabbi, "if I had I would give you."

"I got already seventy," Mendel said, heavy-hearted. "All I need more is thirty-five."

"God will give you," said the rabbi.

"In the grave, said Mendel. "I need tonight. Come, Isaac."

"Wait," called the rabbi.

He hurried inside, came out with a fur-lined caftan, and handed it to Mendel.

"Yascha," shrieked his wife, "not your new coat!"

"I got my old one. Who needs two coats for one body?"

"Yascha, I am screaming—"

"Who can go among poor people, tell me, in a new coat?"

"Yascha," she cried, "what can this man do with your coat? He needs tonight the money. The pawnbrokers are asleep."

"So let him wake them up."

"No." She grabbed the coat from Mendel.

He held on to a sleeve, wrestling her for the coat. Her I know, Mendel thought. "Shylock," she muttered. Her eyes glittered.

The rabbi groaned and tottered dizzily. His wife cried out as Mendel yanked the coat from her hands.

"Run," cried the rabbi.

"Run, Isaac."

They ran out of the house and down the steps.

"Stop, you thief," called the rabbi's wife.

The rabbi pressed both hands to his temples and fell to the floor.

"Help!" his wife wept. "Heart attack! Help!"

But Mendel and Isaac ran through the streets with the rabbi's new fur-lined caftan. After them noiselessly ran Ginzburg.

It was very late when Mendel bought the train ticket in the only booth open.

There was no time to stop for a sandwich so Isaac ate his peanuts and they hurried to the train in the vast deserted station.

"So in the morning," Mendel gasped as they ran, "there comes a man that he sells sandwiches and coffee. Eat but get change. When reaches California the train, will be waiting for you on the station Uncle Leo. If you don't recognize him he will recognize you. Tell him I send best regards."

But when they arrived at the gate to the platform it was shut, the light out.

Mendel, groaning, beat on the gate with his fists.

"Too late," said the uniformed ticket collector, a bulky, bearded man with hairy nostrils and a fishy smell.

He pointed to the station clock. "Already past twelve."

"But I see standing there still the train," Mendel said, hopping in his grief.

"It just left—in one more minute."

"A minute is enough. Just open the gate."

"Too late I told you."

Mendel socked his bony chest with both hands. "With my whole heart I beg you this little favor."

"Favor you had enough already. For you the train is gone. You shoulda been dead already at midnight. I told you that yesterday. This is the best I can do."

"Ginzburg!" Mendel shrank from him.

"Who else?" The voice was metallic, eyes glittered, the expression amused.

"For myself," the old man begged, "I don't ask a thing. But what will happen to my boy?"

Ginzburg shrugged slightly. "What will happen happens. This isn't my responsibility. I got enough to think about without worrying about somebody on one cylinder."

"What then is your responsibility?"

"To create conditions. To make happen what happens. I ain't in the anthropomorphic business."

"Whatever business you in, where is your pity?"

"This ain't my commodity. The law is the law."

"Which law is this?"

"The cosmic universal law, goddamit, the one I got to follow myself."

"What kind of law is it?" cried Mendel. "For God's sake, don't you understand what I went through in my life with this poor boy? Look at him. For thirty-nine years, since the day he was born, I wait for him to grow up, but he don't. Do you understand what this means in a father's heart? Why don't you let him go to his uncle?" His voice had risen and he was shouting.

Isaac mewled loudly.

"Better calm down or you'll hurt somebody's feelings," Ginzburg said with a wink toward Isaac.

"All my life," Mendel cried, his body trembling, "what did I have? I was poor. I suffered from my health. When I worked I worked too hard. When I didn't work was worse. My wife died a young woman. But I didn't ask from anybody nothing. Now I ask a small favor. Be so kind, Mr. Ginzburg."

The ticket collector was picking his teeth with a match stick.

"You ain't the only one, my friend, some got it worse than you. That's how it goes in this country."

"You dog you." Mendel lunged at Ginzburg's throat and began to choke. "You bastard, don't you understand what it means human?"

They struggled nose to nose. Ginzburg, though his astonished eyes bulged, began to laugh. "You pipsqueak nothing. I'll freeze you to pieces."

His eyes lit in rage and Mendel felt an unbearable cold like an icy dagger invading his body, all of his parts shriveling.

Now I die without helping Isaac.

A crowd gathered. Isaac yelped in fright.

Clinging to Ginzburg in his last agony, Mendel saw reflected in the ticket collector's eyes the depth of his terror. But he saw that Ginzburg, staring at himself in Mendel's eyes, saw mirrored in them the extent of his own awful wrath. He beheld a shimmering, starry, blinding light that produced darkness.

Ginzburg looked astounded. "Who me?"

His grip on the squirming old man slowly loosened, and Mendel, his heart barely beating, slumped to the ground.

"Go." Ginzburg muttered, "take him to the train."

"Let pass," he commanded a guard.

The crowd parted. Isaac helped his father up and they tottered down the steps to the platform where the train waited, lit and ready to go.

Mendel found Isaac a coach seat and hastily embraced him. "Help Uncle Leo, Isaakil. Also remember your father and mother."

"Be nice to him," he said to the conductor. "Show him where everything is."

He waited on the platform until the train began slowly to move. Isaac sat on the edge of his seat, his face strained in the direction of his journey. When the train was gone, Mendel ascended the stairs to see what had become of Ginzburg.

What You Hear from 'Em?

Sometimes people misunderstood Aunt Munsie's question, but she wouldn't bother to clarify it. She might repeat it two or three times, in order to drown out some fool answer she was getting from some fool white woman, or man, either. "What you hear from 'em?" she would ask. And, then, louder and louder: "What you hear from 'em? *What you hear from 'em?*" She was so deaf that anyone whom she thoroughly drowned out only laughed and said Aunt Munsie had got so deaf she couldn't hear it thunder.

It was, of course, only the most utterly fool answers that ever received Aunt Munsie's drowning-out treatment. She was, for a number of years at least, willing to listen to those who mistook her " 'em" to mean any and all of the Dr. Tolliver children. And for more years than that she was willing to listen to those who thought she wanted just *any* news of her two favorites among the Tolliver children—Thad and Will. But later on she stopped putting the question to all insensitive and frivolous souls who didn't understand that what she was interested in hearing—and *all* she was interested in hearing—was when Mr. Thad Tolliver and Mr. Will Tolliver were going to pack up their families and come back to Thornton for good.

They had always promised her to come back—to come back sure enough, once and for all. On separate occasions, both Thad and Will had actually given her their word. She had not seen them together for ten years, but each of them had made visits to Thornton now and then with his own family. She would see a big car stopping in front of her house on a Sunday afternoon and see either Will or Thad with his wife and children piling out into the dusty street—it was nearly always summer when they came—and then see them filing across the street, jumping the ditch, and unlatching the gate to her yard. She always met them in that pen of a yard, but long before they had jumped the ditch she was clapping her hands and calling out, "Hai-ee! Hai-ee, now! Look-a-here! Whee! Whee! Look-a-here!" She had got so blind that she was never sure whether it was Mr. Thad or Mr. Will until she had her arms around his waist. They had always looked a good deal alike, and their city clothes made them look even more alike nowadays. Aunt Munsie's eyes were so bad, besides being so full of moisture on those occasions, that she really recognized them by their girth. Will had grown a regular wash pot

355

of a stomach and Thad was still thin as a rail. They would sit on her porch for twenty or thirty minutes—whichever one it was and his family—and then they would be gone again.

Aunt Munsie would never try to detain them—not seriously. Those short little old visits didn't mean a thing to her. He—Thad or Will—would lean against the banister rail and tell her how well his children were doing in school or college, and she would make each child in turn come and sit beside her on the swing for a minute and receive a hug around the waist or shoulders. They were timid with her, not seeing her any more than they did, but she could tell from their big Tolliver smiles that they liked her to hug them and make over them. Usually, she would lead them all out to her back yard and show her pigs and dogs and chickens. (She always had at least one frizzly chicken to show the children.) They would traipse through her house to the back yard and then traipse through again to the front porch. It would be time for them to go when they came back, and Aunt Munsie would look up at *him*—Mr. Thad or Mr. Will (she had begun calling them "Mr." the day they married)—and say, "Now, look-a-here. When you comin' back?"

Both Thad and Will knew what she meant, of course, and whichever it was would tell her he was making definite plans to wind up his business and that he was going to buy a certain piece of property, "a mile north of town" or "on the Old River Road," and build a jim-dandy house there. He would say, too, how good Aunt Munsie's own house was looking, and his wife would say how grand the zinnias and cannas looked in the yard. (The yard was all flowers—not a blade of grass, and the ground packed hard in little paths between the flower beds.) The visit was almost over then. There remained only the exchange of presents. One of the children would hand Aunt Munsie a paper bag containing a pint of whiskey or a carton of cigarettes. Aunt Munsie would go to her back porch or to the pit in the yard and get a fern or a wandering Jew, potted in a rusty lard bucket, and make Mrs. Thad or Mrs. Will take it along. Then the visit was over, and they would leave. From the porch Aunt Munsie would wave goodbye with one hand and lay the other hand, trembling slightly, on the banister rail. And sometimes her departing guest, looking back from the yard, would observe that the banisters themselves were trembling under her hand—so insecurely were those knobby banisters attached to the knobby porch pillars. Often as not Thad or Will, observing this, would remind his wife that Aunt Munsie's porch banisters and pillars had come off a porch of the house where he had grown up. (Their father, Dr. Tolliver, had been one of the first to widen his porches and remove the gingerbread from his house.) The children and their mother would wave to Aunt Munsie from the street. Their father would close the gate, resting his hand a moment on its familiar wrought-iron frame, and wave to her before he jumped the ditch. If the children had not gone too far ahead, he might even draw their attention to the iron fence which, with its iron gate, had been around the yard at the Tolliver place till Dr. Tolliver took it down and set out a hedge, just a few weeks before he died.

But such paltry little visits meant nothing to Aunt Munsie. No more did the letters that came with "her things" at Christmas. She was supposed to get her daughter, Lucrecie, who lived next door, to read the letters, but in late years she had taken to putting them away unopened, and some of the presents, too. All she wanted to hear from *them* was when they were coming back for good, and she had learned that the Christmas letters never told her that. On her daily route with her slop wagon through the square, up Jackson Street, and down Jefferson, there were only four or five houses left where she asked her question. These were houses where the amount of pig slop was not worth stopping for, houses where one old maid, or maybe two, lived, or a widow with one old bachelor son who had never amounted to anything and ate no more than a woman. And so—in the summertime, anyway—she took to calling out at the top of her lungs, when she approached the house of one of the elect, "What you hear from 'em?" Sometimes a Miss Patty or a Miss Lucille or a Mr. Ralph would get up out of a porch chair and come down the brick walk to converse with Aunt Munsie. Or sometimes one of them would just lean over the shrubbery planted around the porch and call, "Not a thing, Munsie. Not a thing lately."

She would shake her head and call back, "Naw. Naw. Not a thing. Nobody don't hear from 'em. Too busy, they be."

Aunt Munsie's skin was the color of a faded tow sack. She was hardly four feet tall. She was generally believed to be totally bald, and on her head she always wore a white dust cap with an elastic band. She wore an apron, too, while making her rounds with her slop wagon. Even when the weather got bad and she tied a wool scarf about her head and wore an overcoat, she put on an apron over the coat. Her hands and feet were delicately small, which made the old-timers sure she was of Guinea stock that had come to Tennessee out of South Carolina. What most touched the hearts of old ladies on Jackson and Jefferson Streets were her little feet. The sight of her feet "took them back to the old days," they said, because Aunt Munsie still wore flat-heeled, high button shoes. Where ever did Munsie find such shoes any more?

She walked down the street, down the very center of the street, with a spry step, and she was continually turning her head from side to side, as though looking at the old houses and trees for the first time. If her sight was as bad as she sometimes let on it was, she probably recognized the houses only by their roof lines against the Thornton sky. Since this was nearly thirty years ago, most of the big Victorian and ante-bellum houses were still standing, though with their lovely gingerbread work beginning to go. (It went first from houses where there was someone, like Dr. Tolliver, with a special eye for style for keeping up with the times.) The streets hadn't yet been broadened—or only Nashville Street had—and the maples and elms met above the streets. In the autumn, their leaves covered the high banks and filled the deep ditches on either side. The dark macadam surfacing itself was barely wide enough for two automobiles to pass. Aunt Munsie, pulling her slop wagon, which was a long, low, four-wheeled vehicle about the size and shape of a coffin, paraded down the center of the street without any regard for, if with any awareness of, the traffic problems she sometimes made. Seizing the wagon's heavy, sawed-off-looking tongue, she hauled it after her with a series of impatient jerks, just as though that tongue were the arm of some very stubborn, overgrown white child she had to nurse in her old age. Strangers in town or trifling high-school boys would blow their horns at her, but she was never known to so much as glance over her shoulder at the sound of a horn. Now and then a pedestrian on the sidewalk would call out to the driver of an automobile, "She's so deaf she can't hear it thunder."

It wouldn't have occurred to anyone in Thornton—not in those days—that something ought to be done about Aunt Munsie and her wagon for the sake of the public good. In those days, everyone had equal rights on the streets of Thornton. A vehicle was a vehicle, and a person was a person, each with the right to move as slowly as he pleased and to stop where and as often as he pleased. In the Thornton mind, there was no imaginary line down the middle of the street, and, indeed, no one there at that time had heard of drawing a real line on *any* street. It was merely out of politeness that you made room for others to pass. Nobody would have blown a horn at an old colored woman with her slop wagon—nobody but some Yankee stranger or a trifling high-school boy or maybe old Mr. Ralph Hadley in a special fit of temper. When citizens of Thornton were in a particular hurry and got caught behind Aunt Munsie, they leaned out their car windows and shouted: "Aunt Munsie, can you make a little room?" And Aunt Munsie didn't fail to hear *them*. She would holler, "Hai-ee, no! Whee! Look-a-here!" and jerk her wagon to one side. As they passed her, she would wave her little hand and grin a toothless, pink-gummed grin.

Yet, without any concern for the public good, Aunt Munsie's friends and connections among the white women began to worry more and more about the danger of her being run down by an automobile. They talked among themselves and they talked to her about it. They wanted her to give up collecting slop, now she had got so blind and deaf. "Pshaw," said Aunt Munsie, closing her eyes contemptuously. "Not me." She meant by that that no one would dare run into her or her wagon. Sometimes when she crossed the square on a busy Saturday morning or on a first Monday, she would hold one hand with the palm turned outward and stop all traffic until she was safely across and in the alley beside the hotel.

Thornton wasn't even then what it had been before the Great World War. In every other house there was a stranger or a mill hand who had moved up from factory town. Some of the biggest old places stood empty, the way Dr. Tolliver's had until it burned. They stood empty not because nobody wanted to rent them or buy them but because the heirs who had gone off somewhere making money could never be got to part with "the home place." The story was that Thad Tolliver nearly went crazy when he heard their old house had burned, and wanted to sue the town, and even said he was going to help get the Republicans into office. Yet Thad had hardly put foot in the house since the day his daddy died. It was said the Tolliver house had caught fire from the Major Pettigru house, which had burned two nights before. And no doubt it had. Sparks could have smoldered in that roof of rotten shingles for a long time before bursting into flame. Some even said the Pettigru house might have caught from the Johnston house, which had burned earlier that same fall. But Thad knew and Will knew and everybody knew the town wasn't to blame, and knew there was no firebug. Why, those old houses stood there empty year after year, and in the fall the leaves fell from the trees and settled around the porches and stoops, and who was there to rake the leaves? Maybe it was a good thing those houses burned, and maybe it would have been as well if some of the houses that still had people in them burned, too. There were houses in Thornton the heirs had never left that looked far worse than the Thornton or the Pettigru or the Johnston house ever had. The people who lived in them were the ones who gave Aunt Munsie the biggest fool answers to her question, the people whom she soon quit asking her question of or even passing the time of day with, except when she couldn't help it, out of politeness. For, truly, to Aunt Munsie there were things under the sun worse than going off and getting rich in Nashville or in Memphis or even in Washington, D.C. It was a subject she and her daughter Lucrecie sometimes mouthed at each other about across their back fence. Lucrecie was shiftless, and she liked shiftless white people like the ones who didn't have the ambition to leave Thornton. She thought their shiftlessness showed they were *quality*. "Quality?" Aunt Munsie would echo, her voice full of sarcasm. "Whee! Hai-ee! You talk like *you* was *my* mammy, Crecie. Well, if there be quality, there be quality *and* quality. There's quality and there's *has-been* quality, Crecie." There was no end to that argument Aunt Munsie had with Crecie, and it wasn't at all important to Aunt Munsie. The people who still lived in those houses—the ones she called has-been quality—meant little more to her than the mill hands, or strangers from up North who ran the Piggly Wiggly, the five-and-ten-cent store, and the roller-skating rink.

There was this to be said, though, for the has-been quality: they knew *who* Aunt Munsie was, and in a limited, literal way they understood what she said. But those *others*—why, they thought Aunt Munsie a beggar, and she knew they did. They spoke of her as Old What You Have for Mom, because that's what they thought she was saying when she called out, "What you hear from 'em?" Their ears were not attuned to that soft "r" she put in "from" or the elision that made "from 'em" sound to them like "for Mom." Many's the time Aunt Munsie had seen or sensed the presence of one of those *other* people, watching from next door, when Miss Leonora Lovell, say, came down her front walk and handed her a little parcel of scraps across the ditch. Aunt Munsie knew what they thought of her—how they laughed at her and felt sorry for her and despised her all at once. But, like the has-been quality, they didn't matter, never had, never would. Not ever.

Oh, they mattered in a way to Lucrecie. Lucrecie thought about them and talked about them a lot. She called them "white trash" and even "radical Republicans." It made Aunt Munsie grin to hear Crecie go on, because she knew Crecie got all her notions from her own has-been-quality people. And so it didn't matter, except that Aunt Munsie knew that Crecie truly had all sorts of good sense and had only been carried away and spoiled by such folks as she had worked for, such folks as had really raised Crecie from the time she was big enough to run errands for them, fifty years back. In her heart, Aunt Munsie knew that even Lucrecie didn't matter to her the way a daughter might. It was because while Aunt Munsie had been raising a family of white children, a different sort of white people from hers had been raising her own child, Crecie. Sometimes, if Aunt Munsie was in her chicken yard or out in her little patch of cotton when Mr. Thad or Mr. Will arrived, Crecie would come out to the fence and say, "Mama, some of your chillun's out front."

Miss Leonora Lovell and Miss Patty Bean, and especially Miss Lucille Satterfield, were all the time after Aunt Munsie to give up collecting slop. "You're going to get run over by one of those crazy drivers, Munsie," they said. Miss Lucille was the widow of old Judge Satterfield. "If the Judge were alive, Munsie," she said, "I'd make him find a way to stop you. But the men down at the courthouse don't listen to the women in this town any more. Not since we got the vote. And I think they'd be most too scared of you to do what I want them to do." Aunt Munsie wouldn't listen to any of that. She knew that if Miss Lucille had come out there to her gate, she must have *something* she was going to say about Mr. Thad or Mr. Will. Miss Lucille had two brothers and a son of her own who were lawyers in Memphis, and who lived in style down there and kept Miss Lucille in style here in Thornton. Memphis was where Thad Tolliver had his Ford and Lincoln agency, and so Miss Lucille always had news about Thad, and indirectly about Will, too.

"Is they doin' any good? What you hear from 'em?" Aunt Munsie asked Miss Lucille one afternoon in early spring. She had come along just when

Miss Lucille was out picking some of the jonquils that grew in profusion on
the steep bank between the sidewalk and the ditch in front of her house.

"Mr. Thad and his folks will be up one day in April, Munsie," Miss Lucille
said in her pleasantly hoarse voice. "I understand Mr. Will and his crowd
may come for Easter Sunday."

"One day, and gone again!" said Aunt Munsie.

"We always try to get them to stay at least one night, but they're busy
folks, Munsie."

"When they comin' back sure enough, Miss Lucille?"

"Goodness knows, Munsie. Goodness knows. Goodness knows when any
of them are coming back to stay." Miss Lucille took three quick little steps
down the bank and hopped lightly across the ditch. "They're prospering so,
Munsie," she said, throwing her chin up and smiling proudly. This fragile
lady, this daughter, wife, sister, mother of lawyers (and, of course, the darling of all their hearts), stood there in the street holding a handful of jonquils
before her as if it were her bridal bouquet. "They're *all* prospering so, Munsie. Mine *and* yours. You ought to go down to Memphis to see them now and
then, the way I do. Or go up to Nashville to see Mr. Will. I understand he's
got an even finer establishment than Thad. They've done well, Munsie—
yours *and* mine—and we can be proud of them. You owe it to yourself to go
and see how well they're fixed. They're rich men by our standards in Thornton, and they're going farther—*all* of them."

Aunt Munsie dropped the tongue of her wagon noisily on the pavement.
"What I want to go see 'em for?" she said angrily and with a lowering brow.
Then she stooped and, picking up the wagon tongue again, she wheeled her
vehicle toward the middle of the street, to get by Miss Lucille, and started
off toward the square. As she turned out into the street, the brakes of a car,
as so often, screeched behind her. Presently everyone in the neighborhood
could hear Mr. Ralph Hadley tooting the insignificant little horn on his
mama's coupé and shouting at Aunt Munsie in his own tooty voice, above the
sound of the horn. Aunt Munsie pulled over, making just enough room to let
poor old Mr. Ralph get by but without once looking back at him. Then, before Mr. Ralph could get his car started again, Miss Lucille was running
along beside Aunt Munsie, saying, "Munsie, you be careful! You're going to
meet your death on the streets of Thornton, Tennessee!"

"Let 'em," said Aunt Munsie.

Miss Lucille didn't know whether Munsie meant "Let 'em run over me;
I don't care" or meant "Let 'em just dare!" Miss Lucille soon turned back,
without Aunt Munsie's ever looking at her. And when Mr. Ralph Hadley did
get his motor started, and sailed past in his mama's coupé, Aunt Munsie
didn't give him a look, either. Nor did Mr. Ralph bother to turn his face to
look at Aunt Munsie. He was on his way to the drugstore, to pick up his
mama's prescriptions, and he was too entirely put out, peeved, and upset to

endure even the briefest exchange with that ugly, uppity old Munsie of the Tollivers.

Aunt Munsie continued to tug her slop wagon on toward the square. There was a more animated expression on her face than usual, and every so often her lips would move rapidly and emphatically over a phrase or sentence. Why should she go to Memphis and Nashville and see how rich they were? No matter how rich they were, what difference did it make; they didn't own any land, did they? Or at least none in Cameron County. She had heard the old Doctor tell them—tell his boys and tell his girls, and tell the old lady, too, in her day—that nobody was rich who didn't own land, and nobody stayed rich who didn't see after his land firsthand. But of course Aunt Munsie had herself mocked the old Doctor to his face for going on about land so much. She knew it was only something he had heard his own daddy go on about. She would say right to his face that she hadn't ever seen *him* behind a plow. And was there ever anybody more scared of a mule than Dr. Tolliver was? Mules or horses, either? Aunt Munsie had heard him say that the happiest day of his life was the day he first learned that the horseless carriage was a reality.

No, it was not really to own land that Thad and Will ought to come back to Thornton. It was more that if they were going to be rich, they ought to come home, where their granddaddy had owned land and where their money counted for something. How could they ever be rich anywhere else? They could have a lot of money in the bank and a fine house, that was all— like that mill manager from Chi. The mill manager could have a yard full of big cars and a stucco house as big as you like, but who would ever take him for rich? Aunt Munsie would sometimes say all these things to Crecie, or something as nearly like them as she could find words for. Crecie might nod her head in agreement or she might be in a mood to say you could live on just being quality better than on being rich in Thornton. "Quality's better than land or better than money in the bank here," Crecie would say.

Aunt Munsie would sneer at her and say, "It never were."

Lucrecie could talk all she wanted about the old times! Aunt Munsie knew too much about what they were like, for both the richest white folks and the blackest field hands. Nothing about the old times was as good as these days, and there were going to be better times yet when Mr. Thad and Mr. Will Tolliver came back. Everybody lived easier now than they used to, and were better off. She could never be got to reminisce about her childhood in slavery, or her life with her husband, or even about those halcyon days after the old Mizziz had died and Aunt Munsie's word had become law in the Tolliver household. Without being able to book read or even to make numbers, she had finished raising the whole pack of towheaded Tollivers just as the Mizziz would have wanted it done. The Doctor told her she *had* to—he didn't ever once think about getting another wife, or taking in some cousin, not after his "Molly darling"—and Aunt Munsie *did*. But, as Crecie said, when a time was past in her mama's life, it seemed to be gone and done with in her head, too.

Lucrecie would say frankly she thought her mama was "hard about people and things in the world." She talked about her mama not only to the Blalocks, for whom she had worked all her life, but to anybody else who gave her an opening. It wasn't just about her mama, though, that she would talk to anybody. She liked to talk, and she talked about Aunt Munsie not in any ugly, resentful way but as she would about when the sheep-rains would begin or where the fire was last night. (Crecie was twice the size of her mama, and black the way her old daddy had been, and loud and good-natured the way he was—or at least the way Aunt Munsie wasn't. You wouldn't have known they were mother and daughter, and not many of the young people in town did realize it. Only by accident did they live next door to each other; Mr. Thad and Mr. Will had bought Munsie her house, and Crecie had heired hers from her second husband.) *That* was how she talked about her mama—as she would have about any lonely, eccentric, harmless neighbor. "I may be dead wrong, but I think Mama's kind of hardhearted," she would say. "Mama's a good old soul, I reckon, but when something's past, it's gone and done with for Mama. She don't think about day before yestiddy—yestiddy, either. I don't know, maybe that's the way to be. Maybe that's why the old soul's gonna outlive us all." Then, obviously thinking about what a picture of health she herself was at sixty, Crecie would toss her head about and laugh so loud you might hear her all the way out to the fair grounds.

Crecie, however, knew her mama was not honest-to-God mean and hadn't ever been mean to the Tolliver children, the way the Blalocks liked to make out she had. All the Tolliver children but Mr. Thad and Mr. Will had quarreled with her for good by the time they were grown, but they had quarreled with the old Doctor, too (and as if they were the only ones who shook off their old folks this day and time). When Crecie talked about her mama, she didn't spare anything, but she was fair to her, too. And it was in no hateful or disloyal spirit that she took part in the conspiracy that finally got Aunt Munsie and her slop wagon off the streets of Thornton. Crecie would have done the same for any neighbor. She had small part enough, actually, in that conspiracy. Her part was merely to break the news to Aunt Munsie that there was now a law against keeping pigs within the city limits. It was a small part but one that no one else quite dared to take.

"They ain't no such law!" Aunt Munsie roared back at Crecie. She was slopping her pigs when Crecie came to the fence and told her about the law. It had seemed the most appropriate time to Lucrecie. "They ain't never been such a law, Crecie," Aunt Munsie said. "Every house on Jackson and Jefferson used to keep pigs."

"It's a brand-new law, Mama."

Aunt Munsie finished bailing out the last of the slop from her wagon. It was just before twilight. The last, weak rays of the sun colored the clouds behind the mock orange tree in Crecie's yard. When Aunt Munsie turned around from the sty, she pretended that that little bit of light in the clouds hurt her eyes, and turned away her head. And when Lucrecie said that everybody had until the first of the year to get rid of their pigs, Aunt Munsie was in a spell of deafness. She headed out toward the crib to get some corn for the chickens. She was trying to think whether anybody else inside the town still kept pigs. Herb Mallory did—two doors beyond Crecie. Then Aunt Munsie remembered Herb didn't pay town taxes. The town line ran between him and Shad Willis.

That was sometime in June, and before July came, Aunt Munsie knew all there was worth knowing about the conspiracy. Mr. Thad and Mr. Will had each been in town for a day during the spring. They and their families had been to her house and sat on the porch; the children had gone back to look at her half-grown collie dog and the two hounds, at the old sow and her farrow of new pigs, and at the frizzliest frizzly chicken Aunt Munsie had ever had. And on those visits to Thornton, Mr. Thad and Mr. Will had also made their usual round among their distant kin and close friends. Everywhere they went, they had heard of the near-accidents Aunt Munsie was causing with her slop wagon and the real danger there was of her being run over. Miss Lucille Satterfield and Miss Patty Bean had both been to the mayor's office and also to see Judge Lawrence to try to get Aunt Munsie "ruled" off the streets, but the men in the courthouse and in the mayor's office didn't listen to the women in Thornton any more. And so either Mr. Thad or Mr. Will—how would which one of them it was matter to Munsie?—had been prevailed upon to stop by Mayor Lunt's office, and in a few seconds' time had set the wheels of conspiracy in motion. Soon a general inquiry had been made in the town as to how many citizens still kept pigs. Only two property owners besides Aunt Munsie had been found to have pigs on their premises, and they, being men, had been docile and reasonable enough to sell what they had on hand to Mr. Will or Mr. Thad Tolliver. Immediately afterward—within a matter of weeks, that is—a town ordinance had been passed forbidding the possession of swine within the corporate limits of Thornton. Aunt Munsie had got the story bit by bit from Miss Leonora and Miss Patty and Miss Lucille and others, including the constable himself, whom she did not hesitate to stop right in the middle of the square on a Saturday noon. Whether it was Mr. Thad or Mr. Will who had been prevailed upon by the ladies she never ferreted out, but that was only because she did not wish to do so.

The constable's word was the last word for her. The constable said yes, it was the law, and he admitted yes, he had sold his own pigs—for the constable was one of those two reasonable souls—to Mr. Thad or Mr. Will. He didn't say which of them it was, or if he did, Aunt Munsie didn't bother to remember it. And after her interview with the constable, Aunt Munsie never again exchanged words with any human being about the ordinance against pigs. That afternoon, she took a fishing pole from under her house and drove the old sow and the nine shoats down to Herb Mallory's, on the outside of town. They were his, she said, if he wanted them, and he could pay her at killing time.

It was literally true that Aunt Munsie never again exchanged words with anyone about the ordinance against pigs or about the conspiracy she had discovered against herself. But her daughter Lucrecie had a tale to tell about what Aunt Munsie did that afternoon after she had seen the constable and before she drove the pigs over to Herb Mallory's. It was mostly a tale of what Aunt Munsie said to her pigs and to her dogs and her chickens.

Crecie was in her own back yard washing her hair when her mama came down the rickety porch steps and into the yard next door. Crecie had her head in the pot of suds, and so she couldn't look up, but she knew by the way Mama flew down the steps that there was trouble. "She come down them steps like she was wasp-nest bit, or like some young'on who's got hisself wasp-nest bit—and her all of eighty, I reckon!" Then, as Crecie told it, her mama scurried around in the yard for a minute or so like she thought Judgment was about to catch up with her, and pretty soon she commenced slamming at something. Crecie wrapped a towel about her soapy head, squatted low, and edged over toward the plank fence. She peered between the planks and saw what her mama was up to. Since there never had been a gate to the fence around the pigsty, Mama had taken the wood ax and was knocking a hole in it. But directly, just after Crecie had taken her place by the plank fence, her mama had left off her slamming at the sty and turned about so quickly and so exactly toward Crecie that Crecie thought the poor, blind old soul had managed to spy her squatting there. Right away, though, Crecie realized it was not *her* that Mama was staring at. She saw that all Aunt Munsie's chickens and those three dogs of hers had come up behind her, and were all clucking and whining to know why she didn't stop that infernal racket and put out some feed for them.

Crecie's mama set one hand on her hip and rested the ax on the ground. "Just look at yuh!" she said, and then she let the chickens and the dogs—and the pigs, too—have it. She told them what a miserable bunch of creatures they were, and asked them what right they had to always be looking for handouts from her. She sounded like the boss-man who's caught all his pickers laying off before sundown, and she sounded, too, like the preacher giving his sinners Hail Columbia at camp meeting. Finally, shouting at the top of her voice and swinging the ax wide and broad above their heads, she sent the dogs howling under the house and the chickens scattering in every direction. "Now, g'wine! G'wine widja!" she shouted after them. Only the collie pup, of the three dogs, didn't scamper to the farthest corner underneath the house. He stopped under the porch steps, and not two seconds later he was poking his long head out again and showing the whites of his doleful brown eyes. Crecie's mama took a step toward him and then she halted. "You want to know what's the commotion about? I reckoned you would," she said with profound contempt, as though the collie were a more reasonable soul than the other animals, and as though there were nothing she held in such thorough disrespect as reason. "I tell you what the com- motion's about," she said. "They *ain't* comin' back. They ain't never comin' back. They ain't never had no notion of comin' back." She turned her head to one side, and the only explanation Crecie could find for her mama's next words was that that collie pup did look so much like Miss Lucille Satterfield.

"Why don't I go down to Memphis or up to Nashville and see 'em some- time, like *you* does?" Aunt Munsie asked the collie. "I tell you why. Becaze I ain't nothin' to 'em in Memphis, and they ain't nothin' to me in Nashville. *You* can go!" she said, advancing and shaking the big ax at the dog. "A collie dog's a collie dog anywhar. But Aunt Munsie, she's just their Aunt Munsie here in Thornton. I got mind enough to see *that*." That collie slowly pulled his head back under the steps, and Aunt Munsie watched for a minute to see if he would show himself again. When he didn't, she went and jerked the fishing pole out from under the house and headed toward the pigsty. Crecie remained squatting beside the fence until her mama and the pigs were out in the street and on their way to Herb Mallory's.

That was the end of Aunt Munsie's keeping pigs and the end of her daily rounds with her slop wagon, but it was not the end of Aunt Munsie. She lived on for nearly twenty years after that, till long after Lucrecie had been put away, in fine style, by the Blalocks. Ever afterward, though, Aunt Mun- sie seemed different to people. They said she softened, and everybody said it was a change for the better. She would take paper money from under her carpet, or out of the chinks in her walls, and buy things for up at the church, or buy her own whiskey when she got sick, instead of making somebody bring her a nip. On the square she would laugh and holler with the white folks the way they liked her to and the way Crecie and all the other old- timers did, and she even took to tying a bandanna about her head—took to talking old-nigger foolishness, too, about the Bell Witch, and claiming she remembered the day General N. B. Forrest rode into town and saved all the cotton from the Yankees at the depot. When Mr. Will and Mr. Thad came to see her with their families, she got so she would reminisce with them about their daddy and tease them about all the silly little things they had done when they were growing up: "Mr. Thad—him still in kilts, too—he says, 'Aunt Munsie, reach down in yo' stockin' and git me a copper cent. I want some store candy.' " She told them about how Miss Yola Ewing, the sewing woman, heard her threatening to bust Will's back wide open when he broke the lamp chimney, and how Miss Yola went to the Doctor and told him he ought to run Aunt Munsie off. Then Aunt Munsie and the Doctor had had a big laugh about it out in the kitchen, and Miss Yola must have eavesdropped on them, because she left without finishing the girls' Easter dresses.

Indeed, these visits from Mr. Thad and Mr. Will continued as long as Aunt Munsie lived, but she never asked them any more about when they were sure enough coming back. And the children, though she hugged them more than ever—and, toward the last, there were the children's children to be hugged—never again set foot in her back yard. Aunt Munsie lived on for nearly twenty years, and when they finally buried her, they put on her tombstone that she was aged one hundred years, though nobody knew how old she was. There was no record of when she was born. All anyone knew was that in her last years she had said she was a girl helping about the big house when freedom came. That would have made her probably about twelve years old in 1865, according to her statements and depictions. But all agreed that in her extreme old age Aunt Munsie, like other old darkies, was not very reliable about dates and such things. Her spirit softened, even her voice lost some of the rasping quality that it had always had, and in general she became not very reliable about facts.

Old Doc Rivers

Horses. These definitely should be taken into consideration in estimating Rivers' position, along with the bad roads, the difficult means of communication of those times.

For a physician everything depended on horses. They were a factor determining his life.

Rivers prided himself on his teams. It was something to look at when he came down the street in the rubber-tired sulky with the red wheels. He'd sit there peering out under the brim of his hat with that smile of his always on his face, confident, a little disdainful, but not unfriendly.

He knew them all. . . .

Hello, Frank, how's the wife?

Not so good, Doc.

The old trouble, eh? Tell you what I'll do. I'll drive around and take her up to the hospital this afternoon.

Can't get her to do it, Doc.

Scared?

Guess you hit it.

All right, you old rascal; have a cigar. And he'd turn away, with the horses pawing and shaking their heads right and left, ready to go.

A young man and a bachelor, this was the happiest period of his life, when he was exhilarated by an occupation, the sun, the cold, the motion of the horses, their haunches working muscularly before him as he sat and smoked. Maybe it was that and a mad rush to get from place to place; it came and went in a moment. He saw it, realized it, there was nothing else and—he had the rest of his life to live.

This is how he practiced. . . .

Come in, Jerry—making a pass at him with his open hand—How's the old soak?

Fer Christ's sake, Doc, lay off me. I'm sick.

Who's sick? Have a drap of the auld Crater. He nearly always had a jug of it just behind his desk. Did a dog bite you?

Look a' this damned neck of mine. Jesus, what the hell's the matter with you? Easy, I says.

Shut up! You white-livered Hibernian.

Aw, Doc, for Christ's sake, gimme a break.

What's the matter, did I do anything to you?

Listen, Doc, ain't ya gonna put something on it?

On what? Keep those pants buttoned. Sit down. Grab onto these arms. And don't let go until I'm through or I'm likely to slit you in half.

Yeow! Jesus, Mary and Joseph! Whadje do to me, Doc?

I think your throat's cut, Jerry. Here, drink this. Go lie down over there a minute. I didn't think you were so yellow.

What! Lie down? What for? Whadda you think I am, a woman? Wow! Have you got any more of the liquor? Say, you're some man, Doc. You're some man. What do you get?

That's all right, Jerry, bring it around next week.

That's some relief.

The phone rang. It was one of the first in the region. Wanted at the hospital.

Hey, Maggie!—to the dour old Irish woman who sullenly cared for his world: Tell John to drive around to the side door.

Wait a minute now, wait a minute. There's a woman out there has been wantin' to see you for three days. She looks real sick. She's been here all morning waitin' for you.

Get her in.

Doctor . . .

Yes, I know—he could see that her color was bad. Where is it? In your belly?

Yes, Doctor.

He made a quick examination, slipping on a rubber glove without removing his coat, washing his hands after at the basin in the corner of the room. The whole thing hadn't taken six minutes.

Leaning over his desk he scribbled two notes.

Take thirty drops of it tonight, in a little water. And here, here's a note to Sister Rose. Get up to the hospital in the morning. Don't eat any breakfast.

But, Doctor, what's the matter with me?

Now, now. Tomorrow morning. Don't worry, Mother. It'll be all right. Good-bye, and he pushed her out of the door.

John's waiting for you, said big Margaret as he was struggling with his coat, his hat, a cigar, stopping in the corner of the porch to light. A few moments later he was into the carriage and off.

He leaned back, seeing nothing. The horses trotted up the Plank Road. Past the railroad cut. It was a dark spring night. The cherry blossoms were out on the McGee property. Past the nurseries. Down the steep hill by the swamp. The turn. By the Cadmus farm. The County Bridge; clattering over the board. Over the creek. The creek was flowing swiftly, an outgoing tide, a few lights streaking it, a few sounds rising, a faint ripple and a cool air.

Naturally, he must have given value for value, good services for money received. He had a record of thirty years behind him, finally, for getting there (provided you could find him) anywhere, anytime, for anybody—no distinctions; and for doing something, mostly the right thing, without delay and of his own initiative, once he was there.

He was ready, energetic and courageous. The people were convinced that he knew his stuff—if anyone knew it. And they would pay him well for his services—if they paid him at all.

But what could he do? What did he do? What kind of a doctor was he, really?

Thinking it over, it occurred to me to drop in at the hospital in the small nearby city where he took many of his operative cases to see for myself exactly what he had been about all these years. To satisfy myself, then, as to the man's scope I went to the St. Michael's Hospital of which I am speaking and induced the librarian to get out the older record books for me to look at.

As usual in such cases, something other than the thing desired first catches the eye.

These were heavy ledgers, serious and interesting in appearance with their worn leather covers and gold lettering across the front: Registry of Cases treated at St. Michael's Hospital, etc., etc. There were a dozen of them in all from the year 1898 on. I felt a catch at the throat before the summary of so much human misery.

Opening at random, there it lay, the whole story of the hospital, what had been done and the result, along with the doctors' names and other like information, listed in tall columns. These were carefully written in through the months and years in longhand of many characters, minute and tall, precise and free, in blue, in green, black, purple and even red; with stub pens, sharp pens and even pencil, across two full pages with two narrower fly leaves between.

I chose the years 1905 and 1908 and began to thumb over the leaves looking for Rivers' name. But my eye fell instead upon the list of patients' occupations. Such a short time ago and yet some of these entries struck me as odd: Liveryman, coachman, bartender! Nothing in years has so impressed me with the swiftness of time's flight.

In the doctors' column, there was Rivers, dead surely of the effects of his addiction, but here another who had shot himself in despair at the outcome, it is said, of an affair with the wife of another physician on the same page, his friend. While this one had divorced his wife and married once again—a younger woman. Another at sixty had quietly laid himself down upon his office couch and said good-bye and died. This one had left town hurriedly taking himself to the coast, possibly to escape jail—leaving a wife and child behind him. Some had grown old in the profession and been forgotten though they were still alive. One of these, ninety and more, totally deaf, still morosely wandered the streets and scarcely anyone remembered that he had been a doctor. Queer, all that since 1908.

What had Rivers really accomplished?

Surgically, there were, to be sure, more than enough of the usual scraping, and appendicitis was common. But here is a list of some of his undertakings; I copy from the records: endometritis, salpingitis, contracture of the hand, ruptured spleen, hernia, laceration (some accident, no doubt). There were malignancies of the bowel, excisions of the thyroid, breast amputations; here an ununited fracture of the humerus involving the insertion of a plate and marked "Cured" in the final column. There were normal maternity cases, Caesarean sections, ruptured ectopic pregnancies. He treated fistulas, empyema, hydrocele. He performed hysterectomies, gastroenterostomies, gall bladder resections. He even tackled a deviated nasal septum. There were fractures of all the bones of the body, nearly, and many of those of the head, simple and compound.

And at the far edge of the right-hand page, you would see the brief legend "Cured" as often following his name as that of any other doctor.

On the medical side, the old familiar "neurasthenia" which meant that they never did discover what was the matter with the patient; but also nephritis, pneumonia, endocarditis, rheumatism, malaria and typhoid fever. Most left the hospital cured.

And who were they? Plumber, nurseryman, farmer, saloonkeeper (with hob-nail liver), painter, printer, housewife, that's the way it would go. It was a long and interesting list of the occupations of the region from tea merchant to no occupation at all.

Acute alcoholism and D.T. were frequent entries.

It was not money. It came of his sensitivities, his civility; it was that that made him do it, I'm sure; the antithesis rather of that hog-like complacency that comes to so many men following the successful scamper for cash. Nervous, he accepted his life at its own terms and never let it beat him—to no matter what extremity he was driven.

But sometimes I know he had to quit an operation half way through and have another finish it for him. Or perhaps he would retire for a moment (we all knew why), return, change his gloves, and continue. The transformation in him would be striking. From a haggard old man he would be changed "like that" into a resourceful and alert operator.

Going further, I asked several men who had been in the habit of standing opposite him across the operating table their opinion of him as a surgeon—what had been the secret of his success.

Again, I began to pick up odd pieces of news. Dr. Jamison, who had been an intern in the hospital during several of Rivers' most active years, recalled how he would awaken sometimes in his room on the first floor at night to find Rivers asleep outside the covers on his bed beside him snoring like a good fellow. And once on a trip to the state hospital for mental diseases at Nashawan, one of the attendants of the place had come up to the group to ask them if the person he had found in a semi-conscious condition leaning against the wall down the corridor was one of their party. It was Rivers; something had gone wrong with his usual arrangements and he was coked to the eyes.

In sum, his ability lay first in an uncanny sense for diagnosis. Then, he didn't flounder. He made up his mind and went to it. Furthermore, he was not, as might be supposed, radical and eccentric in his surgical technique but conservative and thoroughgoing throughout. He was not nervous but cool and painstaking—so long as he had the drug in him. His principles were sound, nor was he exhibitionistic in any sense of the word.

And what a psychologist he was. There was a boy down in Kingsland who had had diarrhoea for about a week. Several doctors had seen him and pre-scribed medicine but the child had been eating almost anything he wanted. Finally they called in Rivers. He pulled down the kid's pants, took one look and said, Hell, what he needs is a circumcision. And he did it, there and then, kept food away from him a day or two (because of the operation) and of course the kid got well. That's how smart he was.

Only twice did I personally assist him at operations.

The first case was that of a man called Milliken, an enormous, hulking fellow in his late thirties, swarthy, hairy-chested and with arms and legs on him fit for the strong man in the circus. He ran a milk route at one end of the town. It was acute appendicitis.

When we got to the little house where he lived, a double house I recall, the only room big enough to handle him in was the parlor. We rigged up a table in the usual way. Rivers said we were ready and told the big boy to climb on up. Which he did.

I forgot to mention that Milliken was a great drinker. He also forgot to mention it to me at the time.

Go ahead with the ether, said Rivers.

Well, it didn't take me long—not more than twenty minutes—to find out that ether wouldn't touch this fellow anyway you gave it—unless it might be by a tube. There are individuals like that, powerfully muscled men and alcoholics.

By this time Rivers and his assistant were ready.

Wait a minute, Doc, managed to mumble the patient. For, strange to say, the man had been docile up to that point so that we thought he was under. But it was not so.

I could see that Rivers was losing patience but I was already pouring a stream of ether upon the mask. They were ready for the incision, scrubbed up, the sheet in place, just waiting.

Rivers was fidgeting and I wasn't in a particularly pleasant mood myself. Finally he spoke sharply to me asking if I didn't know how to give an anesthetic. I could feel my face flush but I didn't say anything. Instead I took out the chloroform and began to give that, carefully. Rivers looked approval but said nothing. We all waited a moment or two for this to take effect. By this time, we were all sweating and mad—at the patient, each other, and ourselves.

The outcome was that, after three attempts at an incision—at which time an earthquake occurred under our grips, Rivers gave it up and turned to me.

Here, he said, Gimme that mask. Come up here and assist Willie. I'll show you how to get this man under.

I wanted to scrub. He said, No, put on the gloves. I obeyed. There was nothing else to do. Asepsis had gone to the winds long since in our efforts to keep the man from walking out of the room.

Rivers just took the chloroform bottle and poured the stuff into that Bohunk. I expected to see him turn black and pass out.

But he didn't.

After a few minutes, we were told by Rivers to go ahead.

His assistant just touched the skin with his knife and up flew the man's knees. I was tickled to death.

Go ahead, go ahead, cried Rivers, excitedly, hold him down and go to it.

That's what we did. One man held the head and arms. I finally quit entirely as an assistant, lay on my stomach across the man's thighs and grasped the legs of the table on the other side. One man, alone, did the actual work. It is to his credit that he did it well.

It must have been a month after that I saw the patient, one day, standing in front of the fire house. Curious, I went up to him to find out if he felt anything while the operation had been going on.

At first he didn't know me, but when I told him who I was, expecting to get a crack in the eye maybe for my trouble, he came up with a start:

Did I feel anything? said he. My God, every bit of it, every bit of it. But he was a well man by that time.

It was the case though of an old German harness maker of East Hazelton, Frankel by name, which first raised doubts in my mind as to Rivers' actual condition. I received the call one day and went to the address given, where I knew the old man and his wife lived above the store.

They had the kitchen already rigged up as an operating room, a plain deal table with a smaller one at the foot of it with blankets and a sheet over them for the old man to lie on. There were sterile dressings, the instruments were boiling on the gas stove and everything was in good order as far as I could make out.

As soon as I had entered, Rivers called into the hall for the old fellow to come on along, we were ready for him. He had been in bed in the front of the house and I shall never forget my surprise and the shock to my sense of propriety when I saw Frankel, whom I knew, coming down the narrow, dark corridor of the apartment in his bare feet and an old-fashioned nightgown that reached just to his knees. He was holding his painful belly with both hands while his scared wife accompanied him solicitously on one side.

The old fellow was too sick for that sort of thing but Rivers just motioned him without a word uttered to climb up on the table where they put another sheet over him and I was told to start the anesthetic. I did so, silent, and not too well pleased with the way things were going.

Rivers asked the wife if she had any more of that good whiskey about the place. She brought it out. He poured himself nearly a tumblerful, filled the glass with water at the sink and, while he was drinking, held up the flask with the other hand toward his confrere and to me, gesturing. We refused. With that he finished his glass, plugged the cork in the bottle and dropped it into the side pocket of his coat which hung nearby on a chair.

He was in his undershirt and suspenders, sleeves rolled up. From this time forward, things went ahead normally and properly, more or less, according to the usual operating-room technique of the time.

Rivers made the incision. He took one look and shrugged his shoulders. It was a ruptured appendix with advanced general peritonitis. He shoved in a drain and let it go at that, the right thing to do. But the patient died next day.

I tell you there was a howl about the town: another decent citizen done to death by that dope fiend Rivers. Several of my friends cautioned me to watch my step. You may be sure, in any case, that I thought carefully over what had occurred but I did not come to any immediate conclusion.

And yet the man could be—often was—kindly, alert, courteous. Most interesting it is to hear that he played the violin excellently and would often spend an evening, in the early days, playing duets with the one musician of any note that could be encountered in the neighborhood—the organist at the nearby cathedral.

When little Virginia Shippen, aged five, had a kidney complication, following scarlet fever, Rivers came in day and night, did—as he thought— everything that could be done to save her. Still she remained unconscious, dropsical; the kidneys had ceased to function. One evening Rivers told them that he was through—that she would be dead by morning.

At this point, the mother asked if he would object if she made a suggestion. She wanted to try flaxseed poultices over the kidney regions. Go ahead, said Rivers.

The next day the child's kidneys had started slowly to function, sanguineous, muddy stuff, but she was conscious and her fever had dropped. Rivers was delighted, praised the mother and told her that she had taught him something. The child grew up and lived thirty years thereafter.

He was short with women:

Well, Mary, what is it?

I have a pain in my side, doctor.

How long have you had it, Mary?

Today, doctor. It's the first time.

Just today.

Yes, doctor.

Climb up on the table. Pull up your dress. Throw that sheet over you. Come on, come on. Up with you. Come on now, Mary. Pull up your knees.

Ooh!

He could be cruel and crude. And like all who are so, he could be sentimentally tender also, and painstaking without measure.

A young woman, one of my early friends and patients, spoke to me of his kindness to her. Her foster parents—for she was an adopted child—would never have anyone else. For months she went to him, two and three times a week, while he with the greatest gentleness and patience treated her. It was a nasopharyngeal condition of some sort, difficult to manage. Little by little, he brought her along till she was well, charging them next to nothing for his services.

Money was never an end with him.

The end was, he made this girl, who was frail and gentle, one of his life-long admirers.

But on another occasion in the drug store one day a boy about ten came up to him with a sizable abscess on his neck. They had not been able to find the doctor in his office so the boy had followed him there.

Come here, said Rivers, Let's see. And with that he took a scalpel out of his vest pocket, and made a swipe at the thing.

But the boy was too quick. He jerked back and the knife caught him low. He turned and ran, bleeding and yelling, out of the door. Rivers chuckled and paid no further attention to the incident.

Naturally there were certain favorite places which he'd visit more often than others. First of all was the Jeanette Mansion in Crestboro, two miles above Hazelton north along the ridge, where a number of French families had settled sixty or eighty years previously.

They were rather a different class, these French, from some of the other inhabitants of the region and showed it by keeping a great deal to themselves in their large manor houses surrounded by the billowy luxuriance of tall trees.

A fence, the beginning of all culture, invariably surrounded the property as a frame, giving a sense of propriety and measure. Ease and retirement seemed to blossom here, though naturally this was often an appearance only.

Not, I think, that these things meant anything consciously to Rivers, but they were there and he passed among them. In that way they must have influenced him more than a little. For he liked it all, obviously. Though, of course, it was the people really who attracted him.

He was a Frenchman, an Alsatian—I can't think of his name, said my informer, old Dr. Trowbridge. When you get older, your memory is not so good. Wait a minute. No, well, anyway, he went back to France. So and so lives in the house now. He had several daughters—they were a very gay family.

I had been asking the old doctor how it was that Rivers began to take the dope. Oh, he must have been taking something before he came here. I don't know how else to explain his eccentricity. Anyway, when he went to Europe, to Freiburg to study with Seibert, the pathologist (I don't think he studied very much), this man, oh, what is his name? he had gone back to France—had to give Rivers the money to return to America.

Jeannette, that's it—he was a high liver. He built himself a greenhouse in the back and put all kinds of plants in it. He must have spent hundreds and hundreds of dollars on it. He would sit out there and play cards with his friends. Not difficult surely to understand the attraction this had for the tormented doctor. For, if Jeannette was a voluptuary, his friend Rivers was no laggard before any lead which he could find it in his conscience to propose.

To play cards, to laugh, talk and partake with the Frenchman of his imported wines and liquors was good. After a snowstorm, of a Sunday morning, to sit there at ease—out of reach of patients—in a tropical environment and talk, sip wines and enjoy a good cigar—that was something. It was a quaint situation, too, in that crude environment of those days, so altogether foreign, incongruous and delightfully aloof.

It would take a continental understanding—reinforced as it is by centuries of culture—to comprehend and to accept the complexities and contradictions of a nature such as Rivers'. Not in the provincial bottom of the New Jersey of that time had the doctor found such another release.

The man was now at the height of his popularity and power.

Intelligence he had and force—but he also had nerves, a refinement of the sensibilities that made him, though able, the victim of the very things he best served. This was the man himself whom the drug retrieved.

He was far and away by natural endowment the ablest individual of our environment, a serious indictment against all the evangelism of American life which I most hated—at the same time a man trying to fill his place among those lacking the power to grasp his innate capabilities.

I don't believe Jeannette doped. It cannot have been other than as to a last hope, a veritable island of safety, that Rivers went to the mansion. The only influence that might possibly have saved him, as they say, had it but been known. In any case, they were gay and the time passed; at the mansion he was free, enlivened—then when that was finished, he was again beaten.

The mansion was relaxation to him, but he couldn't live there and his restlessness would in the end pass beyond it.

No doubt, there would be periods when he didn't hit the dope for months at a time. Then he'd get taking it again. Finally he'd feel himself slipping and he'd head off—overnight sometimes—leaving his practice as it might lie—for the woods.

This flight to the woods, or something like it, is a thing we most of us have yearned for at one time or another, particularly those of us who live in the big cities. As Rivers did. For in their jumble we have lost touch with ourselves, have become indeed not authentic persons, but fantastic shapes in some gigantic fever dream. He, at least, had the courage to break with it and to go.

With this pressure upon us, we eventually do what all herded things do; we begin to hurry to escape it, then we break into a trot, finally into a mad run (watches in our hands), having no idea where we are going and having no time to find out.

He wanted to plunge into something bigger than himself. Primitive, physically sapping. Maine gave it. To hunt the deer. He'd bring them home and give cuts of venison around to all his friends.

But that, too, ended pretty badly. After his eyes had been affected, by abuse and illness, he one day by accident shot his best friend in the woods, a guide he always followed, shot him through the temples as dead as a door nail.

Characteristic of the man is that he made amends to the unfortunate's family faithfully as best he could, everything that was asked of him, to the last penny. And then, when the last payment had been made, he invited a young doctor of his acquaintance to dinner with him in New York—for a rousing celebration.

Rivers made a hobby one time of catching rattlesnakes, which abound in the mountains of North Jersey. He enjoyed the sport and the danger, apparently, while there was a scientific twist to it in that the venom they collected was to be used for laboratory work in New York.

A patient of mine gave me an impression of his office as it looked in those days:

There were six of us kids, brothers and sisters. I myself must have been about ten years old. We used to go up and sit there Sunday mornings. We'd be crazy for it. We used to like to look at his trophies. He had 'em too, moose and deer heads up on the wall and fish of all kinds.

He was a great hunter. I remember one time he was telling my father how he was bitten by a rattler, on the arm. Being a doctor, he knew what he was up against. He asked his guide to take his knife and cut the place out. But the guide didn't have the nerve. So the Doc took his own hunting knife in the other hand and sliced it wide open and sucked the blood out of it. I suppose he took a shot of dope first to steady himself. We were in the office with my father and he rolled up his sleeve and showed us the cut—right down the middle of his arm.

It was about this time too that he once had Charlie Hensel in to see him, one evening when there were quite a few others besides, out in the waiting room. Put on the gloves, Charlie, he said—he always had a couple of pairs of them lying around the place somewhere—and let's see what you can do.

But Charlie was good in those days and he knew the Doc was in no shape for him to be roughing it up with. He shook his head and said, No, not tonight, Doc.

That nettled Rivers. Scared? he said. What's the matter, a young fella like you? Come, put'em on.

All right, said Charlie in his sweet, easy voice. Just as you say. He told me the story shortly after it happened.

So they started in to spar after pushing back the desk and clearing a little space for themselves.

Charlie tapped the old boy lightly on the face a couple of times keeping away from the body. At this the Doc let go a hot one for Charlie's middle.

Come on, come on, he kept saying.

But Charlie could see that the Doc was getting winded so he tapped him again and was going to say he guessed that would be enough for tonight when the Doc drove in a swift one which caught Charlie on the temple just as he was going to drop his hands. Come on, come on, he said one more, a young fella like you.

So Charlie, wanting to end the business, feinted, just easy and then lifted the Doc one under the chin that sent him staggering backward to the wall. There he sat down unexpectedly in the consultation chair they had placed back out of the way. It shook the building.

The trouble with you, Charlie—the trouble with hitting you, Charlie, said the Doc slowly after a while, is that you ain't got any belly at all. Which was true enough. Charlie was very narrow across the middle then—like a sailor.

He'd have spells when his brother even could do nothing with him. He would go completely mad. He put in several sessions at the State Insane Asylum—six months or more—on at least two occasions.

When he'd been there a month or so, he'd begin to ask the Superintendent, who was a friend of his, whether he didn't think he could go out to work again. You're as good a doctor as I am, old man, would say this one finally. If you think you can make it, go ahead. And back he'd turn again to the old grind.

Then one winter he got so low with typhoid fever that it looked as if this time the game was up. They wanted a nurse; he refused to have one. And nobody wanted him as a patient either. He was completely gone with dope and the disease. Finally he himself asked for a girl he had known some years before at Blockley Hospital, a nurse he had once seen there and admired.

She took on the case.

He married her when he was able to be up and about again, and they went to Europe on a honeymoon. No doubt, she loved him.

Yes, I can remember his wife, said a lady to me. When she first came out she was a pretty thing, just like anybody else. But I can still see her one day when she came into the store knocking against the counters, first on one side then on the other; she was covered with diamonds, her hands and her neck—she didn't seem to know where she was going. Her face didn't seem to be bigger than the palm of my hand.

A great many of his more respectable friends left him now. They'd still call him—if he was right—but he was too greatly distrusted.

You know how it used to be, said one of my best friends to me one day much to my surprise. You'd get some doctor and fool around with him for a while and get another and they'd all say something different and you wouldn't know where the hell you were. And this is the story he told me:

Well, this happened many years ago. I was sick and my old man was worried. Finally the druggist tipped us off. Get Rivers, he said. He's a dope but when he's right you can't beat him. And I tell you what I'll do—because he knew the old man well and he himself had been something of a rounder in his day—I'll call up Rivers and get him down here at the store. And, if he's right, I'll send him up.

So he did.

Later in the day when the Doc came into the room he took one look at me. This boy's got typhoid fever, he said. Just like that—that's how he did it. And I'll tell you what I'll do. To prove it, I'll take his blood now and send it in to my brother—he was doing nothing but blood work at that time—and I'll let you know in a few days.

Sure enough, he was right. He had the jump on the thing. The result was I had a light case and we had Rivers for years after that as our family physician.

He'd sit at the table writing a prescription and you could see his head fall down lower and lower—he'd go to sleep right there, right in front of your eyes. My old man would shake him every once in a while and finally he'd get up and go out.

When he started to hit the dope, his brother did his best to get him into some hospital in the city. He knew he was good and, if he could get him in there in a proper atmosphere, he thought he could save him. But the old boy was too foxy. He liked it out here, his friends, the life or whatever it was and they couldn't move him.

The thing, one of the main things, that got the other doctors down on him was his habit of going off—just disappearing sometimes. He liked to go fishing, and he was a crack shot. He'd have important cases, or anything. But that didn't make any difference. You'd call him up to find out why he hadn't been there and they'd say, He's gone away for a few days. We don't know where.

All you could do was get another doctor.

A couple of years after that, one summer when my old man had gone off on a trip somewhere, he sent me down to the only boarding house in town— you know where I mean. He'd left me in the house alone the year before and he wasn't any too satisfied with some of the things pulled off while he was away. Well, this time Rivers heard of it and wanted me to come over and live with him.

I don't know how he got me out of there, but he did. The old gal who ran the place didn't want to let me go, knowing my father and all that. But Rivers persuaded her that I was sick, I guess, and needed treatment and that the best way for me was to live at his house where he could keep his eye on me. So I got my things together in two minutes, you can bet, and into his buggy I hopped and over we went.

My old man hasn't forgiven him for that to this day.

Sunday mornings were the times. It was a regular show. Because most of his patients were poor people and they could come only on Sunday. I'm telling you you never saw an office like it. He had the right idea, he was for humanity—put it any way you like. They'd be sitting all over the place, out in the hall, up the stairs, on the porch, anywhere they could park themselves.

When it was somebody that didn't know me, he'd say I was a young doctor. I was just seventeen then. He'd give me a white coat and tell me to come on. Jesus! Naturally I thought he was great. And I'll tell you in all those four months I never used to see any of those butcheries they'd talk about. Everything he did was O.K. I suppose I'd think different now, but then I thought he was a wonder.

I do remember one woman, though. God, it was a crime. You can imagine what I mean. Here I was, a kid never knowing anything at all. I was having the time of my life. Yes, everything, you're right. I held her while he did the job. I often think of it.

That was the romantic period of my life, those four months I lived with him.

He never kept any track of money. There wasn't a book around the place. Any money he got he shoved it in his pocket. But he never paid for anything, either.

Clever? That boy was there! He'd go over to his desk and you'd see him fumbling around with some instruments. And right in front of you he'd give himself a shot and, unless you were wise, you wouldn't see him do it.

He was foxy too. He'd stall for a few minutes to give it time to act. That was when he had anything important to do. He'd wait a few minutes, then he'd come out steely-eyed and as quiet and steady as the best of them.

That was the difference between him and her. It made her crazy. She didn't know how to control it, but it steadied him down.

Many's the time he'd wake me up in the middle of the night to go out with him. Down at Johnny Kessler's was one of his hangouts where he'd go for soft-shell crabs and clam chowder.

Once he gave me some tickets for a show in New York. Some dirty racket, I've forgotten. He told me to get some of my friends and go in and have a good time. He gave us the tickets and started us off on his own liquor. It was the first show of that kind I'd ever taken in.

When I came home next morning, he himself took care of me, undressed me and put me to bed.

I can remember one night while I was living here, he waked me up at two o'clock in the morning. It was in summer, one of those hot, muggy nights. I'd been operated on too, the day before, he'd taken out my tonsils or something and I was feeling rotten. But that didn't make any difference, I had to go out with him just the same.

We got the old buggy and started out. We went down in the meadows, at two A.M. mind you, down to Mooney's saloon, the old halfway house, you know where it is. He went in and left me there. The mosquitos nearly ate me alive. He had a case in there or something, maybe he took a few drinks. I don't know what.

Anyway, I sat there slapping mosquitoes. The old man came out after a while and told me the Doc was asleep and that they didn't want to wake him. So I, kid like, not wanting to make a fuss or anything, I said all right and just sat there. He left me there in that buggy till five A.M. Jesus!

Then he came out and we went home. When we got there, he said, Let's have some lamb chops! So out we went again, to the butcher's. He went to the door and of course it was closed. So he went up on the porch around at the side and stamped and banged until that fellow had to get up and come down and get him his chops out of the ice box.

Then we went home and he cooked them in the kitchen. And, say, he could cook. He was a wonderful cook. He could make a piece of meat taste like nothing in the world.

We ate the chops and then I went to bed.

When Doc wasn't in his office, he wasn't home, that's all.

When practice was light in summer and there'd be nothing else to do, as it happens sometimes to us all, he'd call his coachman and say, Hitch 'em up, Johnny—or Jake, or whoever it might be that was driving for him at the time—and start out, nobody at first knew whither.

Where are we headin', Doc?

He nodded to the left, down the hill.

It was a clear June day—the kids were still in school—about two in the afternoon. John let the horses jog lazily down the macadam.

Someone hailed him: Well, Doc, where you sneakin' off to? Swimmin'? The Doc gave the man a broad wink as much as to say: Go to hell.

Down near the track there was a bunch of willows by the ice house where the road turns before straightening out to go through the cat-tails. Maybe he saw them, maybe he didn't, you never knew.

Hello, Doc. Where ye goin'?

He just nodded his head. They just smiled and nodded in reply.

Killy-fish rippled the road ditch, a diminutive tempest, as the carriage and the hoof beats of the horses slightly shook the ground in passing.

Without further sign from the Doc, John turned to the left at Mooney's halfway house and continued up the road. Along this road, so I have been told—and the house is still there—lived a woman who kept a regular hang-out for Rivers. It might have been a common joint, I don't know, but that isn't the way I heard it.

Certainly it was in an unusually isolated location, one of the old places, like the mansions on the hill only smaller, more suitable to farming. She was a descendant of the original builders.

Hello, Jimmie, how are you? Come in, bring your cigar with you.

That's the way it began. That's the way it always began. He would be just starting a stogie.

Hello, Doc, how's the boy? would say her brother. He ran the farm for her since her husband walked out.

I hope he's sunk in the mud, was all she'd say when that subject came up for comment.

By this time John would have turned the horses around and be on his way home.

The house is still there in much the same condition as formerly, quite close to the road with the farm buildings piled up in the rear, mostly given over to pigeons now. Rivers was known to about live there at one time.

Anyhow, you could see the chickens walking around in the yard all day. They had a colored man who had grown up on the place to take care of the few remnants of the garden that still remained; he went by the windows to-ward the middle of the afternoon and you could hear him call the chickens and see them run.

What could the attraction have been? Just one thing. Someone else, something else, to take him out of it. She was a good drinker. She gave him a rest.

But certainly she had, and I guess he knew it pretty well too, quite a bit put away. You know how these old farmers sometimes are. The increase in land valuations grow to be enormous; they have no need to move to become wealthy selling off sections of the original farm to the Polacks and promoters. She was one of those, hearing of cities and seeing trains crawling right before their eyes night and day, who remain isolated—peculiarly childish. Hot and eccentric.

Rivers would find an abandoned corner like that to wander into.

The drink alone would have been enough in itself to attract him. But she was a woman. The loafers around the bar at Donnelley's were all right. She was a woman. Maybe he never thought much of that but she *was* just the same.

Plenty of woman.

His sensitiveness, his refinement, his delicacy—found perhaps a release in this backhanded fashion. Can you believe it?

Jesus, she could put up a fight if she wanted to.

She didn't give a good God damn for the whole blankin' world—if you could believe her when she was drunk. And she said it—many times—to her brother and the Doc who put her to bed before he went home.

Then he'd have to come back next day and get her out of it—if they could find him. That's how they came to call him the first time.

Come on, Jimmie, let's get married, she would say.

Sure, where's the priest? and you could tell by his voice that you wouldn't ask him that many times before you wouldn't see him again ever.

Then he quit her. They'd drunk up all her booze, or her brother put a stop to the affair but, anyway, he quit.

I saw her just once many years later when she was completely abandoned.

It was the night we had her up at the Police Station for running through the gates at the railroad crossing. There were five in the car. It was a marvel the train didn't crash them. I was police physician at that time. They wanted me to pass on her, whether or not she was drunk.

She shoved her face close up against mine and yelled at me: Have you a sister, have you a brother? Then tell me I'm drunk. Her breath reeked half across the room. Look at me! Then she went into an unrepeatable string of filth and profanity. And that's what I think of youse. I said it. You heard me.

It was the first and only time I saw her—if indeed she was the one of whom I had heard spoken. She must, at least, have been a good bit more attractive formerly.

As far as I know, he took all the ordinary hypnotics—morphine, heroin and cocaine also. What dose he ever got up to, it's hard to say. I've seen three grains of morphine do no more than make a woman—lying in a maternity ward—normally quiet.

Of course, it got him finally; he began to slip badly in the latter years, made pitiful blunders. But the final phase was marked by that curious idolatry that sometimes attracts people to a man by the very danger of his name.

It lived again in the way many people, not all, still clung to Rivers the more he went down and down.

They seemed to recreate him in their minds, the beloved scapegoat of their own aberrant desires—and believed that he alone could cure them.

He became a legend and indulged himself the more.

But he did do awful things. It is said that he had made the remark that all a woman needed was half her organs—the others were just a surgeon's opportunity. Half the girls of Creston were without the half of theirs, through his offices, if you could believe his story.

It amused me to hear Jack Hardt describe how old Rivers would drop in at their tiny farm out in the reeds along the turnpike by the cedar swamp; a very small place, just a few feet of ground rescued from the bog with room only for a chicken coop, a doghouse, a barn and a hay rick. The old man used to make a fairly decent living off it, though, formerly, selling salt hay. I remember Jack's telling me how the hired man would sleep on the hay in winter with the snow seeping through on them between the boards and the one in the middle sweating from the body heat of his companions.

Rivers was a frequent caller at that place and always welcome there. The boy knew him well. The Doc would go out into the old privy they had at the back of the yard, and stay there for an hour or more sometimes. The kids would go out and peep at him asleep on the seat.

He'd do the same anywhere. One woman up on the hill who did not know him well had him in to see her. He asked if she had a spare room with a bed in it. She said, Yes, not thinking what was in his mind. He went in and stayed. She was frightened to death. She frantically called up several friends but she could interest no one. Rivers had lain down on the bed and there he slept until nearly five in the afternoon, when his man called to fetch him.

The man knew to a dot when to come. In the morning after Rivers failed to show up, he had simply driven off. When the drug had worn itself out, he was there.

Rivers just got up, said nothing, and went home.

Sometimes, though, it was not so harmless.

How did he get away with it?

It is a little inherent in medicine itself—mystery, necromancy, cures—charms of all sorts, and he knew and practiced this black art. Toward the last of his life he had a crooked eye and was thought to be somewhat touched.

An impressionable lady once caused him an unpleasant half hour because of these things. It appears that he had for some reason taken a flier with her in hypnotism and unexpectedly succeeded in putting her under. But he could not rouse her to normal consciousness again when he was through with the experiment and finally becoming himself frightened, called frantically for his friend Willie to come down and help him get her out of the office. The two men, no doubt as mystified as the patient herself at the turn of affairs, were thoroughly scared before—after great efforts—they succeeded in bringing the lady to herself once more.

My wife remembers him staring in at our front door through the screen. He had come to ask if I had any death certificates. She couldn't tell which eye was looking at her. But she noted the wistfulness of his stoop, his eager smile, his voice, his gestures. She felt sorry for him.

But most feared him—in short, dared not attack him even when they knew he had really killed someone.

A cure for disease? He knew what that amounted to. For of what shall one be cured? Work, in this case, through sheer intuitive ability flooded him under. Drugs righted him.

Frightened, under stress, the heart beats faster, the blood is driven to the extremities of the nerves, floods the centers of action and a man feels in a flame. That's what Rivers wanted, must have wanted. The reaction from such a state required its tonics also.

That awful fever of overwork which we feel especially in the United States—he had it. A trembling in the arms and thighs, a tightness of the neck and in the head above the eyes—fast breath, vague pains in the muscles and in the feet. Followed by an orgasm, crashing the job through, putting it over in a fever heat. Then the feeling of looseness afterward. Not pleasant. But there it is. Then cigarettes, a shot of gin. And that's all there is to it. Women the same, more and more.

He had no time, had to be fast, he had to improvise and did—to a marvel.

When a street laborer was clipped once by a trolley car, his arm almost severed near the shoulder, Rivers was the first to get there. Such cases were always his particular delight. With one look he took in the situation as usual, made up his mind, and remarking that the arm could be of no possible further use to the man, amputated it there and then—with a pair of bandage scissors.

Such deeds took the popular fancy and the rumor of them spread like magic.

It's funny too, the answer of the Sisters in the hospital when some of the doctors wanted to prevent him from operating there—principally because he would pass out, finally, in the middle of a case and someone else would have to go in and clean it up for him. The Sisters would say in reply to such complainers: What do you wish us to do? So long as people go to the man, we will keep a bed free for them here. Do you want us to go back on them?

It was an unanswerable argument.

He was one of the few that ever in these parts knew the meaning of all, to give himself completely. He never asked why, never gave a damn, never thought there was anything else. He was like that, things had an absolute value for him.

But one of the younger doctors, a first-rate physician who began practicing in the town a month or two prior to my arrival, had it in for Rivers. My
wife would sometimes say to me, If you know he is killing people, why do
you doctors not get together and have his license taken away from him?

I would answer that I didn't know. I doubted that we could prove anything. No one wanted to try.

Dr. Grimley, though, did want to do something that day.

He had had a Hungarian girl, who was scared as hell of the knife, under
his care with a strangulated hernia. Grimley tried his best to reduce it but
without success. He knew the danger and urged her by every means at his
command to go to the hospital and have the operation. She refused.

He very properly told her that, unless she did as he told her, he would no
longer handle the case and that she would die.

The next day, she called him again. As soon as he entered the room, he
could see that it was all over. She had called in Rivers. He had told her that
he could cure her. God knows what condition he was in at the time. He
pressed upon the sac until it burst. The next day she died.

Grimley was wild. I met him at the corner by the drug store. Though a
very quiet man he was fairly foaming at the mouth. He wanted to have Rivers arrested, he wanted to have him prosecuted for malpractice and to put
him out of the way once and for all—said he'd do it.

He never did.

In reality, it was a population in despair, out of hand, out of discipline,
driven about by each other blindly, believing in the miraculous, the
drunken, as it may be. Here was, to many, though they are diminishing fast,
something before which they could worship, a local shrine, all there was left,
a measure of the poverty which surrounded them. They believed in him:
Rivers, drunk or sober. It is a plaintive, failing story.

Typical of their behavior is the tale of a very sober and canny butcher
whom I knew well who had a small daughter that had what seemed to me to
be typical epileptic fits. They called me in and I told the parents there was
little I could do for them.

Later I saw them again and they confessed to me frankly that they had
taken the child to Dr. Rivers. I wished them luck.

A year later, I had occasion to talk to them again of the child. She had
not had a convulsion for several months. Rivers had cured her. How, I do
not know.

Yes, the father said, it took us quite a while to get him working but once
he really got his mind down on the case, it didn't take him long till he had
her where he wanted her. They believed it and it was so.

People sought him out, they'd wait months for him finally—though he
did, of his own volition, give up maternity cases toward the end. When

everyone else failed, they believed he'd see them through: a powerful fetish. He would save them.

The end was recounted to me by a young patient of mine, a teller in the bank. His father had always had Rivers. So when the old man fell and broke his arm, they called up the Doc who came and deliberately hopped himself up right before the patient—undisguisedly, so indifferent had he become.

That finished it. It was the look in his eyes. He's crazy, said the patient. Take him away. I don't want him fooling around me. I'll get another doctor.

But it would not be just to say that this was really the end, for that gives a wrong impression. Rivers was through, yes, in some ways, but he did not quit by any means. The truth is that during his last years he bought a good-sized lot on the square before the Municipal Building in the center of town. Here he built a fine house, had a large garden, lawns and a double garage, where he kept two cars always ready for service.

Here he continued to practice for several years while his wife bred small dogs—Blue Poms, I think, for her amusement and for sale, one or more of which Rivers would often take out in the car with him on his calls, holding them on his lap, for in those days he himself never sat at the wheel.

Leaving the Yellow House

The neighbors—there were in all six white people who lived at Sego Desert Lake—told one another that old Hattie could no longer make it alone. The desert life, even with a forced-air furnace in the house and butane gas brought from town in a truck, was still too difficult for her. There were women even older than Hattie in the county. Twenty miles away was Amy Walters, the gold miner's widow. But she was a hardier old girl. Every day of the year she took a bath in the icy lake. And Amy was crazy about money and knew how to manage it, as Hattie did not. Hattie was not exactly a drunkard, but she hit the bottle pretty hard, and now she was in trouble and there was a limit to the help she could expect from even the best of neighbors.

They were fond of her, though. You couldn't help being fond of Hattie. She was big and cheerful, puffy, cosmic, boastful, with a big round back and stiff, rather long legs. Before the century began she had graduated from finishing school and studied the organ in Paris. But now she didn't know a note from a skillet. She had tantrums when she played canasta. And all that remained of her fine fair hair was frizzled along her forehead in small gray curls. Her forehead was not much wrinkled, but the skin was bluish, the color of skim milk. She walked with long strides in spite of the heaviness of her hips, pushing on, round-backed, with her shoulders and showing the flat rubber bottoms of her shoes.

Once a week, in the same cheerful, plugging but absent way, she took off her short skirt and the dirty aviator's jacket with the wool collar and put on a girdle, a dress, and high-heeled shoes. When she stood on these heels her fat old body trembled. She wore a big brown Rembrandt-like tam with a ten-cent-store brooch, eye-like, carefully centered. She drew a straight line with lipstick on her mouth, leaving part of the upper lip pale. At the wheel of her old turret-shaped car, she drove, seemingly methodical but speeding dangerously, across forty miles of mountainous desert to buy frozen meat pies and whiskey. She went to the Laundromat and the hairdresser, and then had lunch with two martinis at the Arlington. Afterward she would often visit Marian Nabot's Silvermine Hotel at Miller Street near skid row and pass the rest of the day gossiping and drinking with her cronies, old divorcees like herself who had settled in the West. Hattie never gambled any more and she didn't care for the movies. And at five o'clock she drove back at the same speed, calmly, partly blinded by the smoke of her cigarette. The fixed cigarette gave her a watering eye.

The Rolfes and the Paces were her only white neighbors at Sego Desert Lake. There was Sam Jervis too, but he was only an old gandy-walker who did odd jobs in her garden, and she did not count him. Nor did she count among her neighbors Darly, the dudes' cowboy who worked for the Paces, nor Swede, the telegrapher. Pace had a guest ranch, and Rolfe and his wife were rich and had retired. Thus there were three good houses at the lake, Hattie's yellow house, Pace's, and the Rolfes'. All the rest of the population—Sam, Swede, Watchta the section foreman, and the Mexicans and Indians and Negroes—lived in shacks and boxcars. There were very few trees, cottonwoods and box elders. Everything else, down to the shores, was sagebrush and juniper. The lake was what remained of an old sea that had covered the volcanic mountains. To the north there were some tungsten mines; to the south, fifteen miles, was an Indian village—shacks built of plywood or railroad ties.

In this barren place Hattie had lived for more than twenty years. Her first summer was spent not in a house but in an Indian wickiup on the shore. She used to say that she had watched the stars from this almost roofless shelter. After her divorce she took up with a cowboy named Wicks. Neither of them had any money—it was the Depression—and they had lived on the range, trapping coyotes for a living. Once a month they would come into town and rent a room and go on a bender. Hattie told this sadly, but also gloatingly, and with many trimmings. A thing no sooner happened to her than it was transformed into something else. "We were caught in a storm," she said, "and we rode hard, down to the lake and knocked on the door of the yellow house"—now her house. "Alice Parmenter took us in and let us sleep on the floor." What had actually happened was that the wind was blowing—there had been no storm—and they were not far from the house anyway; and Alice Parmenter, who knew that Hattie and Wicks were not married, offered them separate beds; but Hattie, swaggering, had said in a loud voice, "Why get two sets of sheets dirty?" And she and her cowboy had slept in Alice's bed while Alice had taken the sofa.

Then Wicks went away. There was never anybody like him in the sack; he was brought up in a whorehouse and the girls had taught him everything, said Hattie. She didn't really understand what she was saying but believed that she was being Western. More than anything else she wanted to be thought of as a rough, experienced woman of the West. Still, she was a lady, too. She had good silver and good china and engraved stationery, but she kept canned beans and A-1 sauce and tuna fish and bottles of catsup and fruit salad on the library shelves of her living room. On her night table was the Bible her pious brother Angus—the other brother was a heller—had given her; but behind the little door of the commode was a bottle of bourbon. When she awoke in the night she tippled herself back to sleep. In the glove compartment of her old car she kept little sample bottles for emergencies on the road. Old Darly found them after her accident.

The accident did not happen far out in the desert as she had always feared, but very near home. She had had a few martinis with the Rolfes one evening, and as she was driving home over the railroad crossing she lost control of the car and veered off the crossing onto the tracks. The explanation she gave was that she had sneezed, and the sneeze had blinded her and made her twist the wheel. The motor was killed and all four wheels of the car sat smack on the rails. Hattie crept down from the door, high off the road-bed. A great fear took hold of her—for the car, for the future, and not only for the future but spreading back into the past—and she began to hurry on stiff legs through the sagebrush to Pace's ranch.

Now the Paces were away on a hunting trip and had left Darly in charge; he was tending bar in the old cabin that went back to the days of the pony express, when Hattie burst in. There were two customers, a tungsten miner and his girl.

"Darly, I'm in trouble. Help me. I've had an accident," said Hattie.

How the face of a man will alter when a woman has bad news to tell him! It happened now to lean old Darly; his eyes went flat and looked unwilling, his jaw moved in and out, his wrinkled cheeks began to flush, and he said, "What's the matter—what's happened to you now?"

"I'm stuck on the tracks. I sneezed. I lost control of the car. Tow me off, Darly. With the pickup. Before the train comes."

Darly threw down his towel and stamped his high-heeled boots. "Now what have you gone and done?" he said. "I told you to stay home after dark."

"Where's Pace? Ring the fire bell and fetch Pace."

"There's nobody on the property except me," said the lean old man. "And I'm not supposed to close the bar and you know it as well as I do."

"Please, Darly. I can't leave my car on the tracks."

"Too bad!" he said. Nevertheless he moved from behind the bar. "How did you say it happened?"

"I told you, I sneezed," said Hattie.

Everyone, as she later told it, was as drunk as sixteen thousand dollars: Darly, the miner, and the miner's girl.

Darly was limping as he locked the door of the bar. A year before, a kick from one of Pace's mares had broken his ribs as he was loading her into the trailer, and he hadn't recovered from it. He was too old. But he dissembled the pain. The high-heeled narrow boots helped, and his painful bending

looked like the ordinary stooping posture of a cowboy. However, Darly was
not a genuine cowboy, like Pace who had grown up in the saddle. He was a
late-comer from the East and until the age of forty had never been on
horseback. In this respect he and Hattie were alike. They were not genuine
Westerners.

Hattie hurried after him through the ranch yard.

"Damn you!" he said to her. "I got thirty bucks out of that sucker and I
would have skinned him out of his whole pay check if you minded your business. Pace is going to be sore as hell."

"You've got to help me. We're neighbors," said Hattie.

"You're not fit to be living out here. You can't do it any more. Besides,
you're swacked all the time."

Hattie couldn't afford to talk back. The thought of her car on the tracks
made her frantic. If a freight came now and smashed it, her life at Sego
Desert Lake would be finished. And where would she go then? She was not
fit to live in this place. She had never made the grade at all, only seemed to
have made it. And Darly—why did he say such hurtful things to her? Because he himself was sixty-eight years old, and he had no other place to go,
either; he took bad treatment from Pace besides. Darly stayed because his
only alternative was to go to the soldiers' home. Moreover, the dude women
would still crawl into his sack. They wanted a cowboy and they thought he
was one. Why, he couldn't even raise himself out of his bunk in the morning.
And where else would he get women? "After the dude season," she wanted
to say to him, "you always have to go to the Veterans' Hospital to get fixed up
again." But she didn't dare offend him now.

The moon was due to rise. It appeared as they drove over the upgraded
dirt road toward the crossing where Hattie's turret-shaped car was sitting on
the rails. Driving very fast, Darly wheeled the pickup around, spraying dirt
on the miner and his girl, who had followed in their car.

"You get behind the wheel and steer," Darly told Hattie.

She climbed into the seat. Waiting at the wheel, she lifted up her face
and said, "Please God, I didn't bend the axle or crack the oil pan."

When Darly crawled under the bumper of Hattie's car the pain in his ribs
suddenly cut off his breath, so instead of doubling the tow chain he fastened
it at full length. He rose and trotted back to the truck on the tight boots.
Motion seemed the only remedy for the pain; not even booze did the trick
any more. He put the pickup into towing gear and began to pull. One side
of Hattie's car dropped into the roadbed with a heave of springs. She sat with
a stormy, frightened, conscience-stricken face, racing the motor until she
flooded it.

The tungsten miner yelled, "Your chain's too long."

Hattie was raised high in the air by the pitch of the wheels. She had to
roll down the window to let herself out because the door handle had been

jammed from inside for years. Hattie struggled out on the uplifted side crying, "I better call the Swede. I better have him signal. There's a train due."

"Go on, then," said Darly. "You're no good here."

"Darly, be careful with my car. Be careful."

The ancient sea bed at this place was flat and low, and the lights of her car and of the truck and of the tungsten miner's Chevrolet were bright and big at twenty miles. Hattie was too frightened to think of this. All she could think was that she was a procrastinating old woman, she had lived by delays; she had meant to stop drinking, she had put off the time, and now she had smashed her car—a terrible end, a terrible judgment on her. She got to the ground and, drawing up her skirt, she started to get over the tow chain. To prove that the chain didn't have to be shortened, and to get the whole thing over with, Darly threw the pickup forward again. The chain jerked up and struck Hattie in the knee and she fell forward and broke her arm.

She cried, "Darly, Darly, I'm hurt. I fell."

"The old lady tripped on the chain," said the miner. "Back up here and I'll double it for you. You're getting nowheres."

Drunkenly the miner lay down on his back in the dark, soft red cinders of the roadbed. Darly had backed to slacken the chain.

Darly hurt the miner, too. He tore some skin from his fingers by racing ahead before the chain was secure. Without complaining, the miner wrapped his hand in his shirttail saying, "She'll do it now." The old car came down from the tracks and stood on the shoulder of the road.

"There's your goddamn car," said Darly to Hattie.

"Is it all right?" she said. Her left side was covered with dirt, but she managed to pick herself up and stand, round-backed and heavy, on her still legs. "I'm hurt, Darly." She tried to convince him of it.

"Hell if you are," he said. He believed she was putting on an act to escape blame. The pain in his ribs made him especially impatient with her. "Christ, if you can't look after yourself any more you've got no business out here."

"You're old yourself," she said. "Look what you did to me. You can't hold your liquor."

This offended him greatly. He said, "I'll take you to the Rolfes. They let you booze it up in the first place, so let them worry about you. I'm tired of your bunk, Hattie."

He raced uphill. Chains, spade, and crowbar clashed on the sides of the pickup. She was frightened and held her arm and cried. Rolfe's dogs jumped at her to lick her when she went through the gate. She shrank from them crying, "Down, down."

"Darly," she cried in the darkness, "take care of my car. Don't leave it standing there on the road. Darly, take care of it, please."

But Darly in his ten-gallon hat, his chin-bent face wrinkled, small and angry, a furious pain in his ribs, tore away at high speed.

"Oh, God, what will I do," she said.

The Rolfes were having a last drink before dinner, sitting at their fire of pitchy railroad ties, when Hattie opened the door. Her knee was bleeding, her eyes were tiny with shock, her face gray with dust.

"I'm hurt," she said desperately. "I had an accident. I sneezed and lost control of the wheel. Jerry, look after the car. It's on the road."

They bandaged her knee and took her home and put her to bed. Helen Rolfe wrapped a heating pad around her arm.

"I can't have the pad," Hattie complained. "The switch goes on and off, and every time it does it starts my generator and uses up the gas."

"Ah, now, Hattie," Rolfe said, "this is not the time to be stingy. We'll take you to town in the morning and have you looked over. Helen will phone Dr. Stroud."

Hattie wanted to say, "Stingy! Why you're the stingy ones. I just haven't got anything. You and Helen are ready to hit each other over two bits in canasta." But the Rolfes were good to her; they were her only real friends here. Darly would have let her lie in the yard all night, and Pace would have sold her to the bone man. He'd give her to the knacker for a buck.

So she didn't talk back to the Rolfes, but as soon as they left the yellow house and walked through the super-clear moonlight under the great skirt of box-elder shadows to their new station wagon, Hattie turned off the switch, and the heavy swirling and battering of the generator stopped. Presently she became aware of real pain, deeper pain, in her arm, and she sat rigid, warming the injured place with her hand. It seemed to her that she could feel the bone sticking out. Before leaving, Helen Rolfe had thrown over her a comforter that had belonged to Hattie's dead friend India, from whom she had inherited the small house and everything in it. Had the comforter lain on India's bed the night she died? Hattie tried to remember, but her thoughts were mixed up. She was fairly sure the deathbed pillow was in the loft, and she believed she had put the death bedding in a trunk. Then how had this comforter got out? She couldn't do anything about it now but draw it away from contact with her skin. It kept her legs warm. This she accepted, but she didn't want it any nearer.

More and more Hattie saw her own life as though, from birth to present, every moment had been filmed. Her fancy was that when she died she would see the film shown. Then she would know how she appeared from the back, watering the plants in the bathroom, asleep, playing the organ, embracing—everything, even tonight, in pain, almost the last pain, perhaps, for she couldn't take much more. How many twists and angles had life to show her yet? There couldn't be much film left. To lie awake and think such thoughts was the worst thing in the world. Better death than insomnia. Hattie not only loved sleep, but she believed in it.

The first attempt to set the bone was not successful. "Look what they've done to me," said Hattie and showed the visitors the discolored breast. After the second operation her mind wandered. The sides of her bed had to be raised, for in her delirium she roamed the wards. She cursed at the nurses when they shut her in. "You can't make people prisoners in a democracy without a trial, you bitches." She had learned from Wicks how to swear. "*He* was profane," she used to say. "I picked it up unconsciously."

For several weeks her mind was not clear. Asleep, her face was lifeless; her cheeks were puffed out and her mouth, no longer wide and grinning, was drawn round and small. Helen sighed when she saw her.

"Shall we get in touch with her family?" Helen asked the doctor. His skin was white and thick. He had chestnut hair, abundant but very dry. He sometimes explained to his patients, "I had a tropical disease during the war."

He asked, "Is there a family?"

"Old brothers. Cousins' children," said Helen. She tried to think who would be called to her own bedside (she was old enough for that). Rolfe would see that she was cared for. He would hire private nurses. Hattie could not afford that. She had already gone beyond her means. A trust company in Philadelphia paid her eighty dollars a month. She had a small savings account.

"I suppose it'll be up to us to get her out of hock," said Rolfe. "Unless the brother down in Mexico comes across. We may have to phone one of those old guys."

In the end, no relations had to be called. Hattie began to recover. At last she could recognize visitors, though her mind was still in disorder. Much that had happened she couldn't recall.

"How many quarts of blood did they have to give me?" she kept asking. "I seem to remember five, six, eight different transfusions. Daylight, electric light . . . " She tried to smile, but she couldn't make a pleasant face as yet. "How am I going to pay?" she said. "At twenty-five bucks a quart. My little bit of money is just about wiped out."

Blood became her constant topic, her preoccupation. She told everyone who came to see her, "—have to replace all that blood. They poured gallons in to me. Gallons. I hope it was all good." And, though very weak, she began to grin and laugh again. There was more hissing in her laughter than formerly; the illness had affected her chest.

"No cigarettes, no booze," the doctor told Helen.

"Doctor," Helen asked him, "do you expect her to change?"

"All the same, I am obliged to say it."

"Life sober may not be much of a temptation to her," said Helen.

Her husband laughed. When Rolfe's laughter was intense it blinded one of his eyes. His short Irish face turned red; on the bridge of his small, sharp nose the skin whitened. "Hattie's like me," he said. "She'll be in business till she's cleaned out. And if Sego Lake turned to whiskey she'd use her last strength to knock her old yellow house down to build a raft of it. She'd float away on whisky. So why talk temperance?"

Hattie recognized the similarity between them. When he came to see her she said, "Jerry, you're the only one I can really talk to about my troubles. What am I going to do for money?" I have Hotchkiss Insurance. I paid eight dollars a month."

"That won't do you much good, Hat. No Blue Cross?"

"I let it drop ten years ago. Maybe I could sell some of my valuables."

"What valuables have you got?" he said. His eye began to droop with laughter.

"Why," she said defiantly, "there's plenty. First there's the beautiful, precious Persian rug that India left me."

"Coals from the fireplace have been burning it for years, Hat!"

"The rug is in *perfect* condition," she said with an angry sway of the shoulders. "A beautiful object like that never loses its value. And the oak table from the Spanish monastery is three hundred years old."

"With luck you could get twenty bucks for it. It would cost fifty to haul it out of here. It's the house you ought to sell."

"The house?" she said. Yes, that had been in her mind. "I'd have to get twenty thousand for it."

"Eight is a fair price."

"Fifteen. . . . " She was offended, and her voice recovered its strength. "India put eight into it in two years. And don't forget that Sego Lake is one of the most beautiful places in the world."

"But where is it? Five hundred and some miles to San Francisco and two hundred to Salt Lake City. Who wants to live way out here but a few eccentrics like you and India? And me?"

"There are things you can't put a price tag on. Beautiful things."

"Oh, bull, Hattie! You don't know squat about beautiful things. Any more than I do. I live here because it figures for me, and you because India left you the house. And just in the nick of time, too. Without it you wouldn't have had a pot of your own."

His words offended Hattie; more than that, they frightened her. She was silent and then grew thoughtful, for she was fond of Jerry Rolfe and he of her. He had good sense and moreover he only expressed her own thoughts. He spoke no more than the truth about India's death and the house. But she told herself, He doesn't know everything. You'd have to pay a San Francisco architect ten thousand just to *think* of such a house. Before he drew a line.

"Jerry," the old woman said, "what am I going to do about replacing the blood in the blood bank?"

"Do you want a quart from me, Hat?" His eye began to fall shut.

"You won't do. You had that tumor, two years ago. I think Darly ought to give some."

"The old man?" Rolfe laughed at her. "You want to kill him?"

"Why!" said Hattie with anger, lifting up her massive face. Fever and perspiration had frayed the fringe of curls; at the back of the head the hair had knotted and matted so that it had to be shaved. "Darly almost killed me. It's his fault that I'm in this condition. He must have *some* in him. He runs after all the chicks—all of them—young and old."

"Come, you were drunk, too," said Rolfe.

"I've driven drunk for forty years. It was the sneeze. Oh, Jerry, I feel wrung out," said Hattie, haggard, sitting forward in bed. But her face was cleft by her nonsensically happy grin. She was not one to be miserable for long; she had the expression of a perennial survivor.

Every other day she went to the therapist. The young woman worked her arm for her; it was a pleasure and a comfort to Hattie, who would have been glad to leave the whole cure to her. However, she was given other exercises to do, and these were not so easy. They rigged a pulley for her and Hattie had to hold both ends of a rope and saw it back and forth through the scraping little wheel. She bent heavily from the hips and coughed over her cigarette. But the most important exercise of all she shirked. This required her to put the flat of her hand to the wall at the level of her hips and, by working her finger tips slowly, to make the hand ascend to the height of her shoulder. That was painful; she often forgot to do it, although the doctor warned her, "Hattie, you don't want adhesions, do you?"

A light of despair crossed Hattie's eyes. Then she said, "Oh, Dr. Stroud, buy my house from me."

"I'm a bachelor. What would I do with a house?"

"I know just the girl for you—my cousin's daughter. Perfectly charming and very brainy. Just got her Ph.D."

"You must get quite a few proposals yourself," said the doctor.

"From crazy desert rats. They chase me. But," she said, "after I pay my bills I'll be in pretty punk shape. If at least I could replace that blood in the blood bank I'd feel easier."

"If you don't do as the therapist tells you, Hattie, you'll need another operation. Do you know what adhesions are?"

She knew. But Hattie thought, *How long must I go on taking care of myself?* It made her angry to hear him speak of another operation. She had a moment of panic, but she covered it up. With him, this young man whose skin was already as thick as buttermilk and whose chestnut hair was as dry as death, she always assumed the part of a child. In a small voice she said, "Yes, doctor." But her heart was in a fury.

Night and day, however, she repeated, "I was in the Valley of the Shadow. But I'm alive." She was weak, she was old, she couldn't follow a train of thought very easily, she felt faint in the head. But she was still here; here was her body, it filled a space, a great body. And though she had worries and perplexities, and once in a while her arm felt as though it was about to give her the last stab of all; and though her hair was scrappy and old, like onion roots, and scattered like nothing under the comb, yet she sat and amused herself with visitors; her great grin split her face; her heart warmed with every kind word.

And she thought, People will help me out. It never did me any good to worry. At the last minute something turned up, when I wasn't looking for it. Marian loves me. Helen and Jerry love me. Half Pint loves me. They would never let me go to the ground. And I love them. If it were the other way around, I'd never let them go down.

Above the horizon, in a baggy vastness which Hattie by herself occasionally visited, the features of India, her *shade*, sometimes rose. India was indignant and scolding. Not mean. Not really mean. Few people had ever been really mean to Hattie. But India was annoyed with her. "The garden is going to hell, Hattie," she said. "Those lilac bushes are all shriveled."

"But what can I do? The hose is rotten. It broke. It won't reach."

"Then dig a trench," said the phantom of India. "Have old Sam dig a trench. But save the bushes."

Am I thy servant still? said Hattie to herself. *No,* she thought, *let the dead bury their dead.*

But she didn't defy India now any more than she had done when they lived together. Hattie was supposed to keep India off the bottle, but often both of them began to get drunk after breakfast. They forgot to dress, and in their slips the two of them wandered drunkenly around the house and blundered into each other, and they were in despair at having been so weak. Late in the afternoon they would be sitting in the living room, waiting for the sun to set. It shrank, burning itself out on the crumbling edges of the mountains. When the sun passed, the fury of the daylight ended and the mountain surfaces were more blue, broken, like cliffs of coal. They no longer suggested faces. The east began to look simple, and the lake less inhuman and haughty. At last India would say, "Hattie—it's time for the lights." And Hattie would pull the switch chain of the lamps, several of them, to give the generator a good shove. She would turn on some of the wobbling eighteenth-century-style lamps whose shades stood out from their slender bodies like dragonflies' wings. The little engine in the shed would shuffle, then spit, then charge and bang, and the first weak light would rise unevenly in the bulbs.

"Hettie!" cried India. After she drank she was penitent, but her penitence too was a hardship to Hattie, and the worse her temper the more British her accent became. *"Where the hell ah you Het-tie!"* After India's death Hattie found some poems she had written in which she, Hattie, was affectionately and even touchingly mentioned. That was a good thing—Literature. Education. Breeding. But Hattie's interest in ideas was very small, whereas India had been all over the world. India was used to brilliant society. India wanted her to discuss Eastern religion, Bergson and Proust, and Hattie had no head for this, and so India blamed her drinking on Hattie. "I can't talk to you," she would say. "You don't understand religion or culture. And I'm here because I'm not fit to be anywhere else. I can't live in New York any more. It's too dangerous for a woman my age to be drunk in the street at night."

And Hattie, talking to her Western friends about India, would say, "She is a lady" (implying that they made a pair). "She is a creative person" (this was why they found each other so congenial). "But helpless? Completely. Why she can't even get her own girdle on."

"Hettie! Come here. Het-tie! Do you know what sloth is?"

Undressed, India sat on her bed and with the cigarette in her drunken, wrinkled, ringed hand she burned holes in the blankets. On Hattie's pride she left many small scars, too. She treated her like a servant.

Weeping, India begged her afterward to forgive her. *"Hattie, please don't condemn me in your heart. Forgive me, dear, I know I am bad. But I hurt myself more in my evil than I hurt you."*

Hattie would keep a stiff bearing. She would lift up her face with its incurved nose and puffy eyes and say, "I am a Christian person. I never bear a grudge." And by repeating this she actually brought herself to forgive India.

But of course Hattie had no husband, no child, no skill, no savings. And what she would have done if India had not died and left her the yellow house nobody knows.

Jerry Rolfe said privately to Marian, "Hattie can't do anything for herself. If I hadn't been around during the forty-four blizzard she and India both would have starved. She's always been careless and lazy and now she can't even chase a cow out of the yard. She's too feeble. The thing for her to do is to go East to her damn brother. Hattie would have ended at the poor farm if it hadn't been for India. But besides the damn house India should have left her some dough. She didn't use her goddamn head."

When Hattie returned to the lake she stayed with the Rolfes. "Well, old shellback," said Jerry, "there's a little more life in you now."

Indeed, with joyous eyes, the cigarette in her mouth and her hair newly frizzed and overhanging her forehead, she seemed to have triumphed again. She was pale, but she grinned, she chuckled, and she held a bourbon old-fashioned with a cherry and a slice of orange in it. She was on rations; the Rolfes allowed her two a day. Her back, Helen noted, was more bent than before. Her knees went outward a little weakly; her feet, however, came close together at the ankles.

"Oh, Helen dear and Jerry dear, I am so thankful, so glad to be back at the lake. I can look after my place again, and I'm here to see the spring. It's more gorgeous than ever."

Heavy rains had fallen while Hattie was away. The sego lilies, which bloomed only after a wet winter, came up from the loose dust, especially around the marl pit; but even on the burnt granite they seemed to grow. Desert peach was beginning to appear, and in Hattie's yard the rosebushes were filling out. The roses were yellow and abundant, and the odor they gave off was like that of damp tea leaves.

"Before it gets hot enough for the rattlesnakes," said Hattie to Helen, "we ought to drive up to Mark's ranch and gather watercress."

Hattie was going to attend to lots of things, but the heat came early that year and, as there was no television to keep her awake, she slept most of the day. She was now able to dress herself, though there was little more that she could do. Sam Jervis rigged the pulley for her on the porch and she remembered once in a while to use it. Mornings when she had her strength she rambled over to her own house, examining things, being important and giving orders to Sam Jervis and Wanda Gingham. At ninety, Wanda, a Shoshone, was still an excellent seamstress and housecleaner.

Hattie looked over the car, which was parked under a cottonwood tree. She tested the engine. Yes, the old pot would still go. Proudly, happily, she listened to the noise of tappets; the dry old pipe shook as the smoke went out at the rear. She tried to work the shift, turn the wheel. That, as yet, she couldn't do. But it would come soon, she was confident.

At the back of the house the soil had caved in a little over the cesspool and a few of the old railroad ties over the top had rotted. Otherwise things were in good shape. Sam had looked after the garden. He had fixed a new catch for the gate after Pace's horses—maybe because he could never afford to keep them in hay—had broken in and Sam found them grazing and drove them out. Luckily, they hadn't damaged many of her plants. Hattie felt a moment of wild rage against Pace. He had brought the horses into her garden for a free feed, she was sure. But her anger didn't last long. It was reabsorbed into the feeling of golden pleasure that enveloped her. She had little strength, but all that she had was a pleasure to her. So she forgave even Pace, who would have liked to do her out of the house, who had always used her, embarrassed her, cheated her at cards, swindled her. All that he did for the sake of his quarter horses. He was a fool about horses. They were ruining him. Racing horses was a millionaire's amusement.

She saw his animals in the distance, feeding. Unsaddled, the mares appeared undressed; they reminded her of naked women walking around with their glossy flanks in the sego lilies which curled on the ground. The flowers were yellowish, like winter wool, but fragrant; the mares, naked and gentle, walked through them. Their strolling, their perfect beauty, the sound of their hoofs on stone touched a deep place in Hattie's nature. Her love for horses, birds, and dogs was well known. Dogs led the list. And now a piece cut from a green blanket reminded Hattie of her dog Richie. The blanket was one he had torn, and she had cut it into strips and placed them under the doors to keep out the drafts. In the house she found more traces of him: hair he had shed on the furniture. Hattie was going to borrow Helen's vacuum cleaner, but there wasn't really enough current to make it pull as it should. On the doorknob of India's room hung the dog collar.

Hattie had decided that she would have herself moved into India's bed when it was time to die. Why should there be two deathbeds? A perilous look came into her eyes, her lips were pressed together forbiddingly. *I follow,* she said, speaking to India with an inner voice, *so never mind.* Presently—before long—she would have to leave the yellow house in her turn. And as she went into the parlor, thinking of the will, she sighed. Pretty soon she would have to attend to it. India's lawyer, Claiborne, helped her with such things. She had phoned him in town, while she was staying with Marian, and talked matters over with him. He had promised to try to sell the house for her. Fifteen thousand was her bottom price, she said. If he couldn't find a buyer, perhaps he could find a tenant. Two hundred dollars a month was the rental she set. Rolfe laughed. Hattie turned toward him one of those proud, dulled looks she always took on when he angered her. Haughtily she said, "For summer on Sego Lake? That's reasonable."

"You're competing with Pace's ranch."

"Why, the food is stinking down there. And he cheats the dudes," said Hattie. "He really cheats them at cards. You'll never catch me playing blackjack with him again."

And what would she do, thought Hattie, if Claiborne could neither rent nor sell the house? This question she shook off as regularly as it returned. *I don't have to be a burden on anybody,* thought Hattie. *It's looked bad many a time before, but when push came to shove, I made it. Somehow I got by.* But she argued with herself: *How many times? How long, O God—an old thing, feeble, no use to anyone?* Who said she had any right to own property?

She was sitting on her sofa, which was very old—India's sofa—eight feet long, kidney-shaped, puffy, and bald. An underlying pink shone through the green; the upholstered tufts were like the pads of dogs' paws; between them rose bunches of hair. Here Hattie slouched, resting, with knees wide apart and a cigarette in her mouth, eyes half-shut but farseeing. The mountains seemed not fifteen miles but fifteen hundred feet away, the lake a blue band; the tealike odor of the roses, though they were still unopened, was already in the air, for Sam was watering them in the heat. Gratefully Hattie yelled, "Sam!"

Sam was very old, and all shanks. His feet looked big. His old railroad jacket was made tight across the back by his stoop. A crooked finger with its great broad nail over the mouth of the hose made the water spray and sparkle. Happy to see Hattie, he turned his long jaw, empty of teeth, and his long blue eyes, which seemed to bend back to penetrate into his temples (it was his face that turned, not his body), and he said, "Oh, there, Hattie. You've made it home today? Welcome, Hattie."

"Have a beer, Sam. Come around the kitchen door and I'll give you a beer."

She never had Sam in the house, owing to his skin disease. There were raw patches on his chin and behind his ears. Hattie feared infection from his touch, having decided that he had impetigo. She gave him the beer can, never a glass, and she put on her gloves before she used the garden tools. Since he would take no money from her—Wanda Gingham charged a dollar a day—she got Marian to find old clothes for him in town and she left food for him at the door of the damp-wood-smelling boxcar where he lived.

"How's the old wing, Hat?" he said.

"It's coming. I'll be driving the car again before you know it," she told him. "By the first of May I'll be driving again." Every week she moved the date forward. "By Decoration Day I expect to be on my own again," she said.

In mid-June, however, she was still unable to drive. Helen Rolfe said to her, "Hattie, Jerry and I are due in Seattle the first week of July."

"Why, you never told me that," said Hattie.

"You don't mean to tell me this is the first you heard of it," said Helen. "You've known about it from the first—since Christmas."

It wasn't easy for Hattie to meet her eyes. She presently put her head down. Her face became very dry, especially the lips. "Well, don't you worry about me. I'll be all right here," she said.

"Who's going to look after you?" said Jerry. He evaded nothing himself and tolerated no evasion in others. Except that, as Hattie knew, he made every possible allowance for her. But who would help her? She couldn't count on her friend Half Pint, she couldn't really count on Marian either. She had had only the Rolfes to turn to. Helen, trying to be steady, gazed at her and made sad, involuntary movements with her head, sometimes nodding, sometimes seeming as if she disagreed. Hattie, with her inner voice, swore at her: *Bitch-eyes. I can't make it the way she does because I'm old. Is that fair?* And yet she admired Helen's eyes. Even the skin about them, slightly wrinkled, heavy underneath, was touching, beautiful. There was a heaviness in her bust that went, as if by attachment, with the heaviness of her eyes. Her head, her hands and feet should have taken a more slender body. Helen, said Hattie, was the nearest thing she had on earth to a sister. But there was no reason to go to Seattle—no genuine business. Why the hell Seattle? It was only idleness, only a holiday. The only reason was Hattie herself; this was their way of telling her that there was a limit to what she could expect them to do for her. Helen's nervous head wavered, but her thoughts were steady. She knew what was passing through Hattie's mind. Like Hattie, she was an idle woman. Why was her right to idleness better?

Because of money? thought Hattie. Because of age? Because she has a husband? Because she had a daughter in Swarthmore College? But an interesting thing occurred to her. Helen disliked being idle, whereas Hattie herself had never made bones about it: an idle life was all she was good for. But for her it had been uphill all the way, because when Waggoner divorced her she didn't have a cent. She even had to support Wicks for seven or eight years. Except with horses, Wicks had no sense. And then when she had had to take tons of dirt from India. *I am the one,* Hattie asserted to herself. *I would know what to do with Helen's advantages. She only suffers from them. And if she wants to stop being an idle woman why can't she start with me, her neighbor?* Hattie's skin, for all its puffiness, burned with anger. She said to Rolfe and Helen, "Don't worry. I'll make out. But if I have to leave the lake you'll be ten times more lonely than before. Now I'm going back to my house."

She lifted up her broad old face, and her lips were childlike with suffering. She would never take back what she had said.

But the trouble was no ordinary trouble. Hattie was herself aware that she rambled, forgot names, and answered when no one spoke.

"We can't just take charge of her," Rolfe said. "What's more, she ought to be near a doctor. She keeps her shotgun loaded so she can fire it if anything happens to her in the house. But who knows what she'll shoot? I don't believe it was Jacamares who killed that Doberman of hers."

Rolfe drove into the yard the day after she moved back to the yellow house and said, "I'm going into town. I can bring you some chow if you like."

She couldn't afford to refuse his offer, angry though she was, and she said, "Yes, bring me some stuff from the Mountain Street Market. Charge it." She had only some frozen shrimp and a few cans of beer in the icebox. When Rolfe had gone she put out the package of shrimp to thaw.

People really used to stick by one another in the West. Hattie now saw herself as one of the pioneers. The modern breed had come later. After all, she had lived on the range like an old-timer. Wicks had had to shoot their

Christmas dinner and she had cooked it—venison. He killed it on the reservation, and if the Indians had caught them, there would have been hell to pay.

The weather was hot, the clouds were heavy and calm in a large sky. The horizon was so huge that in it the lake must have seemed like a saucer of milk. *Some milk!* Hattie thought. Two thousand feet down in the middle, so deep no corpse could ever be recovered. A body, they said, went around with the currents. And there were rocks like eyeteeth, and hot springs, and colorless fish at the bottom which were never caught. Now that the white pelicans were nesting they patrolled the rocks for snakes and other egg thieves. They were so big and flew so slow you might imagine they were angels. Hattie no longer visited the lake shore; the walk exhausted her. She saved her strength to go to Pace's bar in the afternoon.

She took off her shoes and stockings and walked on bare feet from one end of her house to the other. On the land side she saw Wanda Gingham sitting near the tracks while her great-grandson played in the soft red gravel. Wanda wore a large purple shawl and her black head was bare. All about her was—was nothing, Hattie thought; for she had taken a drink, breaking her rule. Nothing but mountains, thrust out like men's bodies; the sagebrush was the hair on their chests.

The warm wind blew dust from the marl pit. This white powder made her sky less blue. On the water side were the pelicans, pure as spirits, slow as angels, blessing the air as they flew with great wings.

Should she or should she not have Sam do something about the vine on the chimney? Sparrows nested in it, and she was glad of that. But all summer long the king snakes were after them and she was afraid to walk in the garden. When the sparrows scratched the ground for seed they took a funny bound; they held their legs stiff and flung back the dust with both feet. Hattie sat down at her old Spanish monastery table, watching them in the cloudy warmth of the day, clasping her hands, chuckling and sad. The bushes were crowded with yellow roses, half of them now rotted. The lizards scrambled from shadow to shadow. The water was smooth as air, gaudy as silk. The mountains succumbed, falling asleep in the heat. Drowsy, Hattie lay down on her sofa. Its pads were like dogs' paws. She gave in to sleep and when she woke it was midnight; she did not want to alarm the Rolfes by putting on her lights so she took advantage of the moon to eat a few thawed shrimps and go to the bathroom. She undressed and lifted herself into bed and lay there feeling her sore arm. Now she knew how much she missed her dog. The whole matter of the dog weighed heavily on her soul. She came close to tears, thinking about him, and she went to sleep oppressed by her secret.

I suppose I had better try to pull myself together a little, thought Hattie nervously in the morning. *I can't just sleep my way through.* She knew what her difficulty was. Before any serious question her mind gave way. It scattered or diffused. She said to herself, *I can see bright, but I feel dim. I guess I'm not so lively any more. Maybe I'm becoming a little touched in the head, as Mother was.* But she was not so old as her mother when she did those strange things. At eighty-five, her mother had to be kept from going naked in the street. *I'm not as bad as that yet. Thank God! Yes, I walked into the men's wards, but that was when I had a fever, and my nightie was on.*

She drank a cup of Nescafé and it strengthened her determination to do something for herself. In all the world she had only her brother Angus to go to. Her brother Will had led a rough life; he was an old heller, and now he drove everyone away. He was too crabby, thought Hattie. Besides he was angry because she had lived so long with Wicks. Angus would forgive her. But then he and his wife were not her kind. With them she couldn't drink, she couldn't smoke, she had to make herself small-mouthed, and she would have to wait while they read a chapter of the Bible before breakfast. Hattie could not bear to sit at table waiting for meals. Besides, she had a house of her own at last. Why should she have to leave it? She had never owned a thing before. And now she was not allowed to enjoy her yellow house. *But I'll keep it*, she said to herself rebelliously. *I swear to God I'll keep it. Why, I barely just got it. I haven't had time.* And she went out on the porch to work the pulley and do something about the adhesions in her arm. She was sure now that they were there. *And what will I do?* she cried to herself. *What will I do? Why did I ever go to Rolfe's that night—and why did I lose control on the crossing?* She couldn't say, now, "I sneezed." She couldn't even remember what had happened, except that she saw the boulders and the twisting blue rails and Darly. It was Darly's fault. He was sick and old himself. *He* couldn't make it. He envied her, the house, and her woman's peaceful life. Since she returned from the hospital he hadn't even come to visit her. He only said, "Hell, I'm sorry for her, but it was her fault." What hurt him most was that she had said he couldn't hold his liquor.

Fierceness, swearing to God did no good. She was still the same procrastinating old woman. She had a letter to answer from Hotchkiss Insurance and it drifted out of sight. She was going to phone Claiborne the lawyer, but it slipped her mind. One morning she announced to Helen that she believed she would apply to an institution in Los Angeles that took over the property of old people and managed it for them. They gave you an apartment right on the ocean, and your meals and medical care. You had to sign over half of your estate. "It's fair enough," said Hattie. "They take a gamble. I may live to be a hundred."

"I wouldn't be surprised," said Helen.

However, Hattie never got around to sending to Los Angeles for the brochure. But Jerry Rolfe took it on himself to write a letter to her brother Angus about her condition. And he drove over also to have a talk with Amy

Walters, the gold miner's widow at Fort Walters—as the ancient woman called it. The Fort was an old tar-paper building over the mine. The shaft made a cesspool unnecessary. Since the death of her second husband no one had dug for gold. On a heap of stones near the road a crimson sign FORT WALTERS was placed. Behind it was a flagpole. The American flag was raised every day.

Amy was working in the garden in one of dead Bill's shirts. Bill had brought water down from the mountains for her in a homemade aqueduct so she could raise her own peaches and vegetables.

"Amy," Rolfe said, "Hattie's back from the hospital and living all alone. You have no folks and neither has she. Not to beat around the bush about it, why don't you live together?"

Amy's face had great delicacy. Her winter baths in the lake, her vegetable soups, the waltzes she played for herself alone on the grand piano that stood beside her wood stove, the murder stories she read till darkness obliged her to close the book—this life of hers had made her remote. She looked delicate, yet there was no way to affect her composure, she couldn't be touched. It was very strange.

"Hattie and me have different habits, Jerry," said Amy. "And Hattie wouldn't like my company. I can't drink with her. I'm a teetotaller."

"That's true," said Rolfe, recalling that Hattie referred to Amy as if she were a ghost. He couldn't speak to Amy of the solitary death in store for her. There was not a cloud in the arid sky today, and there was no shadow of death on Amy. She was tranquil, she seemed to be supplied with a sort of pure fluid that would feed her life slowly for years to come.

He said, "All kinds of things could happen to a woman like Hattie in that yellow house, and nobody would know."

"That's a fact. She doesn't know how to take care of herself."

"She can't. Her arm hasn't healed."

Amy didn't say that she was sorry to hear it. In the place of those words came a silence which might have meant that. Then she said, "I might go over there a few hours a day, but she would have to pay me."

"Now, Amy, you must know as well as I do that Hattie has no money—not much more than her pension. Just the house."

At once Amy said, no pause coming between his words and hers, "I would take care of her if she'd agree to leave the house to me."

"Leave it in your hands, you mean?" said Rolfe. "To manage?"

"In her will. To belong to me."

"Why, Amy, what would you do with Hattie's house?" he said.

"It would be my property, that's all. I'd have it."

"Maybe you would leave Fort Walters to her in your will," he said.

"Oh, no," she said. "Why should I? I'm not asking Hattie for her help. I don't need it. Hattie is a city woman."

Rolfe could not carry this proposal back to Hattie. He was too wise ever to mention her will to her.

But Pace was not so careful of her feelings. By mid-June Hattie had begun to visit his bar regularly. She had so many things to think about she couldn't stay at home. When Pace came in from the yard one day—he had been packing the wheels of his horse-trailer and was wiping grease from his fingers—he said with his usual bluntness, "How would you like it if I paid you fifty bucks a month for the rest of your life, Hat?"

Hattie was holding her second old-fashioned of the day. At the bar she made it appear that she observed the limit; but she had started drinking at home. One before lunch, one during, one after lunch. She began to grin, expecting Pace to make one of his jokes. But he was wearing his scoop-shaped Western hat as level as a Quaker, and he had drawn down his chin, a sign that he was not fooling. She said, "That would be nice, but what's the catch?"

"No catch," he said. "This is what we'd do. I'd give you five hundred dollars cash, and fifty bucks a month for life, and you let me sleep some dudes in the yellow house, and you'd leave the house to me in your will."

"What kind of a deal is that?" said Hattie, her look changing. "I thought we were friends."

"It's the best deal you'll ever get," he said.

The weather was sultry, but Hattie till now had thought that it was nice. She had been dreamy but comfortable, about to begin to enjoy the cool of the day; but now she felt that such cruelty and injustice had been waiting to attack her, that it would have been better to die in the hospital than be so disillusioned.

She cried, "Everybody wants to push me out. You're a cheater, Pace. God! I know you. Pick on somebody else. Why do you have to pick on me? Just because I happen to be around?"

"Why, no, Hattie," he said, trying now to be careful. "It was just a business offer."

"Why don't you give me some blood for the bank if you're such a friend of mine?"

"Well, Hattie, you drink too much and you oughtn't to have been driving anyway."

"I sneezed, and you know it. The whole thing happened because I sneezed. Everybody knows that. I wouldn't sell you my house. I'd give it to the lepers first. You'd let me go away and never send me a cent. You never pay anybody. You can't even buy wholesale in town any more because nobody trusts you. I'm stuck, that's all, just stuck. I keep on saying that this is my only home in all the world, this is where my friends are, and the weather is always perfect and the lake is beautiful. But I wish the whole damn empty old place were in Hell. It's not human and neither are you. But I'll be here the day the sheriff takes away your horses—you never mind! I'll be clapping and applauding!"

He told her then that she was drunk again, and so she was, but she was more than that, and though her head was spinning she decided to go back to the house at once and take care of some things she had been putting off. This very day she was going to write to the lawyer, Claiborne, and make sure that Pace never got her property. She wouldn't put it past him to swear in court that India had promised him the yellow house.

She sat at the table with pen and paper, trying to think how to put it.

"I want this on record," she wrote. "I could kick myself in the head when I think of how he's led me on. I have been his patsy ten thousand times. As when that drunk crashed his Cub plane on the lake shore. At the coroner's jury he let me take the whole blame. He said he had instructed me when I was working for him never to take in any drunks. And this flier was drunk. He had nothing on but a T shirt and Bermuda shorts and he was flying from Sacramento to Salt Lake City. At the inquest Pace said I had disobeyed his instructions. The same was true when the cook went haywire. She was a tramp. He never hires decent help. He cheated her on the bar bill and blamed me and she went after me with a meat cleaver. She disliked me because I criticized her for drinking at the bar in her one-piece white bathing suit with the dude guests. But he turned her loose on me. He hints that he did certain services for India. She would never have let him touch one single finger. He was too common for her. It can never be said about India that she was not a lady in every way. He thinks he is the greatest sack-artist in the world. He only loves horses, as a fact. He has no claims at all, oral or written, on this yellow house. I want you to have this over my signature. He was cruel to Pickle-Tits who was his first wife, and he's no better to the charming woman who is his present one. I don't know why she takes it. It must be despair." Hattie said to herself, *I don't suppose I'd better send that.*

She was still angry. Her heart was knocking within; the deep pulses, as after a hot bath, beat at the back of her thighs. The air outside was dotted with transparent particles. The mountains were as red as furnace clinkers. The iris leaves were fan sticks—they stuck out like Jiggs's hair.

She always ended by looking out of the window at the desert and lake. *They drew you from yourself. But after they had drawn you, what did they do with you? It was too late to find out. I'll never know. I wasn't meant to. I'm not the type,* Hattie reflected. *Maybe something too cruel for women, young or old.*

So she stood up and, rising, she had the sensation that she had gradually become a container for herself. You get old, your heart, your liver, your lungs seem to expand in size, and the walls of the body give way outward, swelling, she thought, and you take the shape of an old jug, wider and wider toward the top. You swell up with tears and fat. She no longer even smelled to herself like a woman. Her face with its much-slept-upon skin was only faintly like her own—like a cloud that has changed. It was a face. It became a ball of yarn. It had drifted open. It had scattered.

I was never one single thing anyway, she thought. *Never my own. I was only loaned to myself.*

But the thing wasn't over yet. And in fact she didn't know for certain that it was ever going to be over. You only had other people's word for it that death was such-and-such. How do I know? she asked herself challengingly. Her anger had sobered her for a little while. Now she was again drunk. . . . *It was strange. It is strange. It may continue being strange.* She further thought, *I used to wish for death more than I do now. Because I didn't have anything at all. I changed when I got a roof of my own over me. And now? Do I have to go? I thought Marian loved me, but she already has a sister. And I thought Helen and Jerry would never desert me, but they've beat it. And now Pace has insulted me. They think I'm not going to make it.*

She went to the cupboard—she kept the bourbon bottle there; she drank less if each time she had to rise and open the cupboard door. And, as if she were being watched, she poured a drink and swallowed it.

The notion that in this emptiness someone saw her was connected with the other notion that she was being filmed from birth to death. That this was done for everyone. And afterward you could view your life. A here-after movie.

Hattie wanted to see some of it now, and she sat down on the dogs'-paw cushions of her sofa and, with her knees far apart and a smile of yearning and of fright, she bent her round back, burned a cigarette at the corner of her mouth and saw—the Church of Saint Sulpice in Paris where her organ teacher used to bring her. It looked like country walls of stone, but rising high and leaning outward were towers. She was very young. She knew music. How she could ever have been so clever was beyond her. But she did know it. She could read all those notes. The sky was gray. After this she saw some entertaining things she liked to tell people about. She was a young wife. She was in Aix-les-Bains with her mother-in-law, and they played bridge in a mud bath with a British general and his aid. There were artificial waves in the swimming pool. She lost her bathing suit because it was a size too big. How did she get out? Ah, you got out of everything.

She saw her husband, James John Waggoner IV. They were snow-bound together in New Hampshire. "Jimmy, Jimmy, how can you fling a wife away?" she asked him. "Have you forgotten love? Did I drink too much—did I bore you?" He had married again and had two children. He had gotten tired of her. And though he was a vain man with nothing to be vain about—no looks, not too much intelligence, nothing but an old Philadelphia family—she had loved him. She too had been a snob about her Philadelphia connections. Give up the name of Waggoner? How could she? For this reason she had never married Wicks. "How dare you," she had said to Wicks, "come without a shave in a dirty shirt and muck on you, come and ask me to marry! If you want to propose, go and clean up first." But his dirt was only a pretext.

Trade Waggoner for Wicks? she asked herself again with a swing of her shoulders. She wouldn't think of it. Wicks was an excellent man. But he was a cowboy. Socially nothing. He couldn't even read. But she saw this on her film. They were in Athens Canyon, in a cratelike house, and she was reading aloud to him from *The Count of Monte Cristo*. He wouldn't let her stop. While walking to stretch her legs, she read, and he followed her about to catch each word. After all, he was very dear to her. Such a man! Now she saw him jump from his horse. They were living on the range, trapping coyotes. It was just the second gray of evening, cloudy, moments after the sun had gone down. There was an animal in the trap, and he went toward it to kill it. He wouldn't waste a bullet on the creatures but killed them with a kick, with his boot. And then Hattie saw that this coyote was all white—snarling teeth, white scruff. "Wicks, he's white! White as a polar bear. You're not going to kill him, are you?" The animal flattened to the ground. He snarled and cried. He couldn't pull away because of the heavy trap. And Wicks killed him. What else could he have done? The white beast lay dead. The dust of Wicks's boots hardly showed on its head and jaws. Blood ran from the muzzle.

And now came something on Hattie's film she tried to shun. It was she herself who had killed her dog, Richie. Just as Rolfe and Pace had warned her, he was vicious, his brain was turned. She, because she was on the side of all dumb creatures, defended him when he bit the trashy woman Jacamares was living with. Perhaps if she had had Richie from a puppy he wouldn't have turned on her. When she got him he was already a year and a half old and she couldn't break him of his habits. But she thought that only she understood him. And Rolfe had warned her, "You'll be sued, do you know that? The dog will take out after somebody smarter than that Jacamares's woman, and you'll be in for it."

Hattie saw herself as she swayed her shoulders and said, "Nonsense."

But what fear she had felt when the dog went for her on the porch. Suddenly she could see, by his skull, by his eyes that he was evil. She screamed at him, "Richie!" And what had she done to him? He had lain under the gas range all day growling and wouldn't come out. She tried to urge him out with the broom, and he snatched it in his teeth. She pulled him out, and he left the stick and tore at her. Now, as the spectator of this, her eyes opened, beyond the pregnant curtain and the air-wave of marl dust, summer's snow, drifting over the water. "Oh, my God! Richie!" Her thigh was snatched by his jaws. His teeth went through her skirt. She felt she would fall. Would she go down? Then the dog would rush at her throat—then black night, bad-odored mouth, the blood pouring from her neck, from torn veins. Her heart shriveled as the teeth went into her thigh, and she couldn't delay another second but took her kindling hatchet from the nail, strengthened her grip on the smooth wood, and hit the dog. She saw the blow. She saw him die at once. And then in fear and shame she hid the body. And at night she buried him in the yard. Next day she accused Jacamares. On him she laid the blame for the disappearance of her dog.

She stood up; she spoke to herself in silence, as was her habit. *God, what shall I do? I have taken life. I have lied. I have borne false witness. I have stalled. And now what shall I do? Nobody will help me.*

And suddenly she made up her mind that she should go and do what she had been putting off for weeks, namely, test herself with the car, and she slipped on her shoes and went outside. Lizards ran before her in the thirsty dust. She opened the hot, broad door of the car. She lifted her lame hand onto the wheel. Her right hand she reached far to the left and turned the wheel with all her might. Then she started the motor and tried to drive out of the yard. But she could not release the emergency brake with its rasplike rod. She reached with her good hand, the right, under the steering wheel and pressed her bosom on it and strained. No, she could not shift the gears and steer. She couldn't even reach down to the hand brake. The sweat broke out on her skin. Her efforts were too much. She was deeply wounded by the pain in her arm. The door of the car fell open again and she turned from the wheel and with her stiff legs hanging from the door she wept. What could she do now? And when she had wept over the ruin of her life she got out of the old car and went back to the house. She took the bourbon from the cupboard and picked up the ink bottle and a pad of paper and sat down to write her will.

"My Will," she wrote, and sobbed to herself.

Since the death of India she had numberless times asked the questions, To Whom? Who will get this when I die? She had unconsciously put people to the test to find out whether they were worthy. It made her more severe than before.

Now she wrote, "I Harriet Simmons Waggoner, being of sound mind and not knowing what may be in store for me at the age of seventy-two (born 1885), living alone at Sego Desert Lake, instruct my lawyer, Harold Claiborne, Paiute County Court Building, to draw my last will and testament upon the following terms."

She sat perfectly still now to hear from within who would be the lucky one, who would inherit the yellow house. For which she had waited. Yes, waited for India's death, choking on her bread because she was a rich woman's servant and whipping girl. But who had done for her, Hattie, what she had done for India? And who, apart from India, had ever held out a hand to her? Kindness, yes. Here and there people had been kind. But the word in her head was not kindness, it was succor. And who had given her that? *Succor?* Only India. If at least, next best after succor, someone had given her a shake and said, "Stop stalling. Don't be such a slow, old, procrastinating sit-stiller." Again, it was only India who had done her good. She had offered her succor. "Het-tie!" said that drunken mask. "Do you know what sloth is? Demn you! poky old demned thing!"

But I was waiting, Hattie realized. *I was waiting, thinking, "Youth is terrible, frightening. I will wait it out. And men? Men are cruel and strong. They want things I haven't got to give." There were no kids in me,* thought Hattie. *Not that I wouldn't have loved them, but such my nature was. And who can blame me for having it? My nature?*

She drank from an old-fashioned glass. There was no orange in it, no ice, no bitters or sugar, only the stinging, clear bourbon.

So then, she continued, looking at the dry sun-stamped dust and the last freckled flowers of red wild peach, *to live with Angus and his wife? And to have to hear a chapter from the Bible before breakfast? Once more in the house—not of a stranger, perhaps, but not far from it either?* In other houses, in someone else's house, to wait for mealtimes was her lifelong punishment. She always felt it in the throat and stomach. And so she would again, and to the very end. However, she must think of someone to leave the house to.

And first of all she wanted to do right by her family. None of them had ever dreamed that she, Hattie, would ever have something to bequeath. Until a few years ago it had certainly looked as if she would die a pauper. So now she could keep her head up with the proudest of them. And, as this occurred to her, she actually lifted up her face with its broad nose and victorious eyes; if her hair had become shabby as onion roots, if, at the back, her head was round and bald as a newel post, what did it matter? Her heart experienced a childish glory, not yet tired of it after seventy-two years. She, too, had amounted to something. *I'll do some good by going,* she thought. *Now I believe I should leave it to, to . . .* She returned to the old point of struggle. She had decided many times and many times changed her mind. She tried to think, *Who would get the most out of this yellow house?* It was a tearing thing to go through. If it had not been the house but, instead, some brittle thing she could hold in her hand, then her last action would be to throw and smash it, and so the thing and she herself would be demolished together. But it was vain to think such thoughts. To whom should she leave it? Her brothers? Not they. Nephews? One was a submarine commander. The other was a bachelor in the State Department. Then began the roll call of cousins. Merton? He owned an estate in Connecticut. Anna? She had a face like a

hot-water bottle. That left Joyce, the orphaned daughter of her cousin Wil-
fred. Joyce was the most likely heiress. Hattie had already written to her and
had her out to the lake at Thanksgiving, two years ago. But this Joyce was
another odd one; over thirty, good, yes, but placid, running to fat, a
scholar—ten years in Eugene, Oregon, working for her degree. In Hattie's
opinion this was only another form of sloth. Nevertheless, Joyce yet hoped
to marry. Whom? Not Dr. Stroud. He wouldn't. And still Joyce had vague
hope. Hattie knew how that could be. At least have a man she could
argue with.

She was now more drunk than at any time since her accident. Again she
filled her glass. *Have ye eyes and see not? Sleepers awake!*

Knees wide apart she sat in the twilight, thinking. Marian? Marian didn't
need another house. Half Pint? She wouldn't know what to do with it.
Brother Louis came up for consideration next. He was an old actor who had
a church for the Indians at Athens Canyon. Hollywood stars of the silent
days sent him their negligees; he altered them and wore them in the pulpit.
The Indians loved his show. But when Billy Shawah blew his brains out after
his two-week bender, they still tore his shack down and turned the boards
inside out to get rid of his ghost. They had their old religion. No, not Brother
Louis. He'd show movies in the yellow house to the tribe or make a nursery
out of it for the Indian brats.

And now she began to consider Wicks. When last heard from he was
south of Bishop, California, a handy man in a saloon off toward Death Valley.
It wasn't she who heard from him but Pace. Herself, she hadn't actually seen
Wicks since—how low she had sunk then!—she had kept the hamburger
stand on Route 158. The little lunchroom had supported them both. Wicks
hung around on the end stool, rolling cigarettes (she saw it on the film).
Then there was a quarrel. Things had been going from bad to worse. He'd
begun to grouse now about this and now about that. He beefed about the
food, at last. She saw and heard him. "Hat," he said, "I'm good and tired of
hamburger." "Well, what do you think I eat?" she said with that round, de-
fiant movement of her shoulders which she herself recognized as characteristic (*me all over*, she thought). But he opened the cash register and took out
thirty cents and crossed the street to the butcher's and brought back a steak.
He threw it on the griddle. "Fry it," he said. She did, and watched him eat.

And when he was through she could bear her rage no longer. "Now," she
said, "you've had your meat. Get out. Never come back." She kept a pistol
under the counter. She picked it up, cocked it, pointed it at his heart. "If
you ever come in that door again, I'll kill you," she said.

She saw it all. *I couldn't bear to fall so low*, she thought, *to be slave to a
shiftless cowboy.*

Wicks said, "Don't do that, Hat. Guess I went too far. You're right."

"You'll never have a chance to make it up," she cried. "Get out!"

On that cry he disappeared, and since then she had never seen him.

"Wicks, dear," she said. "Please! I'm sorry. Don't condemn me in your heart. Forgive me. I hurt myself in my evil. I always had a thick idiot head. I was born with a thick head."

Again she wept, for Wicks. She was too proud. A snob. Now they might have lived together in this house, old friends, simple and plain.

She thought, *He really was my good friend.*

But what would Wicks do with a house like this, alone, if he was alive and survived her? He was too wiry for soft beds or easy chairs.

And she was the one who had said stiffly to India, "I'm a Christian person. I do not bear a grudge."

Ah yes, she said to herself. *I have caught myself out too often. How long can this go on?* And she began to think, or try to think, of Joyce, her cousin's daughter. Joyce was like herself, a woman alone, getting on in years, clumsy. Probably never been laid. Too bad. She would have given much, now, to succor Joyce.

But it seemed to her now that that too, the succor, had been a story. First you heard the pure story. Then you heard the impure story. Both stories. She had paid out years, now to one shadow, now to another shadow.

Joyce would come here to the house. She had a little income and could manage. She would live as Hattie had lived, alone. Here she would rot, start to drink, maybe, and day after day read, day after day sleep. See how beautiful it was here? It burned you out. How empty! It turned you into ash.

How can I doom a younger person to the same life? asked Hattie. It's for somebody like me. When I was younger it wasn't right. But now it is, exactly. Only I fit in here. It was made for my old age, to spend my last years peacefully. If I hadn't let Jerry make me drunk that night—if I hadn't sneezed! Because of this arm, I'll have to live with Angus. My heart will break there away from my only home.

She was now very drunk, and she said to herself, *Take what God brings. He gives no gifts unmixed. He makes loans.*

She resumed her letter of instructions to lawyer Claiborne: "Upon the following terms," she wrote a second time. "Because I have suffered much. Because I only lately received what I have to give away, I can't bear it." The drunken blood was soaring to her head. But her hand was clear enough. She wrote, "It is too soon! Too soon! Because I do not find it in my heart to care for anyone as I would wish. Being cast off and lonely, and doing no harm where I am. Why should it be? This breaks my heart. In addition to everything else, why must I worry about this, which I must leave? I am tormented out of my mind. Even though by my own fault I have put myself into this position. And I am not ready to give up on this. No, not yet. And so I'll tell you what, I leave this property, land, house, garden, and water rights, to Hattie Simmons Waggoner. Me! I realize this is bad and wrong. Not possible. Yet it is the only thing I really wish to do, so may God have mercy on my soul."

How could this happen? She studied what she had written and finally she acknowledged that she was drunk. "I'm drunk," she said, "and don't know what I'm doing. I'll die, and end. Like India. Dead as that lilac bush."

Then she thought that there was a beginning, and a middle. She shrank from the last term. She began once more—a beginning. After that, there was the early middle, then middle middle, late middle middle, quite late middle. In fact the middle is all I know. The rest is just a rumor.

Only tonight I can't give the house away. I'm drunk and so I need it. And tomorrow, she promised herself, I'll think again. I'll work it out, for sure.

The Black and White

The FIRST OLD WOMAN *is sitting at a milk bar table. Small.*

A SECOND OLD WOMAN *approaches. She is carrying two bowls of soup, which are covered by two plates, on each of which is a slice of bread. She puts the bowls down on the table carefully.*

SECOND

You see that one come up and speak to me at the counter?
  She takes the bread plates off the bowls, takes two spoons from her pocket, and places the bowls, plates and spoons.

FIRST

You got the bread, then?

SECOND

I didn't know how I was going to carry it. In the end I put the plates on top of the soup.

FIRST

I like a bit of bread with my soup.
  They begin the soup. Pause.

SECOND

Did you see that one come up and speak to me at the counter?

FIRST

Who?

SECOND

Comes up to me, he says, hullo, he says, what's the time by your clock? Bloody liberty. I was just standing there getting your soup.

FIRST

It's tomato soup.

SECOND

What's the time by your clock? he says.

FIRST

I bet you answered him back.

SECOND

I told him all right. Go on, I said, why don't you get back into your scrag-hole, I said, clear off out of it before I call a copper.
  Pause.

FIRST

I not long got here.

SECOND

Did you get the all-night bus?

FIRST

I got the all-night bus straight here.

SECOND

Where from?

FIRST

Marble Arch.

SECOND

Which one?

FIRST

The two-nine-four, that takes me all the way to Fleet Street.

SECOND

So does the two-nine-one. [*Pause.*] I see you talking to two strangers as I come in. You want to stop talking to strangers, old piece of boot like you, you mind who you talk to.

FIRST

I wasn't talking to any strangers.

Pause. The FIRST OLD WOMAN *follows the progress of a bus through the window.*
That's another all-night bus gone down. [*Pause.*] Going up the other way. Fulham way. [*Pause.*] That was a two-nine-seven. [*Pause.*] I've never been up that way. [*Pause.*] I've been down to Liverpool Street.

SECOND

That's the other way.

FIRST

I don't fancy going down there, down Fulham way, and all up there.

SECOND

Uh-uh.

FIRST

I've never fancied that direction much.
Pause.

SECOND

How's your bread?
Pause.

FIRST

Eh?

SECOND

Your bread.

FIRST

All right. How's yours?
Pause.

SECOND

They don't charge for the bread if you have soup.

FIRST

They do if you have tea.

SECOND

If you have tea they do. [*Pause.*] You talk to strangers they'll take you in. Mind my word. Coppers'll take you in.

FIRST

I don't talk to strangers.

SECOND

They took me away in the wagon once.

FIRST

They didn't keep you though.

SECOND

They didn't keep me, but that was only because they took a fancy to me.
They took a fancy to me when they got me in the wagon.
The FIRST OLD WOMAN *gazes out of the window.*

FIRST

You can see what goes on from this top table. [*Pause.*] It's better than going
down to the place on the embankment, anyway.

SECOND

Yes, there's not too much noise.

FIRST

There's always a bit of noise.

SECOND

Yes, there's always a bit of life.
Pause.

FIRST

They'll be closing down soon to give it a scrub-round.

SECOND

There's a wind out.
Pause.

FIRST

I wouldn't mind staying.

SECOND

They won't let you.

FIRST

I know. [*Pause.*] Still, they only close hour and half, don't they? [*Pause.*] It's
not long. [*Pause.*] You can go along, then come back.

SECOND

I'm going. I'm not coming back.

FIRST

When it's light I come back. Have my tea.

SECOND

I'm going. I'm going up to the Garden.

FIRST

I'm not going down there. [*Pause.*] I'm going up to the Waterloo Bridge.

SECOND

You'll just about see the last two-nine-six come up over the river.

FIRST

I'll just catch a look of it. Time I get up there.
Pause.
It don't look like an all-night bus in daylight, do it?

About the Authors

EDWARD ALBEE (b. 1928), a major American playwright, made his name with such works as *Who's Afraid of Virginia Woolf* and *Zoo Story.*

TONI CADE BAMBARA (b. 1939), born in New York City, graduated from Queens College and took an M.A. at City College of New York. She has several collections of short stories, including *Gorilla, My Love* and *The Sea Birds Are Still Alive: Collected Stories.*

SAUL BELLOW (b. 1915), who lives and teaches in Chicago, has won three National Book Awards for his novels. He also won the Nobel Prize for literature in 1976.

MICHAEL BLUMENTHAL (b. 1949) teaches writing at Harvard and is the author of four collections of poetry: *Sympathetic Magic, Laps, Days We Would Rather Know,* and *Against Romance.*

PHILIP BOOTH (b. 1925) grew up in New England, where he graduated from Dartmouth and taught at Bowdoin and Wellesley. He has published several books of poetry and has won numerous awards, including the Lamont Prize.

GWENDOLYN BROOKS (b. 1917), a poet and native of Chicago, has been the recipient of many awards, including a Pulitzer Prize for poetry in 1950 for *Annie Allen,* a ballad of African-American life in Chicago.

STERLING BROWN (1901–1989), born in Washington, D.C., graduated from Williams College and received graduate degrees from Harvard. Known primarily for his scholarship in African-American folklore, he is the Poet Laureate of Washington, D.C.

ETHAN CANIN (b. 1960), a student at Harvard Medical School, has short stories collected in the acclaimed *Emperor of the Air* (1988). A new collection of stories is forthcoming.

ANTON CHEKHOV (1860–1904), a major Russian playwright and short story writer, is best known for such plays as *The Cherry Orchard* and *The Three Sisters.* He supported himself through medical school by his writing, and he continued to write during his years as a practicing physician.

LUCILLE CLIFTON (b. 1936), born in Depew, New York, is the author of five collections of poetry and many children's books. She is the former Poet Laureate of Maryland and winner of the Juniper Prize for poetry.

RITA DOVE (b. 1952) was born in Akron, Ohio, and educated at Miami University and the University of Iowa and presently teaches at the University of Virginia. In 1987 she won the Pulitzer Prize for *Thomas and Beulah*, her third collection of poetry.

HENRY DUMAS (1934–1968), born in Arkansas, wrote stories and poems about the African-American experience both in the rural South and the urban North. Two recent collections are *Goodbye, Sweetwater* (stories) and *Knees of a Natural Man* (poems).

STEPHEN DUNN (b. 1939) has several collections of poems, such as *Looking for Holes in the Ceiling* (1974), *Work and Love* (1981), and *Not Dancing* (1984). He has taught writing at Stockton State College, University of Washington, and Columbia University.

ROBERT FROST (1874–1961), the best-known American poet of the twentieth century, wrote of human disillusionment and fear as well as the self-reliance and endurance of individuals living in rural New England.

PETER HARRIS (b. 1947) is professor of English at Colby College. He writes the "Poetry Chronicles" for *Virginia Quarterly Review*.

ERNEST HEMINGWAY (1899–1961), a famous American novelist and short story writer, won many awards, including the Nobel Prize in 1954 for such works as *The Sun Also Rises*, *For Whom the Bell Tolls*, and *Old Man and the Sea*.

EDWIN HONIG (b. 1919), born in Brooklyn, has taught mainly at Harvard and Brown, where he writes poetry and translations of Hispanic literature. He has won many awards, including the PEN.

RANDALL JARRELL (1914–1965) studied at Vanderbilt, where he received a B.A. and M.A., and taught at the University of North Carolina. Known primarily for his poetry, he was part of the Agrarian Group of Southern writers.

TED KOOSER (b. 1939) makes his living in life insurance in Lincoln, Nebraska. He has published several volumes of poetry, including *Sure Signs: New and Selected Poems*, and has held two NEA fellowships.

ELLA LEFFLAND (b. 1931) was born in Martinez, California. She writes short stories and novels, including *Mrs. Munck* and *Love Out of Season*.

URSULA K. LE GUIN (b. 1929) has lived in Portland, Oregon, for the last thirty years. She is the author of *The Left Hand of Darkness* and several other novels of fantasy, science fiction, and satire. She has won many awards, including the Hugo, Nebula, Gandolf, and National Book awards.

DENISE LEVERTOV (b. 1923) is a poet whose work spans more than thirty years. Born in England, she has spent most of her life in the United States. Her most recent collection of poetry is *Breathing the Water* (1987).

AMY LOWELL (1874–1925), one of the prime movers of the Imagist movement, won the Pulitzer Prize posthumously for her verse.

BERNARD MALAMUD (1914–1986) was the author of eight novels, including *The Natural* and *The Assistant*, and four collections of stories, including *The Magic Barrel*, which won the National Book Award.

W. S. MERWIN (b. 1927) has collected his poems in several volumes, including the *First Four Books of Poems*, *The Lice*, and *The Compass Flower*.

SUE MILLER (b. 1943) is the author of *Inventing the Abbotts*, *The Good Mother*, and *Family Pictures*.

LISEL MUELLER (b. 1924) was born in Germany and came to the United States just before World War II. She is the author of *The Private Life*, which won the Lamont Prize, *The Need to Hold Still*, which won the American Book Award, and *Second Language*.

ALICE MUNRO (b. 1931) is a Canadian writer, born in Ontario, whose collected stories, *Dance of the Happy Shades* (1968), and her novel, *The Beggar Maid* (1979), both won the Governor General's Literary Award, Canada's highest award for writers.

HOWARD NEMEROV (1920–1991) was Poet Laureate of the United States from 1988 to 1990. His *Collected Poems of Howard Nemerov* won both the Pulitzer Prize and the National Book Award in 1978. He taught at Washington University, where he was Distinguished Poet in Residence.

FLANNERY O'CONNOR (1925–1964), born in Georgia, studied at the Writer's Workshop at the University of Iowa before her battle with lupus forced her to remain at home. An accomplished writer with a sense of the grotesque and ironic, she is best known for her short story collections *A Good Man Is Hard To Find* and *Everything That Rises Must Converge*.

TILLIE OLSEN (b. 1913), born in Nebraska, worked most of her life in industry and in raising her family. Her stories are collected in *Tell Me a Riddle* and *Other Stories*.

GRACE PALEY (b. 1922), born in New York City, has several collections of short stories drawing on her Jewish experience, the most recent being *Later the Same Day*.

AUGUSTA PERSSE (LADY AUGUSTA GREGORY, 1852–1932) was an Irish playwright and folklorist born in Galway. With W. B. Yeats and others, she founded the Abbey Theatre, which she co-directed. Her Coole Park estate was a retreat for Yeats and many other Irish writers and artists.

HAROLD PINTER (b. 1930), born in London, is England's best-known contemporary playwright, having created such works as *The Caretaker*, *The Birthday Party*, *The Homecoming*, *The Dumb Waiter*, and *Betrayal*, as well as several screenplays and short radio plays.

KATHERINE ANNE PORTER (1890–1980), born in Texas, was an accomplished short story writer who drew often on autobiographical sources. Her *Pale Horse, Pale Rider*, for example, is based on her near-fatal experience with influenza.

SUSAN IRENE REA (b. 1945) graduated with an M.F.A. from Goddard College. She has received several fellowships from the Pennsylvania Council of the Arts and has had works published in many journals, including the *American Scholar* and *Southern Poetry Review*.

EDWIN ARLINGTON ROBINSON (1869–1935) was born in Maine and wrote many of his poems about the people of "Tilbury Town." Three collections of his poems won the Pulitzer Prize, including *Tristram* in 1927.

PHILIP ROTH (b. 1933), born in New Jersey, was educated at Bucknell and the University of Chicago. Since *Goodbye Columbus* (1959 winner of the National Book Award), he has written dozens of novels and short stories, including *Portnoy's Complaint*, *Paternity*, and *Deceptions*.

MAY SARTON (b. 1912) is the author of poetry, novels, and nonfiction. Born in Belgium, she was educated in the United States. She lives alone in York, Maine, the subject of much of her autobiographical writing.

JOHN SAYLES (b. 1950) worked in hospitals and as a laborer before earning a living as a writer. He has written numerous screenplays as well as novels and a short story collection, *The Anarchists' Convention*.

L. J. SCHNEIDERMAN (b. 1932), an internist, is professor of Community and Family Medicine at the University of California, San Diego, Medical School. He is the author of plays, short stories, and the novel *Sea Nymphs by the Hour*.

RICHARD SELZER (b. 1928) has recently retired as a surgeon of the Yale School of Medicine. He is the author of several books, including *Rituals of Surgery, Mortal Lessons, Confessions of a Knife, Letters to a Young Doctor, Taking the World in for Repairs,* and *Imagine a Woman.*

ANNE SEXTON (1928–1974), American poet of the "confessional" school, studied with Robert Lowell and Sylvia Plath, with whom she had much in common.

WILLIAM STAFFORD (b. 1914), educated at the Universities of Kansas and Iowa, taught at Lewis and Clark College in Oregon. *Stories That Could Be True: New and Selected Poems* appeared in 1978, *A Glass Face in the Rain* in 1982.

JOHN STONE (b. 1936) is a cardiologist, poet, and essayist whose work appears often in the Sunday Magazine of the *New York Times.* He teaches at Emory University School of Medicine. His most recent book is *In The Country of Hearts.*

MAY SWENSON (1919–1989), born and raised in Utah, lived and wrote in and around New York City. She was self-taught. Her collections of poems include *Another Animal: Poems, Iconographs* and *New and Selected Things Taking Place.*

AMY TAN (b. 1952) won high acclaim for her first novel, *The Joy Luck Club,* followed by another best-selling novel in 1991, *The Kitchen God's Wife.*

PETER TAYLOR (b. 1917) writes about people of his native Tennessee. His novel *A Summons to Memphis* (1986) won the Pulitzer Prize, and his most recent collection of short stories, *The Old Forest and Other Stories* (1985), has won much praise.

KURT VONNEGUT, JR. (b. 1922), is best known for his science fiction style as he comments on the condition of the modern world. He has written several plays, stories, and novels, the most famous of which is *Slaughterhouse Five* (1970).

ALICE WALKER (b. 1944) won the American Book Award and the Pulitzer Prize for her novel *The Color Purple.* A poet, essayist, biographer, editor, and novelist, her most recent work is *The Temple of My Familiar* (1989).

EUDORA WELTY (b. 1909), born in Mississippi, was educated at the University of Wisconsin. She has received several O. Henry Awards for her short stories and a Pulitzer Prize for fiction for *The Optimist's Daughter* (1973). Her most recent book, *One Writer's Beginnings,* won the MLA Commonwealth Award.

WILLIAM CARLOS WILLIAMS (1883–1963) combined a full-time career as a physician with a major career as a poet. He won many awards, including the National Book Award for *Paterson* and a Pulitzer Prize for *Pictures from Breughel and Other Poems* (1962).

ABOUT THE AUTHORS

WILLIAM BUTLER YEATS (1865–1939), Ireland's greatest poet and one of the major writers of the twentieth century, won the Nobel Prize in 1923, though he created much of his best work after that. Significant volumes of his work include *Collected Poems* (1950) and *Collected Plays* (1952).

Permissions Acknowledgments

427

PERMISSIONS ACKNOWLEDGMENTS

RANDALL JARRELL: "Next Day" reprinted with permission of Macmillan Publishing Company from *The Lost World* by Randall Jarrell. Copyright © Randall Jarrell, 1963, 1965. Originally appeared in *The New Yorker* © 1965 by Randall Jarrell from the book *The Lost World in Randall Jarrell: The Complete Poems*, published by Farrar, Straus & Giroux.

TED KOOSER: "The Very Old" reprinted from *Sure Signs: New and Selected Poems* by Ted Kooser, by permission of the University of Pittsburgh Press. Copyright © 1980 by Ted Kooser.

ELLA LEFFLAND: "The Linden Tree" from *Last Courtesies and Other Stories* by Ella Leffland. Copyright © 1980 by Ella Leffland. Reprinted by permission of HarperCollins Publishers.

URSULA K. LE GUIN: "The Space Crone" from *Dancing at the Edge of the World* by Ursula K. Le Guin. Copyright © 1989 by Ursula K. Le Guin. Used by permission of Grove Press, Inc.

DENISE LEVERTOV: "A Woman Alone" and "The 90th Year" by Denise Levertov: *Life In The Forest*. Copyright © 1978 by Denise Levertov. Reprinted by permission of New Directions Publishing Corporation. World rights.

AMY LOWELL: "A Lady" from *The Complete Poetical Works of Amy Lowell* by Amy Lowell. Copyright © 1955 by Houghton Mifflin Co. Copyright © 1953 by Houghton Mifflin Co., Brinton P. Roberts, and G. D'Andelot, Belin, Esquire. Reprinted by permission of Houghton Mifflin Co.

BERNARD MALAMUD: "Idiots First" and "The Jewbird" from *Idiots First* by Bernard Malamud. Copyright © 1961, 1963 by Bernard Malamud. "In Retirement" from *Rembrandt's Hat* by Bernard Malamud. Copyright © 1973 by Bernard Malamud. Reprinted by permission of Farrar, Straus and Giroux, Inc.

W. S. MERWIN: "Grandfather in the Old Men's Home" and "Grandmother and Grandson" from *The Drunk in the Furnace* by W. S. Merwin. Published by Atheneum. Reprinted by permission of Georges Borchardt Inc. for the author. Copyright © 1956, 1957, 1958, 1959, 1960 by W. S. Merwin.

SUE MILLER: "Appropriate Affect" from *Inventing the Abbots and Other Stories* by Sue Miller. Copyright © 1987 by Sue Miller. Reprinted by permission of HarperCollins Publishers.

LISEL MUELLER: "Monet Refuses the Operation" reprinted by permission of Louisiana State University Press from *Second Language* by Lisel Mueller. Copyright © 1986 by Lisel Mueller.

Index

Albee, Edward, 247
"Ancient Gentility" (William Carlos
    Williams), 312
"Appropriate Affect" (Sue Miller), 271
from *Asphodel, That Greeny Flower*
    (William Carlos Williams), 92

Bambara, Toni Cade, 213
"Bean Eaters, The" (Gwendolyn Brooks),
    90
Bellow, Saul, 388
"Black and White, The" (Harold Pinter),
    415
Blumenthal, Michael, 87
Booth, Philip, 146
Brooks, Gwendolyn, 90
Brown, Sterling, 41

Canin, Ethan, 96, 297
Chekhov, Anton, 326
"Clean, Well-lighted Place, A" (Ernest
    Hemingway), 16
Clifton, Lucille, 43
"Conversation with My Father, A" (Grace
    Paley), 242
"Crazy Jane Talks with the Bishop" (W. B.
    Yeats), 91

"Dillinger in Hollywood" (John Sayles), 336
Dove, Rita, 259
Dumas, Henry, 108
Dunn, Stephen, 261

"Emperor of the Air" (Ethan Canin), 297
"Epstein" (Philip Roth), 117
"Everything That Rises Must Converge"
    (Flannery O'Connor), 192

"Fallback" (Philip Booth), 146
"Fortitude" (Kurt Vonnegut, Jr.), 48
Frost, Robert, 37, 38

"Grandfather in the Old Men's Home"
    (W. S. Merwin), 236
"Grandma's Got a Wig" (Henry Dumas),
    108
"Grandmother and Grandson" (W. S. Mer-
    win), 240
"Grandmother's Stroke" (Stephen Dunn),
    261
Gregory, Lady, 20

Harris, Peter, 237
"He Makes a House Call" (John Stone),
    310
Hemingway, Ernest, 16
Honig, Edwin, 89
"How to be Old" (May Swenson), 46

"Idiots First" (Bernard Malamud), 347
"In Retirement" (Bernard Malamud), 109

Jarrell, Randall, 7
"Jewbird, The" (Bernard Malamud), 205
"Jilting of Granny Weatherall, The"
    (Katherine Ann Porter), 74
"Joy Luck Club, The" (Amy
    Tan), 219

Kooser, Ted, 308

"Lady, A" (Amy Lowell), 44
Le Guin, Ursula K., 31

"Leaving the Yellow House" (Saul Bellow), 388
Leffland, Ella, 134
Levertov, Denise, 39, 257
"Linden Tree, The" (Ella Leffland), 134
Lowell, Amy, 44

"Maggie of the Green Bottles" (Toni Cade Bambara), 213
Malamud, Bernard, 109, 205, 347
"Medicine" (Alice Walker), 88
Merwin, W. S., 236, 240
Miller, Sue, 271
"Misery" (Anton Chekhov), 326
"Miss Rosie" (Lucille Clifton), 43
"Monet Refuses the Operation" (Lisel Mueller), 5
"Mr. Flood's Party" (E. A. Robinson), 35
Mueller, Lisel, 5
Munro, Alice, 281
"My Father-in-law's Contract" (Peter Harris), 237

"Near the Old People's Home" (Howard Nemerov), 309
Nemerov, Howard, 309
"Next Day" (Randall Jarrell), 7
"90th Year, The" (Denise Levertov), 257
"Now, Before the End, I Think" (Edwin Honig), 89

O'Connor, Flannery, 192
"Old" (Anne Sexton), 47
"Old Doc Rivers" (William Carlos Williams), 368
"Old Man's Winter Night, An" (Robert Frost), 37
Olsen, Tillie, 153
"On a Winter Night" (May Sarton), 45

Paley, Grace, 242
Pinter, Harold, 415
"Pleasures of Old Age, The" (Michael Blumenthal), 87
"Porte-Cochere" (Peter Taylor), 184
Porter, Katherine Ann, 74
"Provide, Provide" (Robert Frost), 38

Rea, Susan Irene, 239
Robinson, E. A., 35
Roth, Philip, 109

"Sandbox, The" (Edward Albee), 247
Sarton, May, 45
Sayles, John, 336
Schneiderman, L. J., 262
Selzer, Richard, 321
"Sequel" (L. J. Schneiderman), 262
Sexton, Anne, 47
"Space Crone, The" (Ursula K. Le Guin), 31
"Spelling" (Alice Munro), 281
Stafford, William, 260
Stone, John, 310
"Stroke, The" (Rita Dove), 259
"Stroke" (Susan Irene Rea), 239
"Strokes" (William Stafford), 260
Swenson, May, 46

Tan, Amy, 219
Taylor, Peter, 184, 355
"Tell Me A Riddle" (Tillie Olsen), 153
"To Hell With Dying" (Alice Walker), 315
"Toenails" (Richard Selzer), 321

"Very Old, The" (Ted Kooser), 308
"Virginia Portrait" (Sterling Brown), 41
"Visit of Charity, A" (Eudora Welty), 331
Vonnegut, Kurt, Jr., 48

Walker, Alice, 88, 315
"We are Nighttime Travelers" (Ethan Canin), 96
Welty, Eudora, 9, 331
"What You Hear From 'Em?" (Peter Taylor), 355
Williams, William Carlos, 92, 312, 368
"Woman Alone, A" (Denise Levertov), 39
"Workhouse Ward, The" (Lady Gregory), 20
"Worn Path, A" (Eudora Welty), 9

Yeats, W. B., 91

Literature and Aging
was composed in 10/12 Caledonia with Avant Garde display
on a Xyvision system with Linotronic output
by BookMasters, Inc.;
printed by sheet-fed offset
on 60-pound Glatfelter Natural Smooth acid-free stock,
notch bound into paper covers printed in two colors
on 12-point stock with film lamination
by Edwards Brothers, Inc.;
text designed by Donna Hartwick;
cover designed by Diana Gordy;
and published by
The Kent State University Press
KENT, OHIO 44242